Environmental Epidemiology

Environmental Epidemiology
Study Methods and Application

Edited by

Dean Baker

Center for Occupational and
Environmental Health,
University of California,
Irvine, USA

Mark J. Nieuwenhuijsen

Center for Research in Environmental
Epidemiology (CREAL)
Barcelona, Spain

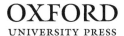

OXFORD
UNIVERSITY PRESS

OXFORD
UNIVERSITY PRESS

Great Clarendon Street, Oxford OX2 6DP

Oxford University Press is a department of the University of Oxford.
It furthers the University's objective of excellence in research, scholarship,
and education by publishing worldwide in

Oxford New York

Auckland   Cape Town Dar es Salaam Hong Kong Karachi
Kuala Lumpur Madrid Melbourne Mexico City Nairobi
New Delhi Shanghai Taipei Toronto
With offices in
Argentina Austria Brazil Chile Czech Republic France Greece
Guatemala Hungary Italy Japan South Korea Poland Portugal
Singapore Switzerland Thailand Turkey Ukraine Vietnam

Oxford is a registered trade mark of Oxford University Press
in the UK and in certain other countries

Published in the United States
by Oxford University Press Inc., New York

ISBN 978-0-19-852792-3

Printed in the United Kingdom by
Lightning Source UK Ltd., Milton Keynes

Preface: for whom this book is intended

Air pollution, water contamination, persistent organic pollutants, pesticides, metals, and radiofrequencies to name a few have all been linked to adverse health effects such as cancer, respiratory disease and reproductive effects. Environmental epidemiology is the study of disease and these environmental determinants of disease in humans on a population level. Risks associated with environmental exposures are generally small, but the exposed population, and hence the population burden of disease, may be large. To detect small risk, the methods need to be refined.

The recent and rapid expansion of environmental epidemiology and health risk assessment looks set to continue in line with growing public, government, and media concern about environmental health issues, and a scientific need to better understand and explain effects of environmental pollutants on health.

Although several books on environmental epidemiology exist, none of these focus primarily on methods and application. In this book, *Environmental epidemiology: methods and application* we discus the methods that form the basis of the field and application in other fields such as health risk assessment. The book brings together contributions from an international renowned group of practitioners.

Environmental epidemiology is a subspecialty of epidemiology, the core science of public health. Although we are assuming that the reader is familiar with the basic concepts of epidemiologic reasoning, we have provided a brief overview. We are also assuming that the reader has some knowledge of environmental science, environmental health and biostatistics.

The aim of the book is to develop an understanding and knowledge of environmental epidemiological methods, and the emphasis is on methodological principles and good practice. The book outlines the basic principles of epidemiology and environmental health, and describes in more detail special environmental epidemiological designs that are rarely described in other textbooks. Furthermore, it describes the principles of health risk assessment and forecasting, and the application of environmental epidemiological study data in these types of studies. The book contains a few chapters on practical issues in the conduct of studies, specifically to guide those not familiar with field work and data analyses and its requirements, and discusses ethical issues and the role of environmental epidemiology in policy making.

The book has been designed to be usable in intermediate level courses in teaching programmes in public health, epidemiology, and environmental sciences. Furthermore, it provides an introduction to environmental epidemiology for researchers of other disciplines such biostatisticians and geneticists, who want to develop an interest in the topic.

There is a Further Information section at the end of the book that will point to introductory as well as advanced-level sources of information that we will not cover in detail. This allows the reader to quickly identify if gaps in her or his background exist, and if so, how these can be remedied. Environmental epidemiology is a *very* multidisciplinary enterprise, and most students embarking on its study will find that they will have some deficiencies one way or the other.

The book will be of interest to anyone concerned with environmental epidemiology. It will be a valuable source for exposure assessors, environmental scientists, epidemiologists, toxicologists, geneticists, biostatisticians, health risk assessors, policy makers and regulators who are dealing with environmental hazards and would need to know the basic principles of assessing the risks.

Dean Baker, MD, MPH and Mark J. Nieuwenhuijsen, PhD

Irvine, CA, USA, January 2008

Contributors

Ben Armstrong, PhD
Reader in Epidemiological Statistics,
Public and Environmental
Health Research Unit,
London School of Hygiene and
Tropical Medicine
UK

Dean Baker, MD, MPH
Professor of Medicine and Director,
Center for Occupational and
Environmental Health,
University of California, Irvine
USA

Nicky G Best, PhD
Professor of Statistics and Epidemiology,
Department of Epidemiology and
Public Health,
Faculty of Medicine,
Imperial College, London
UK

Bert Brunekreef, PhD
Professor of Environmental
Epidemiology and Director,
Institute for Risk Assessment (IRAS),
Utrecht University,
The Netherlands

Paul Cullinan, MD
Reader in Occupational and
Environmental Medicine,
National Heart and Lung Institute,
Imperial College, London
UK

Valentina Gallo, MD, MSc
Research Officer,
Department of Epidemiology and
Public Health,

Faculty of Medicine,
Imperial College, London
UK

Anna Hansell, MD, PhD
Wellcome Intermediate Clinical Fellow,
Department of Epidemiology & Public
Health,
Faculty of Medicine,
Imperial College, London
UK

Maud Huynen, MSc
International Center for Integrative Studies,
Maastricht University,
The Netherlands

Lars Jarup, MD, PhD
Reader in Environmental Medicine and
Public Health,
Department of Epidemiology &
Public Health,
Faculty of Medicine,
Imperial College, London
UK

Klea Katsouyanni MSc, DMed Sc
Professor,
Department of Hygiene and
Epidemiology,
University of Athens Medical School,
Greece

Nino Künzli, MD, PhD
Research Professor,
Center for Research in Environmental
Epidemiology (CREAL),
Institut Municipal d'Investigació Mèdica
(IMIM)
Spain

Pim Martens, PhD
Professor and Director,
International Centre for Integrative Studies
Maastricht University,
The Netherlands

Raymond Neutra, MD, DrPH
Chief Emeritus,
Division of Environmental and Occupational Disease Control,
California State Department of Public Health,
USA

Mark J Nieuwenhuijsen, PhD
Research Professor,
Center for Research in Environmental Epidemiology (CREAL),
Spain

Laura Perez, MSc
Center for Research in Environmental Epidemiology (CREAL),
Institut Municipal d'Investigació Mèdica (IMIM),
Spain

Horacio Riojas-Rodríguez, MD, MSc, PhD
Director,
Division of Environmental Health,
National Institute of Public Health,
Mexico

Primitivo Rojas, MPH
Chief, Community Participation and Education (CPES),
Division of Environmental and Occupational Disease Control,
California State Department of Public Health,
USA

Isabel Romieu, MD, MPH, ScD
Professor of Environmental Epidemiology,
National Institute of Public Health,
Mexico

Lianne Sheppard, PhD
Research Professor,
Biostatistics,
Environmental and Occupational Health Sciences,
School of Public Health and Community Medicine,
University of Washington,
USA

Colin Soskolne, PhD
Professor of Epidemiology,
School of Public Health,
Department of Public Health Sciences,
University of Alberta
Canada

Giota Touloumi, PhD, DMSc
Professor,
Department of Hygiene and Epidemiology,
University of Athens Medical School,
Greece

Paolo Vineis, MD, MPH
Chair in Environmental Epidemiology,
Department of Epidemiology & Public Health,
Faculty of Medicine,
Imperial College, London
UK

Daniel Wartenberg, PhD
Professor,
Department of Epidemiology,
UMDNJ-Robert Wood Johnson Medical School,
USA

Contents

Acknowledgements

We would like to thank all the people that are not specifically mentioned for their contribution to the book. A number of chapters in the book are based on chapters in a previous book called *Environmental Epidemiology*, written for the Office of Global and Integrated Environmental Health of the World Health Organization (WHO/SDE/OEH/99.7), and there may be some residual text in the chapters that a number of people contributed to but who are not specifically mentioned as authors of the chapters. Their contribution, of course, is highly appreciated.

Furthermore, the initial outline of the book was conceived during a meeting at the ISEE conference in Garmisch Partenkirchen in 2001 and we would like to thank all the people who contributed to it then, and have contributed to it since, especially Bert Brunekreef who was instrumental in drafting the outline of the book, and initial efforts to get the book off the ground.

We also would like to thank Stacey Kojaku for all her administrative work, without which the book would not be here.

Specific chapters

Chapters 2, 4, 6 and 9

These chapters, which were substantially updated and revised, are based on chapters by the same author in the book *Environmental Epidemiology*, written for the Office of Global and Integrated Environmental Health of the World Health Organization (WHO/SDE/OEH/99.7). That text, in turn, drew upon the contributions of numerous scientists over the years who participated in WHO committees to develop guidelines for epidemiological studies. We would like to acknowledge the contributions of these scientists to enhancing the methods for environmental epidemiology. We acknowledge the contributions of Neal Pearce to sections in the earlier WHO text on epidemiological principles and measures, which are presented in Chapter 2. We would particularly like to acknowledge the contribution of Tord Kjellström for his leadership in developing the earlier text for the WHO.

Chapter 8

The writing and editing of this chapter was made possible by a grant from the European Community (6th Framework Programme) to Professor Paolo Vineis (grant number 513943) for the Network of Excellence ECNIS – Environmental Cancer Risk, Nutrition and Individual Susceptibility (WP4 and WP8). We also would like to acknowledge Dr. Nicola Vanacore from the National Center of Epidemiology, of the Italian National Institute of Health (Rome) for his expert revision of the neurological examples in the chapter; and Dr. Enrico Petretto, from the Imaging Science Department of the Imperial College (London), for his precious advices on genetics.

Chapter 16

Although the author was an employee of the California Department of Health Services, the opinions expressed and the reasoning used in this chapter does not necessarily represent their policies. He would like to acknowledge the intellectual contributions of Dr. Vincent Delpizzo and Dr. Rob Goble to the risk evaluation guidelines in the California EMF project that deeply influenced this chapter. The writings of Dr. Sander Greenland, who may well disagree with some of the approaches in this chapter, have nonetheless been very influential.

Chapter 1

What is environmental epidemiology?

Bert Brunekreef, Dean Baker, and Mark Nieuwenhuijsen

1.1 Introduction

Environmental epidemiology is a subspecialty of epidemiology, the basic science of public health. Epidemiology is the study of the distribution of health and disease in the population, and of the determinants of this distribution. Environmental epidemiology studies the effects of *environmental* exposures on health and disease in the population. The subject matter of environmental epidemiology is *environmental health:* this, in principle, covers all factors external to the human body which may affect health. However, in section 1.5 it will be explained that several other exposure-related branches have grown out of the main epidemiology tree, and that environmental epidemiology does not try to cover all external factors which may conceivably influence population health, but focuses on physical, chemical and (noninfectious) biological factors in our every day environment.

This chapter begins with some examples of past and present environmental health problems from the developed and developing world, to set the stage. It will then define which environmental factors will be the primary focus of the text and introduce reasons why one might conduct an environmental epidemiology study. The last section of the chapter will then discuss the relationship between environmental epidemiology and related disciplines such as occupational and nutritional epidemiology, and toxicology.

1.2 Classic environmental epidemiological studies

1.2.1 Cholera in nineteenth century London

The investigation of the mid-nineteenth century cholera epidemics in London by John Snow is seen by many as the starting point of modern epidemiology. It is also, clearly, a study in environmental epidemiology.

Worldwide epidemics of cholera claiming hundreds of thousands of lives occurred with some regularity in the nineteenth century. For a long time, the causes were unknown. Early nineteenth century theories suggested that the disease was spread through the air (the so-called miasma or bad air theory), but an 1853 editorial published in the *Lancet* admitted to utter confusion:

> The question: what is cholera? is left unsolved. Concerning this, the fundamental point, all is darkness and confusion, vague theory, and a vain speculation. Is it a fungus, an insect, a miasm, an electrical disturbance, a deficiency of ozone, a morbid offscouring of the intestinal canal? We know nothing; we are at sea, in a whirlpool of conjecture.

Quoted in [1, p. 166]

Cholera epidemics hit London in 1832 and then again in 1848. The latter epidemic prompted a local physician, John Snow, to develop a theory in a pamphlet called 'On the mode of communication of cholera' which was published in 1849. In it, he proposed that the gastrointestinal tract was the main point of entry for the disease, and that contact with excrements from diseased individuals was an important mechanism of transmission.

In his 1849 work, John Snow drew attention to two instances where there had been a large difference in cholera deaths between adjacent city blocks which were essentially indistinguishable (e.g. in terms of air quality) except for the use of drinking water wells which were or were not contaminated by local sewage. He also noted that there were large differences in mortality from cholera in different parts of London that were serviced by drinking water companies that used either upstream (uncontaminated) river Thames water or downtown river water contaminated by sewers discharging into the river. He recommended that drinking water no longer be supplied from river stretches where it could be contaminated by sewage, but medical colleagues and civil authorities were unconvinced, and for many years no practical measures were taken. After the epidemic of 1848–49, public pressure to ensure clean drinking water increased, and a bill was adopted in 1852 requiring water companies to filter their water and to move inlets upstream from the tidal region of the Thames river. However, companies were given until the end of August 1855 to implement these changes [1, p. 256].

It was a time when infectious disease epidemics were of very much concern, and it is no coincidence that John Snow and a number of his colleagues founded the Epidemiological Society of London in 1850. In that same year, discussions continued about the origins of cholera, and in one meeting of the Royal Medical and Surgical Society, Snow discussed an example of drinking water from a local well contaminated by a sewer as a source of a cholera outbreak. Several more outbreaks related to local wells contaminated by sewage were described at the time, not only from London but also from Manchester, and in some of these pumps were shut as a control measure well before the famous Broad Street episode occurred (see below) [1, p. 288].

It was only when the third epidemic hit London in 1853 that more detailed investigations of the occurrence of cholera were conducted. It was then that Snow began to document in detail the death rates due to cholera in city districts served by different water companies. In his analysis of the 1853 epidemic, he noted that mortality rates were much higher in south London areas served by the Southwark and Vauxhall water company, with water inlets in the polluted part of the Thames river, than in areas served by the Lambeth company which took its water from clean upstream inlets. In areas served by both companies, the death rates were intermediate. Whereas this observation was very suggestive, there were also significant differences in affluence between the areas served by Southwark and Vauxhall (mainly poor) and Lambeth (affluent suburban). Snow reasoned that more conclusive evidence was to be expected from a detailed investigation of the areas served by both companies, where adjacent and otherwise similar houses would often be served by either one or the other company.

Snow decided to start a detailed investigation of which company was supplying water to which house. He met a surprising number of obstacles—such as many tenants being unaware of which water company their landlord subscribed to—and was able to solve some of these by measuring the salt content of individual water samples, which happened to be different between the two companies. In the end, however, he was able to establish that the cholera death rate was much higher in homes supplied by the Southwark and Vauxhall company than in homes supplied by the Lambeth company, and that the death rate in areas serviced by both companies could be accurately predicted by the proportion of homes serviced by the respective companies (Table 1.1) [2].

During his intensive investigations in south London, another local outbreak occurred in central London, near Golden and Soho Squares in early September 1854. In a small area, hundreds of residents became ill and died in the course of just a week or so. Snow lived within minutes of the area, and suspected that this local outbreak, as others that had occurred before, was related to a well that had become contaminated. A quick investigation suggested that most of the patients had consumed water from a local well connected to the Broad Street pump, and Snow was able to convince local authorities to remove the handle from the pump. Subsequent investigations showed that the well had been contaminated by a blocked drain connected to a cesspit into which excrements had been put from a baby girl who had died early in the epidemic. The drains were repaired, and 18 days after the handle had been removed from the pump, it was restored [1, p. 310].

One other aspect of Snow's work that still strikes us today is his use of maps to illustrate geographic relationships between environment and disease. His map showing a preponderance of cases close to the Broad Street pump is well known. Figure 1.1 (from [1] with permission), is a version from an enquiry report. The majority of the cholera deaths in the area, he found, had lived closer to and used the Broad street pump than to any of the other 13 pumps in the area. Of note, the map was drawn well after the initial investigation that prompted the removal of the pump handle had been completed.

Table 1.1 Death rates from cholera in London, 1853–4, according to water company supplying the actual house

Water company	Number of houses	Deaths from cholera	Deaths per 10 000 houses
Southwark and Vauxhall	40 046	1263	315
Lambeth	26 107	98	37
Rest of London	256 423	1422	59

Source: J. Snow. *On the Mode of Communication of Cholera*, 2nd ed. London: Churchill, 1855. Reproduced in [2].

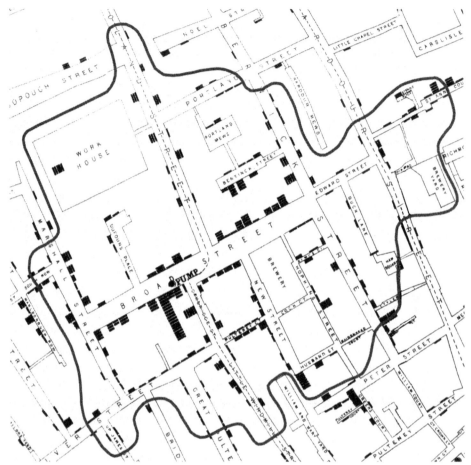

Fig. 1.1 Distribution of the cholera cases around the Broad Street pump. Affected houses are indicated by black rectangles. Source: [1] Reproduced with permission from Vinten-Johansen P, Brody H, Paneth N, Rachman S, Rip M. *Cholera, chloroform, and the science of medicine: A life of John Snow*. New York, NY: Oxford University Press 2003.

1.2.2 **The London smog of 1952**

In London, open coal fires had been used for centuries to heat homes, and public concern about air pollution has a long history there. As far back as 1661, John Evelyn, an English writer, published the booklet 'Fumifugium, or the Inconvenience of Aer and Smoake of London Dissipated'. Periodically, dense winter fogs would descend on London, and with increasing population size and energy consumption, the fogs would mix with smoke to produce 'smog' containing high concentrations of sulphur oxides, acids and soot. Almost certainly, such 'smogs' had produced temporary increases in death rates, but it was not until after World War II that such incidents were more systematically investigated. In early December 1952, an unusually dense fog descended again on London, and after mixing with the smoke of thousands of coal fires, visibility was reduced so much that the city virtually came to a halt. Long-time inhabitants of London were unable to navigate their own city. Even indoors, the fog was dense enough for theaters and movie theaters to close. During the week of the smog, demand for hospital beds far exceeded supply, and death rates soared to three times the normal numbers for the time of the year, which led to a short supply of coffins.

Figure 1.2 [from 3] shows the development of pollution concentrations and death rates over time during the 1952–53 London winter. It is evident that during the 'smog' week of 5–12 December, mortality increased almost immediately after pollution levels increased. For the greater London area, the number of excess deaths was in the order of 4000. For a long period after the smog week, however, death rates did not return to normal levels. In a government report published in 1954, all deaths that occurred after 19 December were not attributed to the smog, but to a flu epidemic that was said to have occurred at the time. Recent analyses of influenza records obtained at the time have suggested that influenza could only have been responsible for a minor part of the estimated extra 8000 deaths [3]. Perhaps, therefore, a much larger number of deaths could be attributed to the smog of 1952.

After the London smog episode and the introduction of the Clean Air Act in 1956, interest in air pollution and health effects reduced for a while, but picked up again in the late 1980s to early 1990s with the introduction of the time series design (see Chapter 8, section 8.1) and publication of the results of the Harvard Six Cities study that showed a clear relationship between levels of air pollution, specifically fine particulate matter, and increased mortality in six cities in the United States (see Figure 6.5 in Chapter 6) [4]. Health effects were seen at much lower levels than previously expected. Air pollution remains one of the largest fields within environmental epidemiology; interest has gone beyond respiratory morbidity and mortality and now includes cancer, cardiovascular morbidity and mortality and effects on pregnancy outcomes. In addition to 'background'

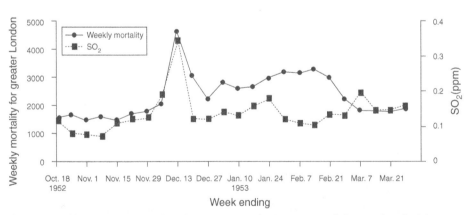

Fig. 1.2 Weekly mortality in London during 1952 and 1953. Source: [3] Reproduced with permission from Bell ML, Davis DL. Reassessment of the lethal London fog of 1952: novel indicators of acute and chronic consequences of acute exposure to air pollution. *Environmental Health Perspectives*. 2001; 109(Suppl 3):389–94.

pollution, traffic-related air pollution has become a topic of interest as a cause of local excess health effects among subjects participating in traffic or living close to busy roads in the developed world.

1.2.3 **Arsenic in well water in Bangladesh**

Well water contaminated with arsenic has probably led to the largest mass poisoning in history in Bangladesh and adjacent west Bengal [5]. To reduce morbidity and mortality due to gastrointestinal disease related to consumption of contaminated surface water, large numbers of tube wells were installed in Bangladesh from the 1970s onwards. The wells typically are connected to aquifers at depths less than 200 meters. In the early 1990s, it was discovered that high arsenic concentrations were present in the water from some of the wells, the arsenic being naturally present in the soil of the area. Health surveys conducted subsequently showed that high proportions of people who consumed well water were affected by the skin lesions that are typical of arsenic poisoning (Figure 1.3). These lesions are thought to occur at least 10 years after exposure has started, so that many more cases are expected to occur.

Cancer rates of the skin, bladder, kidney and lung have also started to increase. As these have latency periods of at least 20 years, it is expected that many cases will appear in the future. In Bangladesh, 35–77 million people are estimated to be exposed to well water with arsenic concentrations over 50 μg/L, a figure that according to US EPA estimates could be associated with a more than 1:100 lifetime cancer risk at a consumption of 1 liter of water per day from the well.

Remediation is complicated as there are tens of thousands of wells, most of which are privately owned. However, cost-effective emergency measures exist, including identification

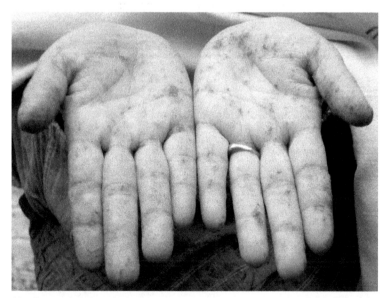

Fig. 1.3 Skin disease that is typical of arsenic poisoning. Reproduced with permission by the World Bank.

of local wells which are not contaminated, or less contaminated—these are painted different colours—and the application of filtration or chemical cleaning procedures.

1.2.4 **The Bhopal incident in India**

Chemical point sources may cause acute and chronic health effects in the population. Not far from Bangladesh, Union Carbide set up a small pesticides factory in Bhopal, India, in 1969. In 1979, the company started manufacturing methyl isocyanate (MIC)—an intermediate chemical used in pesticide production—at the Bhopal factory. It is a little lighter than water but twice as heavy as air; when it escapes into the atmosphere it remains close to the ground. Early in the morning of 3 December 1984, about 27 tonnes of MIC poured out of a tank at the factory for nearly two hours and escaped into the air. MIC spread eight kilometers downwind over the city of nearly 900 000 inhabitants. Up to 3000 people were killed in their sleep or as they fled trying to escape the gas and up to 400 000 were injured. Many people died from choking or circulatory collapse. Pulmonary edema developed in many people in the acute stage or later after a free interval. Complications from the respiratory tract were observed, including pneumothorax, subcutaneous and mediastinal emphysema and bronchopleural fistulas. Many have been suffering adverse health effects ever since. Although several epidemiological investigations have been conducted, the results have been mixed as a result of the methodologies that had to be employed, the population studied and the political situation. This example is discussed further in Chapter 9.

1.3 **Scope of environmental epidemiology**

Now that environmental epidemiology has been illustrated by way of examples, it is time to define what we mean by 'environment' more closely. In principle, 'environment' is all that surrounds us. This includes the water we drink, the air we inhale, the food we eat, the soil we live on, the buildings we dwell in, the work we do, and the society we are part of. All of these environmental factors can impact health in either a positive or a negative way.

Although 'environment' is all-inclusive, in this book a pragmatic choice has been made to focus on the general environment. Hence, there is no discussion of occupational exposures in detail, or nutritional issues unless the food chain serves as vehicle for potentially harmful contaminants. Another restriction is to focus on chemical, physical and mostly noninfectious biological agents, and not address the social environment as a determinant of health status.

Clearly, such demarcations are to some extent artificial. A person who is exposed to sidestream tobacco smoke in the air at home as well as at the office cannot be split into an occupational and an environmental subject. Also, for example, active smoking of cigarettes is generally not considered part of environmental epidemiology, but passive exposure to cigarette smoke from others (environmental tobacco smoke or ETS) is considered to be an issue for environmental epidemiology. The demarcations that have been chosen do by and large reflect the emergence of various subspecialties in epidemiology, as is evident from textbooks, journals and societies catering to these subspecialties. There is, of course, a danger in carving up public health issues in bits and pieces when the subspecialties start to operate in isolation.

The number of *agents* in the environment that may be harmful to health is very large. They can be classified in a number of ways:

* chemical, physical or biological;

* man-made or natural;

* essential or nonessential.

Hundreds of chemical substances have been evaluated for their toxicity. Fact sheets can be found on the Internet, e.g., from the US Agency for Toxic Substances and Disease Registry (ATSDR) at http://www.atsdr.cdc.gov/toxfaq.html. Physical agents that may affect health in the general environment include noise, temperature and various forms of radiation. Apart from infectious agents in the environment, there are many other biogenic substances that may affect health such as toxins produced by fungi, allergens produced by animals or plants, etc.

Agents may be man-made, of natural origin or both. Volcanoes emit sulphur oxides as do power plants that use fossil fuels. Wildfires produce smoke as do man-made fires for heating and cooking. Especially in the chemical industry, substances are being produced that never existed in the ecosystem before. Such uniquely man-made substances may pose special risks because there has been no evolutionary adaptation to their presence in the environment.

Some substances such as iron, calcium, oxygen, etc. are a necessary element for human life and such essential agents have optimal exposures which are optimally compatible with health. Too little or too much can be damaging. Nonessential agents have no known role in human metabolism and although in most cases some exposure can be tolerated without adverse effects on health, exposure is best limited to the lowest levels that are reasonably achievable.

In addition to considering the inherent nature of an agent, it is helpful to consider exposure patterns by *(micro) environments*, *pathways and routes*, and to explicitly consider *time* and *space* as important dimensions. These factors can strongly influence the amount of exposure to an agent and thus are essential components of exposure assessment in conducting environmental epidemiology studies. These issues are considered further in Chapters 2 and 3.

1.4 Reasons to embark on studies in environmental epidemiology

It is helpful to think of studies in environmental epidemiology as measurement of associations between environment and disease. Schematically, we can discern two reasons to embark on a study:

1. Concern about certain established diseases in the population that may have an environmental cause—disease looking for a cause; and

2. Concern about certain environmental factors that may lead to disease in the population—cause looking for disease.

In the first instance, knowledge about disease mechanisms will help to formulate which environmental exposures one may wish to examine. The example of cholera in nineteenth-century London is one in which John Snow used his detailed clinical observations of cholera cases to propose that ingestion rather than inhalation of some harmful entity was likely to be the cause. In the second instance, knowledge about the toxicity or harmfulness of the environmental factor of concern is helpful to formulate hypotheses on which disease end points may conceivably be related to the exposure of interest. The carcinogenic effects of ionizing radiation have been well established in studies among survivors of the atomic bombs dropped on Japan at the end of World War II, and from studies among miners exposed to high concentrations of radon in the mines. Such knowledge prompted studies on the possible relationship between lung cancer and radon exposure in homes built in areas where the ground is rich in radio nuclides [6, 7].

Environmental epidemiological studies are undertaken for a variety of reasons and by different institutions. Often, they aim to establish or improve scientific knowledge of the causal relationship between environmental exposure and disease. Such studies are typically undertaken by a university or research institution. An epidemiological study might also focus on obtaining descriptive data for initial decision-making regarding preventive action. Such investigations may be conducted by local or regional public health agencies in response to community concerns about a perceived environmental exposure or disease epidemic. These investigations must have a practical, problem-solving orientation to address the community's concerns in the shortest possible time period. Community awareness of environmental health issues can also create a demand for epidemiological research. In general, the nature of an environmental epidemiological study is determined by whoever is responsible for conducting the study, the purpose of the study, and the resources available to the investigators.

Epidemiological studies are also often carried out in response to community concern about newly developing or increasing incidence of health effects that are believed to be linked to changes in environmental conditions that have occurred following industrial or agricultural developments. Cases of a disease can occur as an 'epidemic'—for example, a set of congenital malformations may be identified within a community hospital over a short period of time. Similarly, clusters of severe illnesses (e.g., cancer) that were not observed previously in an area often initiate investigation of environmental factors. Methods to evaluate clusters of illnesses are described in Chapter 8, section 8.3, and strategies for working with concerned communities are discussed in Chapter 12.

The need for environmental epidemiology investigations may be particularly urgent in the event of a chemical incident from an industrial facility, such as the Bhopal incident previously described, or a natural disaster such as widespread flooding. Similarly, cumulative exposure or long-term effects following an ecological disaster may require epidemiological investigation. Chapter 9 provides examples of such investigations and describes the epidemiological approaches for both the immediate phase response and longer-term follow up.

Environmental epidemiology has the capacity to provide information that can contribute to rational decision-making and allocation of resources by providing quantitative estimates of the risk reduction that could be anticipated by controlling exposures to environmental hazards. Risk estimates derived from epidemiological studies can, therefore, be used for cost-effectiveness analysis by environmental managers. Regulators often use environmental epidemiological research to inform policy decisions. The role of environmental epidemiology in risk assessment is described in Chapter 14, while Chapter 16 discusses the role of epidemiologists in making environmental health policy.

1.5 Environmental epidemiology and related fields

Environmental epidemiology involves the application of the ideas and methods of many scientific disciplines, including chemistry, meteorology, microbiology, environmental science, and physics to establish human exposure levels. It also uses elements of clinical medicine, biochemistry, and physiology to establish the health impacts. By applying statistical and mathematical methods, environmental epidemiology integrates information collected via the other sciences. The interpretation of this information for preventive action is one of the most challenging and important aspects of environmental epidemiology.

In all epidemiology studies a variety of factors that influence health need to be taken into account, as each of them may contribute independently to the causation of the disease of interest. Environmental epidemiological studies therefore cannot ignore exposure to lifestyle factors such as tobacco smoking, dietary factors or underlying diseases or conditions unrelated or not directly related to the environment, some of which may confound apparent associations between environment and disease. Indeed, significant effort in an environmental epidemiological study is often directed towards accounting for such nonenvironmental factors.

As the field of epidemiology grew larger during the second half of the twentieth century, specializations emerged that tackle specific areas within epidemiology. Some of these are disease-based (e.g., respiratory epidemiology, cancer epidemiology) and some mechanism based (e.g., genetic epidemiology), while others are exposure-based. Although the 'environment' encompasses everything that surrounds us, specific environments and exposures have earned their own specialty within epidemiology. Close cousins of environmental epidemiology are *occupational* and *nutritional* epidemiology, and also *infectious disease* epidemiology.

Occupational epidemiology deals with exposure of workers in the work environment to potentially harmful agents. Practically all of the agents of interest in occupational epidemiology also occur in the general, nonoccupational environment. There are some important differences, however:

1. Occupational epidemiology studies mostly *adult populations* of workers. Usually, worker populations are different from the general populations not only in terms of age, but also in the distribution of gender and health status. Even when engaged in potentially harmful work, workers are, at least initially, usually *more* healthy than the general population of the same age for the simple reason that people who have some chronic illness or impairment are less likely to become employed. This is called the 'healthy worker effect', and it can bias comparisons of health status between worker populations and nonworkers.

2. Exposures in occupational settings are often *higher* than in the general environment. There are many examples of harmful agents (radon, asbestos, etc.) that were first studied in worker populations, but were later found to be of environmental concern as well. Risk assessment for environmental exposures is sometimes based on established exposure–response relationships from occupational studies.

3. Exposures in occupational settings are often also more *specific*, in the sense that one or just a few contaminants or agents related to a specific production process are increased. It is therefore easier to study the effects of such agents without having to worry about confounding by co-pollutants which may also be increased.

4. Exposure assessment tends to rely more often on personal exposure measurement compared to environmental epidemiology. The 'exposure grouping' method is often used to categorize workers by exposure.

5. Employers generally maintain records on personnel (time and location of work), raw materials and products, production processes, and possibly historical environmental monitoring data. It is therefore possible in some instances for investigators to determine the working population at risk and possible levels of exposure to specific agents historically. Equivalent historical records, such as records of residence in a community and past levels of exposure in the communities, are typically more difficult to obtain and less reliable in environmental studies.

6. Other differences have to do with access to study populations or workplaces; as many production facilities are privately owned, studies cannot be conducted without the permission of owners (and, obviously, workers themselves). Even when permission is granted, there may be pressures one way or the other to influence study results, as the stakes for both workers and management can be very high.

Despite these differences between environmental and occupational epidemiology, there are many similarities: there is often interest in effects of the same agents; methods for measuring exposure are often comparable if not exchangeable; modeling of exposure has a prominent place in both fields as large-scale measurements of personal exposures are not often possible.

Nutritional epidemiology deals with diet as a source of health and disease. It is a slightly more distant cousin of environmental epidemiology than occupational epidemiology, because the macro- and micronutrients which are the main focus of nutritional epidemiology are not usually of interest in either occupational or environmental epidemiology. What binds the three is methods of exposure assessment at the conceptual level. In all three, it is difficult to get accurate and precise information about exposure to the agents of interest. Systematic and random error are the result, and pioneering work has been conducted in nutritional epidemiology to think through the statistical concepts to deal with exposure misclassification, and to develop methods of validation of necessarily crude methods of exposure assessment. Also, food consumption can be a major pathway for environmental contaminants to enter the human body, and components such as antioxidants or vitamin content may modify the relationship between environmental pollution and adverse health effects. Methods for measuring food consumption have received much attention in nutritional epidemiology. These methods are useful in environmental epidemiology in combination with assessment of contaminant levels in the food chain, to estimate intake of contaminants with food. Such methods include food frequency questionnaires in which respondents are asked about their habitual diets in detail; diary methods in which subjects are asked to record each food item consumed prospectively over periods of days to weeks; and market basket studies in which subjects report what food items they bought in a certain period of time. In addition, biomarkers of exposure are used, as in other branches of epidemiology, to assess intake of certain substances from all sources combined.

Infectious disease epidemiology deals with the spread of infections and related diseases in populations. Although the basic epidemiological tools and concepts are not different from other branches in epidemiology, there are some special features that separate infectious disease epidemiology from the others. One is that a case can also be a risk factor: someone who has contracted an infectious disease may spread it in their immediate surroundings by various ways of dissemination of the infectious agent. In the case of subclinical infections, an infected person can be a source of exposure to others, leading to new cases, without even being a clinical case themself. Another is that people may become immune to a certain infection through previous contact or immunization. Differences in susceptibility exist for other exposure–response relations in epidemiology as well, but not as extreme as in the case of innate or acquired immunity against specific infections. Thirdly, in the case of acute and life-threatening infectious disease outbreaks, there can be a need for urgency that is seldom matched in other branches of epidemiology. The Broad Street pump cholera outbreak that we discussed before is a classic example, showing the need for enquiry, analysis and decision-making in a matter of days. In infectious disease epidemiology, mathematical models are being developed to study the spread of infections, and to study outbreaks and infectivity. These methods are also specific to this branch of epidemiology.

Toxicology is the science of poisons. Over the years, elaborate batteries of toxicity tests have been developed aimed at identification of adverse effects of chemical substances. Classical studies expose genetically homogenous, inbred strains of experimental animals to various but usually high amounts of the test substance in order to establish at which level animals are killed or suffer clear toxic effects. Studies can be of short duration to establish acute toxicity or be conducted over periods of months or even years to study subchronic or chronic toxicity. Detailed pathological studies are conducted to establish macroscopic causes of death or toxicity, and biochemical studies are being conducted to establish the kinetics of uptake and distribution, and the mechanisms of action. In addition, organ, tissue or cell cultures are being studied to establish in more detail how chemicals affect target organs or components thereof. Increasingly, animal models are being developed that mimic one or another sort of human susceptibility, be it genetic, or related to age or disease state.

In a very limited way, the tools of toxicology are also being used to study toxic effects in humans, by experimental exposure of human subjects to chemicals of interest. Clearly, such studies are restricted to transient, mild effects; to short-term exposures and effects;

and to volunteer subjects in reasonably good health. The clear advantage of toxicology (being mostly experimental) over epidemiology (being mostly observational) is that the causality of the observed effects is not usually in doubt. Epidemiology, being mostly restricted to making observations among free-living, heterogeneous populations, is more prone to producing associations between exposure and disease which may not be causal, but may be related to one or the other sort of bias that can distort observational studies. On the other hand, epidemiology is capable of studying human beings in the real world, so that results, when established to be valid, have immediate applicability to public health policy. Studies among experimental animals, on the contrary, always require extrapolation from animal to man, from high to low dose, and from single chemical exposures to exposures that occur in mixtures (Table 1.2).

It is no wonder, then, that in *risk assessment*, epidemiology and toxicology are complementary. Risk assessment is concerned with making quantitative assessments of the risk associated with a certain level of exposure to a substance or factor in the population (see Chapter 14). The traditional demarcations are those between *hazard assessment*, i.e., establishing that a substance or factor can possibly damage health because of its intrinsic properties; *exposure–response or dose–response assessment*, i.e., establishing at what level of exposure (in epidemiology) or at what dose level (in toxicology) a certain adverse effect on health occurs in which frequency and/or severity; *exposure assessment*, i.e., establishing the distribution of exposure within the population, and *risk characterization*, the final quantitative assessment of which proportion of an exposed population will experience an adverse effect of a certain severity.

Table 1.2 Differences between toxicology and epidemiology

Toxicology	Epidemiology
Experimental	Observational
Animals/tissues/humans	Humans
Single of few subjects	Population
Mechanisms	Black box
Causation	Association
Higher exposures	Low exposures
Defined exposures	Exposures to be estimated
Hazard testing before product introduction	Estimating risk in population
Problems:	
Extrapolation species	Confounding/bias
	Exposure assessment
Low dose extrapolation	Low dose extrapolation
In common:	
Exposure-response	Exposure-response

This chapter has provided some examples of classical environmental epidemiological studies and defined the scope of environmental epidemiology as it will be used in this book, along with the relationship of environmental epidemiology to other exposure-oriented subdisciplines of epidemiology and relevant scientific disciplines. The next chapter provides a review of principles of environmental health and epidemiology for those readers who may not have completed introductory courses in these areas. Thereafter, the book will describe concepts and methods to conduct environmental epidemiological studies and show how these methods are applied in special areas of environmental epidemiology.

1.6 **References**

[1] Vinten-Johansen P, Brody H, Paneth N, Rachman S, Rip M. *Cholera, chloroform, and the science of medicine: A life of John Snow.* New York, NY: Oxford University Press 2003.

[2] Snow J, Frost WH, Richardson BW. *Snow on cholera; being a reprint of two papers.* New York: Hafner Publishing Co. 1965.

[3] Bell ML, Davis DL. Reassessment of the lethal London fog of 1952: novel indicators of acute and chronic consequences of acute exposure to air pollution. *Environmental Health Perspectives.* 2001; **109**(Suppl 3):389–94.

[4] Dockery DW, Pope CA, 3rd, Xu X, Spengler JD, Ware JH, Fay ME, et al. An association between air pollution and mortality in six U.S. cities. *The New England Journal of Medicine.* 1993; 9(329;24):1753–9.

[5] Smith AH, Lingas EO, Rahman M. Contamination of drinking-water by arsenic in Bangladesh: a public health emergency. *Bulletin of the World Health Organization.* 2000; **78**(9):1093–103.

[6] Field RW, Krewski D, Lubin JH, Zielinski JM, Alavanja M, Catalan VS, et al. An overview of the North American residential radon and lung cancer case-control studies. *J Toxicol Environ Health A.* 2006; **69**(7):599–631.

[7] Darby S, Hill D, Auvinen A, Barros-Dios JM, Baysson H, Bochicchio F, et al. Radon in homes and risk of lung cancer: collaborative analysis of individual data from 13 European case-control studies. *BMJ.* 2005; **330**(7485):223.

Chapter 2

Review of environmental health and epidemiological principles

Dean Baker

The objective of this chapter is to review basic concepts and terms of environmental health and epidemiology that will be used in the text. Readers who have completed an introductory course in each of these topics may be able to skip this chapter.

2.1 Basic principles of environmental health

A major aim of environmental epidemiological studies is to determine if exposure to an environmental factor or factors is associated with an effect, or change in health status. If there is an association, it is desirable to be able to show an exposure–response relationship, i.e., a relationship in which an increase in the level of exposure is associated with an increase in the rate of a health effect. This section will review basic principles and terms that are used in environmental health and that are relevant to understanding environmental epidemiology.

The environmental conditions of concern may be chemical, physical (such as ionizing radiation), biological or ergonomic factors. Many examples presented in this book are based on chemical exposures. Nevertheless, when designing epidemiological studies on other types of hazards, one can apply the same principles.

2.1.1 Exposure and dose

Exposure is used to signify the contact that occurs between an environmental hazard and the human body. More precisely, in environmental epidemiology exposure to an environmental substance is generally defined as any contact between a substance in an environmental medium (e.g., water, air, soil) and the surface of the human body (e.g., skin, respiratory tract).

To evaluate the extent of exposure in an epidemiological study it is important to understand the sources, pathways and routes of the substances of interest. The physical course a pollutant takes from the source to a person is often referred to as the *exposure pathway*, while the way a substance enters the body is often referred to as the *exposure route*. For example, the source may be cars that emit air pollutants such as particles and carbon monoxide from the exhaust pipe. Dispersion will take place into the streets and beyond leading to environmental concentrations. Dispersion takes places into so

Box 2.1 Agents and media

- Agents: chemical, biological, physical
- Media (vectors): water, air, soil, food
- Routes of entry: inhalation, ingestion, absorption

called microenvironments such as houses, travel routes and modes, and work places, where people come into contact with the pollutants, and is now referred to as exposure. Exposure routes include inhalation; ingestion; direct skin or eye contact; transplacental blood contact from mother to fetus; or injection directly into the body, such as from a puncture wound. Methods to assess pathways and routes of exposure are discussed in Chapter 3.

The amount of the hazard that enters the body is termed the *dose*; the dose determines whether or not the individual exposed experiences an effect. It is not until a pollutant reaches the internal portion of the body that the exposure can be expressed as a dose. A person could dive into polluted water and be highly exposed to the pollutants therein, but a lung dose would occur only if the person aspirated the water. The concept of dose may be further defined as the *target organ dose*, which is the amount of the agent that reaches the susceptible organ or tissue within the body. The term target organ dose is thus used by investigators to refer to the uptake of an agent by a specific organ, tissue or cell, or the concentration of that agent in the relevant organ, tissue or cell.

Genetic variation in the population influences variation in internal dose and *susceptibility* to an effect. This genetic variation would appear as variability in the distribution of the dose in a subset of the population even if members of the population had similar exposures.

In epidemiology, exposure estimates are usually based on data collected by environmental monitoring instruments or on estimates obtained by direct or indirect methods. These measurement techniques are discussed in Chapter 3. Monitoring data are used to estimate exposure, exposure is used to estimate dose, and dose is used to estimate the biologically effective dose at the target organ. It is important to understand the distinction between these terms as they affect the design and interpretation of an epidemiological study.

Measuring actual exposure is not always possible, and factors leading to exposure may have to be used as *surrogates* of exposure. A challenge for investigators is to decide when some surrogates of exposure, such as the location of a person's residence, is a sufficiently precise indicator of environmental exposure that the surrogate can be used as a measure of exposure in an epidemiological study. The use of surrogate measures and other issues of measuring exposures are discussed in Chapter 3.

2.1.2 **Effect**

In this book the term '*effect*' is used as a generic description of any change in health status or body function that can be shown to be due to exposure to an environmental hazard. This term can apply to an individual as well as to a change in the average experience of a population. Some epidemiologists use the term only in relation to populations.

Health effects of interest in environmental epidemiology cover a wide spectrum—from subjective annoyance to manifest disease or death—and may involve more than one organ system. The health effects associated with a biologically effective dose generally follow a sequence from early biological effects, to altered structure and function, and then to clinical disease or even mortality (Figure 2.1). The likelihood of transition from early biological effects to clinical morbidity or mortality can be affected by ongoing exposure to the hazard and it can be modified or affected by individual susceptibility, such as genetic factors and personal habits, diet, medication use, and simultaneous exposure to other causal factors.

In recent years, following developments in molecular biology and toxicology, interest has focused increasingly on measurable pathophysiological changes and early adverse effects, rather than on overt clinical disease. Examples of early adverse effects include biological indicators or biomarkers for genotoxic effects, immunotoxicity and neurological damage.

Local effects occur at the site of contact with the environmental hazard. Inhalation of chlorine gas, for example, causes severe damage to the tissues of the respiratory tract, which is the first site of bodily contact following inhalation. Irritation of the eyes after exposure to high levels of ambient ozone is another example of a local effect. Effects may also occur at sites other than the point of entry. A chemical, for instance, is transported (usually via the blood) after absorption, to other tissue. A *systemic effect* may then occur in this tissue.

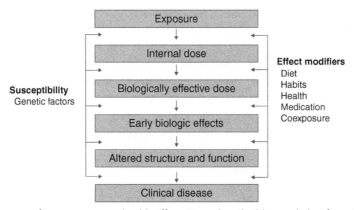

Fig. 2.1 Spectrum from exposure to health effect. Reproduced with permission from JM Links, *Introduction to Environmental Health*.

Health effects can also be classified according to the speed with which they develop in the individual in relation to the beginning and end of the period during which exposure occurs: an *acute effect* is an effect that develops very rapidly after exposure starts whereas a *chronic effect* takes substantial time to develop. These effects can be *temporary* (or *reversible*), meaning that they disappear after exposure ends, or *permanent* (or *irreversible*), meaning that they persist after exposure has ended. Chronic effects are often associated with long-term exposure, but at levels below those at which acute effects are observed. Repeated exposure may cause a reversible effect, but may also induce irreversible damage—for example, permanent hearing loss following repeated noise exposure.

Health effects induced by environmental factors may have a long *latency*, which is the time period between the relevant exposure and the onset of the effect. Follow-up of the atomic bomb survivors in Hiroshima and Nagasaki showed that latency periods for cancer, following exposure to ionizing radiation, ranged from a few years for leukemia to decades for solid tumors [1, 2]. Identification of early subclinical signs of toxicity can be important, particularly if late effects are likely to be severe.

The association between environmental exposures and health effects can be complex, because single environmental factors may cause *multiple effects*. For instance, lead causes biochemical alterations to the heme system eventually leading to anemia, while at the same time affecting the central and peripheral nervous system. Such combined health effects can also be due to *combined exposures* to several hazards. In fact, in many cases of air and water pollution combined exposures do occur. Complex situations may arise if the exposure consists of a mixture of many chemicals, as at some hazardous waste sites. Studying the related health effects can prove extremely difficult. Combined exposures to biological hazards also occur, particularly in areas with poor sanitation and hygiene conditions.

2.1.3 Relationship between exposure and effect

Distinguishing between dose–effect and dose–response relationships is crucial to accurate assessment of the effects of an environmental exposure. A 'dose–effect' relationship describes the relation between dose and type or severity of effect in an individual. For example, Figure 2.2 shows the effects that can occur in adults and children at different concentrations of lead in the blood [3]. The severity of the effects following exposure to a toxic agent increases with increasing dose: from physiological adaptation to irreversible damage.

Characterizing an effect on the basis of what has been observed in a single individual is generally not sufficient, however, since susceptibility varies within a population. Thus exposure–response relationship refers to a population and describes the probability of an effect as a function of the exposure. Exposure–response relationships are the primary focus of epidemiological investigations. It is generally assumed that dose is highly correlated with exposure across an exposed population, so many investigators use the phrase 'dose–response' interchangeably with 'exposure–response', although they are not the same.

In general, the dose–response curve shows how the risk of health effect increases with increasing dose (Figure 2.3). In addition, the shape of a particular dose–response curve

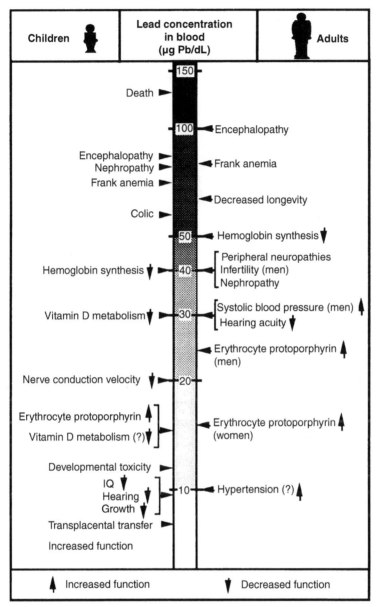

Fig. 2.2 Dose–effect relationship for lead in humans. Reproduced with permission from ATSDR. Case studies in environmental medicine: lead toxicity, 1992. October 2000; cited 1992, available from http://www.atsdr.cdc.gov/HEC/CSEM/lead/cover.html

may indicate the existence of a threshold, i.e., adverse effects do not occur until a certain dose has been reached. For ionizing radiation, some types of effect, such as acute radiation sickness, develop only if exposure to very high doses has occurred, but a radiation dose below which there is no increased risk of cancer has not been identified, meaning that there is no apparent threshold for the risk of cancer.

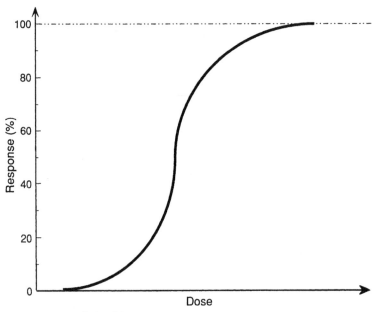

Fig. 2.3 Dose–response relationship.

As previously mentioned, the relation between dose and response may be modified by factors such as age or sex, or by other exposures. For example, young children are particularly susceptible to the central nervous system effects of lead [4], and smoking appears to potentiate the induction of lung cancer associated with exposure to asbestos [5, 6].

As pointed out earlier, the exposure levels encountered in the general population may be relatively low and the dose–response relationships encountered in a study may be weak. The resolution power of a study can then be increased by selectively including subpopulations with highly exposed individuals. Focusing on susceptible individuals can also be a means of detecting effects that would be rarer and hence more difficult to observe in the general population. Other options include increasing the precision of the measurements of exposure and confounding factors. As previously indicated, the specificity of the health risk determination is often crucial. An environmental epidemiology study showing a strong and precise dose–response relationship usually gives convincing evidence for preventive action.

2.1.4 Biomarkers

A *biological marker* or *biomarker* may be defined as any measurable biochemical, physiological, cytological, morphological, or other biological parameter obtainable from human tissues, fluids, or expired gases, that is associated with exposure to an environmental pollutant. The tissues and fluids used to measure biomarkers include, blood, urine, feces, teeth, hair, saliva, amniotic fluids and cells, and semen. In addition, fingernails or toenails and subcutaneous adipose tissue can be used to measure exposure. Blood and urine are the materials most commonly used as biomarkers.

Biomarkers have been used essentially to assess each stage of the spectrum from exposure to preclinical effects, as illustrated in Figure 2.1. *Biomarkers of exposure* include measurements of pollutants or their metabolites in body tissues and fluids, and reflect the pollutant amounts that have entered the human body—thus, they should be considered indicators of dose, but "biomarkers of exposure" has become the generally used term. Table 2.1 shows an example of the use of nicotine and cotinine as indicators of environmental tobacco smoke exposure in infants [7]. The table shows that both plasma nicotine and plasma cotinine increase significantly with environmental exposure to cigarettes. Biomarkers of exposure integrate exposure from all environmental pathways, so it is not possible using only such biomarkers to determine the environmental exposure pathways.

Biomarkers may also reflect early adverse effects or organ system damage. Markers of reproductive effects, for example, include reduced sperm count and somatic cell mutation. Measures, such as DNA-adducts and chromosomal aberrations, have been used as biomarkers of carcinogenesis [8, 9]. *Biomarkers of susceptibility* are used to show whether a person has genetic or environmentally derived variations in metabolism of a chemical that could influence the impact on the target organ. Genetic polymorphism in microsomal enzymes, such as cytochrome P_{450}, which influences the metabolism of many toxic chemicals, is an example of a biomarker of susceptibility. People with certain genetic forms of these enzymes have a reduced ability to metabolize some chemicals. In epidemiological studies, susceptibility biomarkers can improve the precision and strength of exposure–disease associations because they clarify variation that may be due to differences in susceptibility rather than to differences in exposures.

Table 2.1 Nicotine and cotinine as biological markers of exposure to environmental tobacco smoke in infants

(number)		Plasma nicotine [a] (ng ml^{-1})	Plasma cotinine [a] (ng ml^{-1})
Number of smoking parents			
0	221	0.36 ± 0.18	0.41 ± 0.96
1	74	0.47 ± 0.26*	2.78 ± 5.31*
2	41	1.00 ± 1.19*	9.01 ± 8.21*
Daily exposure (cigarettes per day)			
0	301	0.40 ± 0.22	0.96 ± 3.03
1–9	56	0.61 ± 0.51*	4.80 ± 6.78*
10–25	27	1.05 ± 1.32*	8.74 ± 6.21*

[a] Mean ± Standard deviation

* Significantly different from no exposure, $p < 0.01$.

Adapted with permission from M Sorensen, H Bisgaard, M Stage, S Loft. Biomarkers of environmental exposure to to tobacco smoke in infants. *Biomarkers*. 2007 **12**(1):38–46.[7].

2.2 Review of epidemiological principles

Subsequent chapters assume that the reader has a basic understanding of the principles of epidemiology, such as would be learned in an introductory course on epidemiology. This section reviews basic principles and terms that are important for the reader to understand in environmental epidemiology.

2.2.1 Concepts of populations

A fundamental premise in epidemiology is that disease does not occur strictly at random in the human population. It is possible to identify causes of a disease by studying the patterns of disease occurrence among different populations, in particular, by comparing health outcomes of exposed populations with that of unexposed populations. It is important to understand the concepts of population used in epidemiological studies. Figure 2.4 shows the relationship between the key terms used to refer to populations in epidemiological studies. The *general population* refers to all individuals, theoretically in the world, but generally meaning in some specified area such as a country or region.

The *population at risk* consists of the individuals in the general population who could develop the disease of interest. People who already have a disease are not at risk of developing the disease and, therefore, are excluded from the population at risk. Also individuals who previously had an infectious disease, such as measles, and develop immunity against reinfection are not at risk. The population at risk may also be limited to a single gender for gender-specific diseases, such as prostate cancer in males or uterine cancer in females. Even among the population technically at risk of developing a disease, there can be substantial variation in risk, so most investigators may focus on only a subpopulation as the practical population at risk. For example, most studies of breast cancer focus on women although males can develop breast cancer.

It is not necessary and generally not desirable to study the entire population at risk in order to evaluate epidemiological associations between exposure and disease. For example, although the entire population is at risk of developing a heart attack, the risk may be

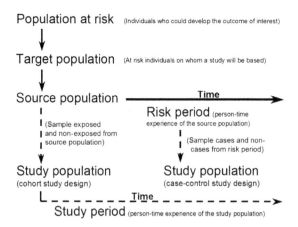

Fig. 2.4 Concepts of populations in epidemiology.

exceedingly small among children. Therefore, an epidemiological study may define a more limited at-risk population. An example would be a study of the occurrence of heart attacks only among persons older than 40 years of age. Populations may also be limited by gender, geography or other characteristics. The resulting selected population at risk is considered the *target population*. The target population is the population to which the interpretation of the study results will most likely be generalized.

The *source population* is the population at risk from which the study participants will be sampled. The source population is closely related to the target population, and many investigators consider these to be synonymous terms. However, in practice, the source population is defined in more operational terms than the target population. Continuing with the above example, the target population may be defined as 40–50 year old males living in a particular region of a particular country, but the source population may be limited to those who have access to medical care if they were to develop a heart attack. Understanding the source population is important because it is the population to which the findings of a study are applicable. Investigators may subsequently consider biological mechanisms, toxicological data and other information to consider whether the findings of a study may be generalized to the source population, the target population or broader population at risk.

A fundamental consideration in epidemiological measurements is not only the number of individuals who develop a health outcome, but also the rate at which the outcome occurs. Therefore, populations concepts in epidemiology incorporate both the number of persons and the time period of the observation. The *risk period* is the total time during which the individuals in the source population are at risk of developing an outcome of interest. The risk period is quantified as the 'person-time' at risk since it incorporates both the number of individuals at risk and the amount of time each individual is at risk. For example, 200 males living at risk over a 10-year period would represent 2000 person-years at risk.

The *study population* consists of individuals sampled from the source population and included in the study. For example, investigators may use a tumor registry to sample males between the ages of 50 and 65 who develop lung cancer within a region over a specific period of time. The source population includes all males between the ages of 50 and 65 living in the region who could develop lung cancer during the specific period of time, while the study population includes only the persons actually recruited into the study.

Several terms are used by investigators to identify individuals in a study population. The most common term used in the epidemiological literature is '*subject*' because individuals in a study population are the subject of the investigation. The term is appropriate for studies that are based on use of existing data, since actual people do not participate in these studies. This term is also used in experimental research. However, it is also common for investigators to use the term '*participant*' for individuals in a study population, especially in clinical or field epidemiological studies that involve data collection on people. The reason this term is being increasingly used in environmental epidemiology is that it expresses more of a sense of partnership between the investigators and the people who participate in a study, than referring to the study population as subjects. This sense of partnership can be important in increasing participation and retention rates in clinical and community-based studies. '*Respondent*' is another term that is used in social science research and sometimes in epidemiological studies that primarily involve collection of questionnaire information. It is also acceptable to refer to people in a study population as '*persons*' or '*individuals*', which is the approach used by some investigators to avoid using any particular label. Because there is not one universally accepted term to refer to people who participate in epidemiological studies, this text will use all of these terms based on whether the term is appropriate for the study design and also in part on the preferences of the chapter authors.

Epidemiological study designs differ in the manner in which the study population is sampled from the source population. In a cohort study, a sample of individuals at risk is drawn from the source population. This study population is followed over time to measure their health outcome occurrence. The person-time follow-up experience of the study population in a cohort study is the *study period*. The study population and study period in a cohort study are directly observable since the individuals are actually under observation. In a case-control study, the study population consists of a sample of cases and non-cases from the risk period of the source population. The full hypothetical study population (source population) in a case-control study is not directly observed, but it is conceptually identical to the study population in a cohort study.

2.2.2 Measurement of health in populations

Epidemiological studies are based on quantification of the occurrence of disease or health outcomes in populations. The most basic measure of disease occurrence is a simple count of the individuals affected. This can be used to show time trends for epidemics and to quantify a specific health problem for a defined geographic area. However, the number of persons who have a disease is generally not informative unless additional information about the population is also available. In order to investigate disease occurrence, the size of the population at risk and the time period during which the number of cases was observed must usually be known. Disease occurrence can then be calculated as a function of the number of health outcome events per unit size of the population for a specified time period.

Occurrence of disease is expressed as *prevalence*, based on the number of cases that exist at a designated point in time, or *incidence*, based on the number of new cases that occur during a given period. Specific definitions of these disease occurrence measures have been developed according to how the cases and populations are observed.

2.2.2.1 Incidence measures

Perhaps the most common measure of disease occurrence is the (person-time) *incidence rate* [10]. This is a measure of the disease occurrence per unit of time. The incidence rate is based on the notion of observing a population over time to determine the number of individuals who develop the health outcome that is being investigated. In Figure 2.5 the study period of a hypothetical population is presented. People enter the study in a particular year, and some of them subsequently develop the disease of interest.

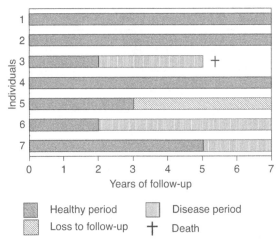

Fig. 2.5 Hypothetical cohort population follow-up status. Adapted from [11]. Reproduced with permission from Beaglehole R, Bonita R, Kjellstrom T. *Basic Epidemiology*. Geneva: WHO 1993.

Some eventually die from the disease, but others from another cause. By the end of the study period, some members of the cohort have died from the disease under study, some are still alive, and others have been 'lost to follow-up' because they died from other causes or because contact with them was lost.

Study participants contribute in formation only during the period in which they can develop the disease and can be studied. Individuals who cease to contribute information include those who die and who therefore cannot develop the disease and those who emigrate and are lost to follow-up during the study. So it is important to consider how much time each person contributes to the study by using the person-time method.

Figure 2.5 illustrates how person-time is measured in a small hypothetical population. In the figure, individuals 1, 2, and 4 are observed during the entire follow-up period and, therefore, each contributes seven person-years at risk of observation. Individuals 3 and 6 were observed for two years before developing disease and each contribute two person-years. They no longer contribute years at risk once they develop the disease. Individual 5 contributes three years of observation before becoming a loss to follow-up, perhaps by moving away. The total period at risk of developing 'disease' in this population is 33 person-years. Because diseased individuals remain at risk of dying, the study period at risk for mortality in this population is 43 person-years (7, 7, 5, 7, 3, 7, 7, years respectively).

The *incidence rate* in a study population is the number of cases divided by the person-time experience of the population. The formulae for the incidence rate and other measures of health and effect are shown in Table 2.3. The formulae are consistent with the notation shown in Table 2.2. So as to not present multiple formulae for each measure, the text will present the formula for the total population (e.g., M_1/Y_T). The structure of the formulae for an exposed population and the nonexposed population are equivalent to those shown for the total population. For example, the incidence rate in an exposed population is $I_1 = a/Y_1$, while the incidence rate in the nonexposed population is $I_0 = b/Y_0$.

Table 2.2 Notation for data for calculating disease incidence

	Exposed	Nonexposed	Total
Cases	a	b	M_1
Non-cases	c	d	M_0
Study population (persons)	N_1	N_0	T
Study period (person-years)	Y_1	Y_0	Y_T
Incidence rate	I_1	I_0	I
Cumulative incidence	R_1	R_0	R

Table 2.3 Measures of health and measures of effect in populations*

Measurements of health	Measures of effect (association)
Incident rate $I = \dfrac{M_1}{Y_T}$	Rate ratio $\qquad RR = \dfrac{I_1}{I_0} = \dfrac{a/Y_1}{b/Y_0}$
Cumulative incidence $R = \dfrac{M_1}{T}$	Risk ratio $\qquad RR = \dfrac{R_1}{R_0} = \dfrac{a/N_1}{b/N_0}$
[new cases]	Odds ratio (case-control) $\qquad OR = \dfrac{a \times d}{b \times c}$
Prevalence $P = \dfrac{M_1}{T}$ [existing cases]	Prevalence ratio $\qquad PR = \dfrac{P_1}{P_0}$
Prevalence odds $P = \dfrac{M_1}{T - M_1} = \dfrac{P}{1-P}$	Prevalence odds ratio $\qquad POR = \dfrac{P_1/(1-P_1)}{P_0/(1-P_0)} \approx \dfrac{I_1 \times \overline{D_1}}{I_0 \times \overline{D_0}}$
	Attributable fraction exposed $\qquad AF_e = \dfrac{I_1 - I_0}{I_1} = \dfrac{RR-1}{RR}$
	Population attributable fraction $\qquad AF_{(pop)} = \dfrac{(I - I_0)}{I}$ $\qquad\qquad\qquad\quad = \dfrac{P_e \times (RR-1)}{P_e \times (RR-1)+1}$

See Table 2.2 for definitions of notations.

Adapted from [12]. Reproduced with permission from Baker D, Kjellström T, Calderon R, Pastides H. *Environmental Epidemiology - A Textbook on Study Methods and Public Health Applications*. Geneva: WHO 1999.

The *cumulative incidence* or risk (also called the incidence proportion) is another important measure of disease occurrence. This is the proportion of study participants who develop the health outcome of interest. Since it is a proportion, it is 'dimensionless'. The relevant time period must be specified, however. The cumulative incidence is conceptually the same as the probability (or risk) of an individual developing the health outcome, as estimated by studying a population.

2.2.2.2 Prevalence measures

The prevalence of a health outcome in a population is based on the number of existing cases at a specific point in time. The prevalence proportion of a health outcome in a population is the number of existing cases at a point in time divided by the size of the population. In common with the cumulative incidence, it is a proportion and therefore dimensionless, but the relevant point in time must be specified. Prevalence is a useful measure of the burden of disease in a population because it indicates the size of the population affected. Prevalence is also an appropriate measure for chronic conditions, such as asthma or diabetes, in which the annual incidence of new cases is very small compared with the number of existing or prevalent cases. The prevalence proportion can also be used to estimate the incidence rate in a population if information about disease duration is available. If we assume that the study population is in a steady state (which is when the incidence rates and disease duration, exposure and covariate prevalence are stable in the population), it can be shown that the prevalence odds are equal to the incidence rate (I) multiplied by the average disease duration, that is: $P/(1-P)=I \times D$ [10].

2.2.3 Comparisons and associations

An epidemiological study generally seeks to estimate the effect of the exposure of interest by comparing disease occurrence in an exposed group with disease occurrence in a nonexposed group. The comparisons result in quantitative estimates of relative risk and risk difference.

2.2.3.1 Relative risk as a measure of effect

The principal measures of effect in cohort studies correspond to the two measures of incident health outcome occurrence described above. The *rate ratio* is the ratio of the incidence rate in the exposed group (a/Y_1) to that in the nonexposed group (b/Y_0). The *risk ratio* is the ratio of the cumulative incidence in the exposed group (a/N_1) to that in the nonexposed group (b/N_0). These two effect measures are generally referred to using the generic term *relative risk*, and each of these three terms are typically abbreviated as 'RR', so the precise meaning of this abbreviation often must be understood from the nature of the study design. For both of these measures of effect, the ratio is equal to 1.0 if no association exists between exposure and health outcome, because the rates or risks are identical in the exposed and unexposed groups.

The *odds ratio* is the primary measure of effect used in case-control studies. In this study design, the investigators sample persons with a specified disease (case) from the population and persons from the same population who are otherwise similar to the cases, but do not have the disease (control). The investigators then determine the past exposure status of the cases and controls, and use this information to estimate the relative risk of disease given their past exposure. In this study design, it is not possible to calculate directly the relative risk, but the relative risk can be estimated by the *odds ratio*, which is the ratio of the exposure odds in cases (a/b) to the exposure odds in controls (c/d), or (ad/bc). If no association exists between exposure and health outcome, the odds ratio is equal to 1.0.

2.2.3.2 Prevalence measures of effect

The *prevalence ratio* is the ratio of the prevalence proportion for the exposed to the prevalence proportion for the unexposed. It is an appropriate effect measure for use in circumstances such as an outbreak of illness due to biological food contamination, for which the period of exposure is short. In such circumstances, the prevalent cases represent the entire number of persons affected. This means that the prevalence ratio is equal to the risk ratio over the entire period of the outbreak.

As noted above, if certain assumptions are met, the prevalence odds is equal to incidence times duration. In this situation, the *prevalence odds ratio* is equal to the incidence rate ratio times the ratio of average disease duration in the two groups. An increased prevalence odds ratio may thus reflect the influence of factors which increase the duration of disease, as well as of those which increase disease incidence. However, if the average duration of disease is the same in the exposed and nonexposed groups (i.e., when exposure has no effect on disease duration), the prevalence odds ratio estimates the incidence rate ratio. The prevalence odds ratio is often used as the effect measure in a prevalence study [13].

2.2.3.3 Rate difference and risk difference as measures of effect

An analogous approach, using the *rate difference* (I_1-I_0) and the *risk difference* (R_1-R_0) rather than ratios, can be used to calculate difference measures of effect. For each of these measures, the rate in the unexposed group is subtracted from the rate in the exposed group. Ratio measures are usually of greater interest than difference measures in epidemiological studies because ratios make assessment of the strength of effect easier. However, difference measures may be of value in certain circumstances, particularly when evaluating the public health impact of an exposure. For example, difference measures can be used to estimate how much disease may potentially be eliminated as a result of an intervention to reduce environmental exposure. If no association exists between exposure and health outcome, the rate difference is equal to zero.

The effect of an exposure on an outcome can also be expressed by calculating the proportion of the disease incidence among the exposed population that can be attributed to the exposure. Known as *attributable fraction*, this measure of effect is based on the assumption that the rate difference represents the incidence of disease among the exposed population that is due to exposure. Consequently, the proportion of the observed incidence among the exposed due to exposure is the rate difference divided by the observed incidence. Furthermore, by dividing each incidence rate in the formula by I_0, the attributable risk can be calculated using only the relative risk measure.

Estimating what proportion of an outcome in a total population is attributable to an exposure—known as *population attributable fraction*—is also possible if the proportion of the total population that has undergone the exposure of interest is known. This measure is estimable because the attributable fraction due to exposure among the 'not exposed' is zero since this group is not exposed. The population attributable risk is therefore the attributable risk among the exposed population multiplied by the proportion of the total population that is exposed. The population attributable fraction can be a useful measure of effect in environmental epidemiology since it provides an indication of the total impact of an exposure on the population. This measure can reveal that exposures associated with a small relative risk of disease can nevertheless have a substantial impact on a population if a large proportion of that population is exposed, as in the case of air or water pollution.

2.2.4 Effect modification

Effect modification occurs when the estimate of the effect of the exposure to the study factor is influenced by the level of another factor in the study population [10]. An example of effect modification is the difference, due to gender, in risk of breast cancer. A study of environmental risk factors for breast cancer would either be restricted to females or, at a minimum, maintain males as a distinct study group, but the potential for effect modification is not always so obvious. The possibility that genetic polymorphisms influence individuals' capacity to metabolize an absorbed toxin, and therefore their susceptibility to environmental exposures, should be taken into consideration. This type of genetic variation is relevant to epidemiological studies because it can result in effect modification in which the same amount of exposure to a toxic substance could result in different levels of effect among different genetic subgroups of the study population. Effect modification due to variation in susceptibility can occur due to environmental as well as genetic factors. For example, gastrointestinal absorption of lead is increased in children with diets deficient in calcium or iron. Therefore, the risk of lead poisoning would be greater among such children than among children with equal lead exposure, but better nutritional status.

Effect modification can also result from biological interaction between multiple environmental exposures, in which the combined effect of the exposures differs from the total effect of the separate exposures. For example, the incidence rate of lung cancer in persons exposed to both asbestos and cigarette smoke is greater than the sum of the incidence rates of lung cancer in individuals exposed to either asbestos or to cigarette smoke, but not to both. Although there is variation across studies, it appears overall that the relative risk of lung cancer following exposure to both asbestos and cigarette smoke is more than additive, but somewhat less than multiplicative of the relative risks attributable to the separate exposures [5].

2.2.5 Validity (systematic error, bias and confounding)

The goal of any environmental epidemiological study is to obtain as accurate an estimate as possible of the quantitative association between an environmental factor and disease occurrence. The basic strategy for enhancing the quality of an epidemiological study consists of designing the study to minimize the potential for error. Additionally, the data and study implementation should be monitored to assess quality and to facilitate evaluation and adjustment for error when analyzing the data. Yet some error is inevitable.

Error is generally classified as random or systematic [10]. *Systematic error* pulls the observed effect estimate systematically towards or away from the true value, while *random error* is the divergence, due to chance, of an observation on a sample from the true population value. *Random error* is due to the variability of data with small numbers but can be reduced by doing a larger study. Systematic error is an inherent feature of the study design and the population under study and cannot be reduced simply by doing a larger study. *Validity* or accuracy is the extent to which the systematic errors are controlled. The term *bias* is used generally to refer to the presence of systematic errors. There are many different types of bias, but three general forms have been distinguished: selection bias; information bias; and confounding [10].

2.2.5.1 Confounding

Confounding occurs if the exposed and nonexposed groups are not comparable due to inherent differences in background disease risk. The differences are usually due to individual characteristics such as age, gender or socioeconomic background, or to exposure to other risk factors. If no other biases are present, the following three conditions are necessary for a factor to be categorized as a confounder:

* it must be a risk factor for the disease in the absence of the exposure under study (it does not have to be an actual cause; it could be a marker for an actual cause);
* it must be associated with exposure in the study population; and,
* it must not be affected by the exposure or disease. (In particular, it cannot be an intermediate factor in the causal pathway between exposure and disease. An intermediate factor is one that is caused by the exposure and which, in turn, causes the disease outcome.) [10]

The bias caused by confounding can be either toward or away from the null value of no apparent association between exposure and health outcome, depending on the relationships between the exposure, confounder, and health outcome. For example, the effectiveness of medical treatment of acute diarrheal disease could be evaluated by comparing sick children who received hospital-based medical treatment with children who received traditional home treatments. Better health outcomes might be observed among the children who received the hospital-based treatment. However, these children may live in a city and may be better nourished than the children who received the traditional home treatment. The seemingly greater efficiency of the hospital-based treatment might therefore be spurious. The apparent effect of the hospital-based treatment would be greater than the true effect because of confounding due to nutritional status.

Alternatively, the children who received hospital-based treatment may have done so because they were considered very ill. In which case, the apparent effect of the hospital-based treatment may be less than the true effect because of confounding due to differences in illness severity between the treatment groups. Multiple confounding factors can also occur and may even act in opposite directions, making clarification of the net bias very difficult.

In epidemiological studies, confounding can be controlled in the study design, or in the analysis, or both. Control of confounding at the design stage can be carried out principally by randomization, restriction or matching [10]. *Randomization*, in which exposure or treatment is randomly assigned to participants by the investigators, is not an option in observational epidemiological studies because the investigator does not assign exposure. *Restriction* entails narrowing the ranges of values of the potential confounders, for example, by restricting the study to white females in a particular age group. However, this approach may limit the number of potential study participants and the amount of information provided by the study. A third strategy is to match study participants on potential confounders (e.g., matching for age, gender, and ethnicity). *Matching* in a case-control study is accomplished by measuring the risk factors in the cases and then selecting controls from the source population for whom the same risk applies (see Chapter 6). Matching can be an effective means of controlling confounding, but it also can be expensive and complicate the analysis and interpretation of study findings.

The most common approach is to control confounding during the data analysis. This involves stratifying data into subgroups according to the levels of the confounders and calculating a summary measure of effect that summarizes the information across strata. Alternatively, multivariate analytical methods can be used to model the effect of exposure while adjusting for confounders. In general, control of confounding requires careful use of *a priori* knowledge, together with assessment of the extent to which the effect estimate changes when the factor is controlled in the analysis. Methods for controlling confounding by stratified analysis and multivariate methods are described in Chapter 7.

2.2.5.2 Selection bias

Whereas confounding is generally due to biases inherent to the source population, *selection bias* arises from the procedures used to select study participants from the source population into the study population. Thus selection bias is not usually a problem in a cohort study involving complete follow-up, since all of the available information from the source population may be used. However, bias can occur in a cohort study if participants are lost to follow-up due to factors associated with both exposure and outcome, or if exposure is an effect modifier for the association of study participation with health outcome. For example, bias could occur in a cohort study of air pollution and lung disease if individuals in polluted areas selectively migrate away from the study area when they develop respiratory symptoms and are consequently lost to follow-up. It is important to recognize that bias in the effect estimate would occur only if loss to follow-up differed between the exposed and the nonexposed; for example, if individuals living in a polluted area with respiratory symptoms were more likely to migrate than nonexposed persons with similar symptoms.

Selection bias is of more concern in case-control studies since these entail sampling from the source population. In particular, selection bias can occur in a case-control study if controls are chosen in a nonrepresentative manner: for example, if exposed individuals were more likely to be selected as controls than nonexposed individuals, as might happen if the controls for lung cancer cases are hospital patients with other diseases (tobacco smoking increases risk of lung cancer and many other diseases).

If appropriate information is available, selection bias can be assessed and controlled using methods similar to those used to assess and control confounding. In particular, selection bias can sometimes be controlled in the analysis by identifying factors relating to participant selection and controlling for them as confounders. For example, persons who have received higher education may be more likely to be selected for or to participate in a study and may have a different disease risk than less-educated persons. If education is negatively or positively related to the exposure of interest, this bias can be partially controlled by collecting information on education and controlling for education in the analysis. The analytical approaches to controlling confounding and selection bias are discussed in Chapter 7.

2.2.5.3 Information bias

Information bias results from misclassification of the study participants with respect to disease or exposure status. Information bias is also called *observation bias, measurement bias,* or *misclassification bias* since information errors commonly arise while measuring or classifying study variables. Two general forms of information bias are recognized, depending on whether the classification error for exposure is independent of the classification error for disease [10]. The distinction is relevant because the consequences of the biases are different.

Nondifferential information bias occurs when the likelihood of misclassification is the same for both groups being compared. In other words, the likelihood of misclassification of disease would be the same among the exposed and nonexposed groups, or misclassification of exposure would be the same among the diseased and nondiseased groups. Of course, in many instances, there is some amount of misclassification in measuring exposure and disease in a study population so the likelihood of misclassification must be considered for all measured variables. Nondifferential misclassification generally biases the effect estimate towards the null value of no apparent effect. So nondifferential information bias tends to produce 'false negative' findings, and is of particular concern in studies that find no association between exposure and disease. An example of probable nondifferential information bias in environmental epidemiology is the use of a person's residence as a surrogate measure of exposure status. For example, the distance of a person's home from a roadway or industrial facility might be used as a measure of potential lead exposure in a case-control study of neurological disease. There would be information bias—equal among cases and controls—if the surrogate distance measured did not accurately reflect true environmental lead exposure.

Differential information bias occurs when the likelihood of misclassification of exposure differs between diseased and nondiseased, or the likelihood of misclassification of disease differs between exposed and nonexposed persons. This type of bias may pull the observed effect estimate toward or away from the null value. For example, in a case-control study, recall of an exposure such as passive smoking in people with a respiratory disease might differ from that of healthy people. Differential information bias might therefore occur and could bias the odds ratio in either direction. Similarly, people living close to a factory may report respiratory symptoms more often than people living some distance from the factory in question, simply because they are more concerned about a possible link between their symptoms and the factory's emissions.

Several common sources of information bias have been recognized. Some of these, such as recall bias and interviewer bias, are of particular concern because the bias may vary among the study groups so that the net effect of the bias is not predictable.

Recall or *reporting bias* refers to differential reporting of information by study participants. For example, persons who have developed lung cancer may be more likely to recall exposure to asbestos or radon than control subjects who have not developed cancer. Several studies have found that persons living in communities near hazardous waste disposal sites tend to report higher prevalences of a wide range of symptoms; a pattern that seems consistent with increased symptom reporting among concerned community residents who are concerned about a potential exposure [see, for example, 14].

Interviewer bias refers to bias in the collection or recording of information by study staff. For example, prior knowledge of the participants' status may influence how study staff obtain or record information. Thus an interviewer might probe the environmental and occupational history of a lung cancer case more closely than that of a control person who does not have cancer. These biases are more likely to occur in historical cohort, case-control and cross-sectional studies than in cohort studies, since an individual's health outcome status may be known before the history of exposure is determined.

Measurement error refers to errors made in measuring study variables. As such, many investigators consider this term to be synonymous with information bias, but it is important to distinguish between the validity of a particular measure of exposure or disease (measurement error) and the validity of a study's effect estimate (information bias). Measurement errors can be systematic, for example, a spirometer that is always incorrectly calibrated, or random, e.g., because of test-to-test variability. Systematic errors reduce a measurement's validity, while random errors reduce measurement precision, but in both instances these errors will result in information bias and reduce the validity of the main effect estimate.

Similarly, measurements of health outcomes, especially biological processes, must take into account systematic variability in effects. *Intraindividual variability* in effects can occur for some conditions or physiological functions that display distinct cyclical (e.g., diurnal or seasonal) variation. This variability must be taken into account when recording measurements relating to conditions and functions. For example, lung function varies in accordance with a diurnal or daily pattern so that measurements taken for an individual in the morning may differ from those taken for the same individual in the evening. The time at which measurements are recorded can therefore be critical. *Interindividual variability* in effects is associated with the range of health outcomes observed in a population following its exposure to an agent; 'resistant' and 'susceptible' persons will be found at the two extremes of distribution.

Chapter 5 provides more detailed information on measurement error and describes strategies to identify and adjust for measurement error.

2.2.6 Precision (random error, statistical power)

As mentioned earlier, random error is variation in measurements due to chance alone. Random error arises due to biological variability, measurement variability, and sampling variability. Sources of biological variability include diurnal variation; changes related to factors such as age, diet, and exercise, and environmental factors such as season or temperature. *Measurement variability* may be due to inaccuracies in the performance or calibration of a measurement instrument, or misreading or incorrect recording of information from an instrument. Further random error may be introduced following mistakes made during data recording, processing, or management. Biological and measurement variability can lead to systematic or random errors.

Sampling variability occurs because the study participants are always a sample of a larger population. If a study was repeated on the same source population, some variability would occur each time in the actual study population sampled from the source population. The primary strategy for increasing precision, given variability in the source population, is to increase the size of the study population. Studying large numbers of participants can be expensive, however. The need for precision must therefore be balanced against considerations of cost and logistics.

An environmental epidemiological study should be large enough to ensure that the estimates of the hypothesized effects will be sufficiently precise, given the anticipated variation among the variables analyzed. Statistical analysis of epidemiological studies is discussed in Chapter 7. As noted in that chapter, the aim of statistical analysis is to estimate the precision of observed effect estimates or other estimates. For example, a statistical analysis of a case-control study would typically present the odds ratio as a measure of effect, with a 95 percent confidence interval as an indication of the precision of the odds ratio estimate. The analysis may also present a p-value as an indication of the likelihood that random error is responsible for the observed association. Although these values cannot be calculated until the data have been collected, estimating the precision of a study by making some reasonable assumptions about the statistical distributions of the variables to be analyzed is possible. Since the precision of a study is very much influenced by its number of participants, these calculations can be used to estimate the number of participants required to achieve the desired statistical power [see, for example, 15].

2.2.6.1 Sampling the population

Studying every member of a population is usually not feasible. Sampling is therefore carried out to enhance efficiency and reduce cost. The quality of the sampling influences not only precision, but also the potential for selection bias and for generalizing the study findings.

The *sampling unit* is the basic unit around which a sampling procedure is planned [16]. In most studies, individuals are selected from a population and then examined for exposure characteristics and health outcome status. The individual is therefore the sampling unit.

The sampling unit does not necessarily consist of people: vital events (births, deaths) or individual records in studies based on existing data could also constitute a sampling unit. In ecological studies, the sampling unit is a group or community.

The totality of the sampling units of the population to be studied is called the *sampling frame*, i.e., the population from which the sample is selected. A sampling frame is a concrete listing of or method to access the source population. The sample (study population) is a subset of the sampling frame. Examples of sampling frames include lists of consecutive hospital admissions, community census enumeration lists and randomized lists of telephone numbers for communities. It is essential to identify a well-defined sampling frame from which a representative sample can be drawn. 'Informal' sampling methods, such as use of volunteers, do not usually result in representative samples.

Methods for sampling persons from populations have been described in several epidemiology and statistical textbooks [see, for example, 16]. While a simple random sample may seem the best means of obtaining a representative sample, in practice obtaining stratified, systematic, cluster or multi-stage samples is usually more efficient. Stratified sampling is more efficient than simple sampling if the distribution of subjects—according to relevant variables, such as age or gender—is not uniform. If the population can be subdivided into subgroups that are more homogeneous with respect to variables of interest than is the population as a whole, study precision can usually be increased through stratification [16].

One of the principal advantages of systematic sampling is that determining the entire sampling frame of potential subjects before beginning the sampling is unnecessary. Moreover, under field conditions, systematic sampling is often simpler than random sampling. Thus sampling births in a hospital by making a systematic sample of every fifth birth would be easier than applying a random selection procedure to each separate birth, with a one-fifth possibility of that birth being selected for recruitment. The disadvantage of systematic sampling, however, is that identifying patterns in the sampling frame that could make the systematic sample unrepresentative can be difficult. Selecting sampling intervals that are not related to exposure or health outcome is therefore important. For example, sampling of births in a hospital should not be based on the day of the week since elective induction of complicated births may be more likely on some days than on others. Systematic samples are also limited in that estimating the variance may be difficult unless it can be assumed that a systematic sample from a randomly ordered population would not differ from a simple random sample. Most studies make this assumption and analyze systematic samples as if they were simple random samples.

Many environmental characteristics or health outcomes are relatively rare. Furthermore, identifying unbiased sampling frames of individuals for environmental epidemiology studies can be difficult. Studies that use more complex, multi-stage sampling approaches to enhance efficiency are therefore likely to become increasingly common. However, maintaining a clear understanding of the relationship between the actual study participants and the source population using these complicated sampling schemes is a considerable challenge.

Box 2.2 Definitions of sampling methods

- *Simple* — Each sampling unit in the population has an equal chance of being included in the sample.

- *Stratified* — The population is divided into strata, or groups of sampling units that have certain characteristics in common, and a random sample of units is drawn from each stratum.

- *Systematic* — The selected sampling units are spaced regularly throughout the sampling frame beginning with a randomly selected unit (*e.g.*, every fifth birth in a hospital).

- *Cluster* — Clusters rather than individual sampling units are first selected from the population and observations are then made on all individual sampling units within the selected clusters.

- *Multi-stage* — Primary sampling units are selected from a population. Secondary sampling units are then sampled from each primary unit, and so on. Multi-stage sampling is similar to cluster sampling, but additional sampling is carried out within the clusters.

2.2.7 Concepts of study design

As summarized so far in this chapter, the objective of an environmental epidemiology study is to assess whether an environmental exposure has an effect on health. This is achieved by comparing the health outcome occurrence of individuals who have been subjected to different exposure levels and, in particular, by comparing the health outcomes of exposed persons with those of unexposed or lesser-exposed persons. The result of such a comparison is quantified by calculating a measure of effect, such as the ratio of the incidence rate among the exposed to that of the unexposed.

Sometimes the environmental hazard that caused the health effect is only vaguely suspected; in other situations it is totally unknown. The first step in investigating the health effect could then be a *descriptive study*, which is a study that defines the population group of interest, estimates the incidence or prevalence of the disease, and identifies possible environmental hazards that might have caused the disease. A descriptive study can be useful in creating hypotheses for further study.

If a specific cause–effect relationship is believed to exist, an *analytical study* can be carried out. In such studies a hypothesis about cause and effect is tested or a quantitative relationship between exposure and effect is evaluated. Analytical studies are based conceptually on following a population over a period of time. Several study design options are available. The various study designs differ in the manner in which the *study population* is sampled from the source population, and the manner in which information is drawn from the risk period. Thus study designs may differ according to whether cases of disease are ascertained for a specified time period (incidence data), or at a particular point in time (prevalence data). Studies based on prevalence data are generally referred to as prevalence or cross-sectional studies. Study designs may also differ according to whether they incorporate all of the information contained in the person-time experience of the study population (cohort studies) or whether they attempt to obtain the same findings by comparing cases of disease with people without disease, selected as a sample of the person-time experience of the source population that generated the cases (case-control studies). Thus the difference between the analytical study types is not the direction of the association between exposure and health outcome, but the relative efficiency, feasibility and quality of data that can be obtained using the alternative approaches. The common types of epidemiological study designs are shown in Table 6.1 of Chapter 6, which describes the methods, strengths, and limitations of the study designs. This section briefly describe common study designs as a background for the next three chapters.

Cross-sectional studies entail the measurement of the prevalence of disease in an at-risk population alongside the simultaneous assessment of exposures and other factors that might modify or confound the relationship between exposure and disease. A comparison population which has been unexposed but is otherwise similar, is also surveyed to provide an 'external' reference; alternatively, an 'internal' approach may be used in which the effects of different degrees of exposure within an entirely exposed population are compared. Cross-sectional surveys are popular because they can be completed rapidly and relatively cheaply and because they have an intuitive appeal. However, such studies have an important drawback because of possible selection bias due to 'survival' whereby those who have suffered effects of exposure may have been selected out of the surveyed population—perhaps through a high mortality or migration out of the area of study. Selection in this way is likely to result in an underestimate of the health effects of an environmental exposure; the opposite may be true if survival (usually migration) is systematically related to low exposures.

In a *case-control (case–referent) study*, cases within the study population are identified by their disease status, either through active case-identification or from routinely collected information. Their exposure histories are then compared with those of 'control' subjects who are selected from the same population but are free of the disease that defines the cases. This study design is an efficient approach for rare diseases, such as many cancers or birth defects, or where the collection of exposure information is expensive or difficult. Case-control studies require considerable attention to case and control definitions and selection and to the assessment of exposure if they are to be free of bias.

Cohort studies are commonly used for the long-term follow-up of populations who have been exposed to an agent of interest. The population may be defined *prospectively* or *retrospectively* (using existing records). This study design allows the estimation of incidence rate(s) of multiple health outcomes across a spectrum of exposure. An unexposed population may be included for comparison, but careful measurement of potential confounding factors is generally required. In any case, substantial effort in needed in cohort studies to ensure high levels of follow-up to reduce the likelihood of selection bias due to loss to follow-up. Sophisticated health care systems that allow the flagging of registered individuals can assist in this respect. Routinely collected, national or regional health statistics may be available for comparison but require consideration of confounding exposures. Chapter 4 provides more information on sources of health outcome data.

Other specialized observational study designs have been developed to address issues of specific relevance in environmental epidemiology. Examples include studies of time-varying exposures and outcomes, such as increased asthma attacks on days with higher air pollution; or spatial clusters of diseases such as cancer. These study designs are discussed in Chapter 8.

Another major type of study design is the *experimental study*. In this type of study a defined population is divided into groups using a randomized sampling procedure and then the investigator will assign or administer an exposure (or treatment) to some of the groups. Because deliberately exposing people to harmful agents is unethical, experimental studies are generally used only to measure the impact of treatments or preventive interventions.

2.2.8 Criteria for causality

An epidemiological study generally aims to determine whether an environmental exposure is causally responsible for disease occurrence. A causal association is one in which a change in the frequency or quality of an exposure or characteristic results in a corresponding change in the frequency of the disease or outcome of interest. However, demonstration of a valid statistical association between exposure occurrence and disease occurrence in a population is not sufficient to conclude that the association is causal; additional criteria should be considered. Hill [17] elaborated a systematic approach to causal inference, although Rothman and others have questioned the value of using causal criteria and have identified limitations of the Hill criteria in particular [18].

The *temporal relationship* is crucial; the cause must precede the effect. This is usually self-evident, but difficulties may arise in studies (usually case-control or cross-sectional studies) when measurements of exposure and effect are made at the same time (e.g., by questionnaire, blood test). In order to evaluate whether the temporal relationship is logical, the induction period (the time period between the causal exposure and disease initiation) must be understood for the disease being studied. For some conditions, such as lung cancer, the induction period may be 15 years or more. Therefore, for carcinogenic agents, the causal exposure must precede clinical disease by at least this induction period.

An association is *plausible* if it is consistent with other knowledge. For instance, laboratory experiments may have shown that a particular environmental exposure can cause cancer in laboratory animals, and this would make the hypothesis that this exposure could cause cancer in humans more plausible. However, biological plausibility is a relative concept. Many epidemiological associations were considered implausible when they were first discovered but subsequently confirmed by experimental studies. An example is the occurrence of severe osteomalacia in a cadmium-polluted area of Japan [19]. Initially, the mechanism of cadmium-induced bone toxicity was not known and the cause was subject to much dispute. Lack of plausibility may simply reflect lack of medical knowledge.

Consistency is shown if several studies give the same result. If a variety of designs are used in different settings, the likelihood that all studies are making the same mistake is minimized. However, a lack of consistency does not exclude a causal association. In certain studies, the exposure levels may be so low that no health effects occur.

The *strength of association* is important in that a strongly elevated relative risk may be more likely to be causal than a weak association that could be influenced by confounding or other biases. However, the fact that an association is weak does not preclude it from being causal; rather, it means that excluding alternative explanations for the observed association is more difficult.

A 'biological gradient' or *exposure–response relationship* can be said to exist when changes in the level of exposure are associated with changes in the prevalence or incidence of the effect. The demonstration of a clear exposure–response relationship provides strong evidence for a causal relationship since it is usually unlikely that confounding or other biases would produce a consistent exposure–response relationship.

Reversibility is also relevant in that when the removal of some possible cause results in an observed reduction in disease risk, the likelihood that the association is causal is strengthened. However, the health effect of exposure may be irreversible (e.g., total deafness caused by gunshot noise), and the reversibility is not a necessary criterion for causation.

Finally, the causal inference is strengthened by data from studies using good study design, and when evidence from several different types of studies is available.

As Rothman and Greenland [18] pointed out, each of the Hill criterion have limitations and exceptions in their application to evaluating epidemiological study findings. These criteria should not be taken as hard and fast rules, nor should they be entirely rejected. Rather they should be considered deductive tests of the causal hypothesis to be used for the rigorous evaluation of a body of epidemiological research.

2.3 **References**

[1] Preston DL, Pierce DA, Shimizu Y, Ron E, Mabuchi K. Dose response and temporal patterns of radiation-associated solid cancer risks. *Health Physics*. 2003 **85**(1):43–6.

[2] Preston DL, Shimizu Y, Pierce DA, Suyama A, Mabuchi K. Studies of mortality of atomic bomb survivors. Report 13: Solid cancer and noncancer disease mortality: 1950–1997. *Radiation Research*. 2003 **160**(4):381–407.

[3] ATSDR. Case studies in environmental medicine: lead toxicity. 1992 October 2000 [cited 1992; Available from: http://www.atsdr.cdc.gov/HEC/CSEM/lead/cover.html

[4] Lanphear B, Hornung R, Khoury J, Yolton K, Baghurst P, Bellinger D, et al. Low-level environmental lead exposure and children's intellectual function: an international pooled analysis. Environmental health perspectives. 2005 **113**(7):884–9.

[5] Case BW. Asbestos, smoking, and lung cancer: interaction and attribution. *Occupational and Environmental Medicine*. 2006 **63**(8):507–8.

[6] Reid A, de Klerk NH, Ambrosini GL, Berry G, Musk AW. The risk of lung cancer with increasing time since ceasing exposure to asbestos and quitting smoking. *Occupational and Environmental Medicine*. 2006 **63**(8):509–12.

[7] Sorensen M, Bisgaard H, Stage M, Loft S. Biomarkers of exposure to environmental tobacco smoke in infants. *Biomarkers*. 2007 **12**(1):38–46.

[8] Wiencke JK. DNA adduct burden and tobacco carcinogenesis. *Oncogene*. 2002 **21**(48):7376–91.

[9] Norppa H, Bonassi S, Hansteen I, Hagmar L, Stromberg U, Rossner P, *et al*. Chromosomal aberrations and SCEs as biomarkers of cancer risk. *Mutat Res*. 2006 **600**(1–2):37–45.

[10] Rothman KJ. *Epidemiology: an introduction*. New York, NY: Oxford University Press 2002.

[11] Beaglehole R, Bonita, R, Kjellström T. *Basic Epidemiology*. Geneva: World Health Organization 1993.

[12] Baker D, Kjellström T, Calderon R, Pastides H. *Environmental Epidemiology - A Textbook on Study Methods and Public Health Applications*. Geneva: World Health Organization 1999 (WHO/SDE/OEH/99.7).

[13] Pearce N. Effect measures in prevalence studies. *Environmental Health Perspectives.* 2004 **112**(10):1047–50.

[14] Baker DB, Greenland S, Mendlein J, Harmon P. A health study of two communities near the Stringfellow Waste Disposal site. *Arch Environ Health.* 1988 **43**(5):325–34.

[15] Delucchi KL. Sample size estimation in research with dependent measures and dichotomous outcomes. *Am J Public Health.* 2004 **94**(3):372–7.

[16] Kelsey JL. *Methods in observational epidemiology*, 2nd edn. New York: Oxford University Press 1996.

[17] Hill AB. The environment and disease: association or causation? *Proc R Soc Med.* 1965 **58**:295–300.

[18] Rothman KJ, Greenland S. Causation and causal inference in epidemiology. *Am J Public Health.* 2005 **95**(Suppl 1):S144–50.

[19] World Health Organization. *Cadmium.* Geneva: WHO 1992.

Chapter 3

Environmental exposure assessment

Mark Nieuwenhuijsen and Bert Brunekreef

3.1 Introduction

Nowadays, health risks associated with environmental exposures are generally small; therefore, exposure assessment needs to be of a high quality to detect a risk when there truly is a risk. Part of the exposure assessment process is to optimize exposure estimates with the aim to detect possible risk and optimize the exposure–response relationship. This can be achieved, for example, by optimizing the distribution of the variance of the exposure estimates [1]. Exposure assessment in environmental epidemiological studies should, and has frequently, made use of both temporal and spatial variability in environmental and exposure levels to optimize the estimates, and determining the main sources of variance in each is one of the important aspects of the assessment.

Exposure variables used in environmental epidemiology generally have to be regarded as, and often are, *approximations* to the 'true' exposure of the study subjects. The accuracy and precision with which 'true' exposure is being approximated may vary widely from one 'surrogate' exposure variable to the next. Exposure misclassification or measurement error can lead to attenuation in health risk estimates or a loss of statistical power, which is discussed in detail in Chapter 5.

3.2 Initial considerations of an exposure assessment strategy

Over recent years, there has been increasing interest in the field of exposure assessment. Investigators know more than ever to what, where and how people are exposed and methods have been improved for assessing the level of exposure, its variability and the determinants. New methods have been developed or newly applied throughout this field, including analytical, measurement, modeling and statistical methods. This has led to a considerable improvement in exposure assessment in epidemiological studies.

All epidemiological studies require exposure estimates or exposure indices to be able to estimate the risk associated with the exposure of interest, but they may differ depending on the study design. The design and interpretation of epidemiological studies is often dependent on the availability of appropriate exposure assessment and therefore needs careful consideration. Quantification of the relation between exposure and health effects requires the use of exposure estimates that are accurate, precise, biologically relevant, for the critical exposure period, and show a range of exposure levels in the population under study. Furthermore, there is generally also a need for the assessment of confounders. Assessment of confounders should be in similar detail as the assessment of exposure, since measurement error in confounders may also affect the health risk estimates (see Chapter 5).

In environmental epidemiology, investigators often deal with large population sizes with the population spread over large distances. This makes estimating exposure more difficult, since the investigators may not be able to visit each subject. Therefore, investigators often rely on some form of area or individual modeling (e.g., geographical information system-based regression modeling) or surrogates of exposure (e.g., distance from road). Small sample sizes, on the other hand, may allow or require more refined exposure assessment such as personal monitoring. The size of the study population could determine how refined the exposure assessment could be. Increasing the study population size could allow for cruder exposure estimates, while smaller population sizes would require more refined exposure estimates to have similar statistical power. Armstrong [2] provided a general framework that can help investigators to decide which measures of exposure to include in their study in order to obtain maximum statistical power, and which validity and reliability substudies to include to assess the quality of the exposure assessment methods used in the full study (discussed in Chapter 5). The premise is that it is theoretically better, but more expensive, to measure 'true' exposure than to measure 'approximate' exposure. When the correlation between the approximate and the true exposure variable is high, the loss of statistical power by using the approximate rather than the true exposure variable is small. So if the cost per subject of measuring approximate exposure is clearly lower than the cost of measuring true exposure, a study using the approximate measure of exposure will be more efficient.

Besides sample size and costs, other considerations to be taken into account in designing an exposure assessment strategy for an epidemiological study are, for example, accessibility to the subjects, and availability of tools and measurement methods and data, particularly for historical assessments. Many environmental epidemiological studies use routinely collected health outcome data from subjects for whom only postcoded (zip code) location of residence is available and no contact with the subjects can be made. Questionnaires, personal monitoring or biomonitoring cannot be used in this situation and one is often restricted to modeling of environmental concentrations in the area or at the location of residence. A disadvantage of this approach is that no or little information is available where subjects spend their time outside the residence, which may be important for obtaining information on total exposure.

The choice of exposure assessment method is often not straightforward and needs careful consideration. It is important to consider what previous studies have done and what is achievable. In the rest of this chapter we will provide an overview of the various methods employed to obtain these exposure indices.

3.3 Source receptor models and pathways and exposure routes

To inform the exposure assessment, it is often important to understand the sources, pathways and routes of the substances of interest; source–receptor models are helpful in achieving this. The physical course a pollutant takes from the source to a subject is often referred to as the exposure pathway, while the way a substance enters the body is often referred to as the exposure route. *Source–receptor models* include the routes and pathways of exposure. Such models are helpful in understanding how people are exposed. In this kind of model it often becomes clear that humans create their own exposure by, e.g., the activities they do and where they spend time. Section 2.1.1 defined the basic terms for exposure pathways and routes, which are also illustrated in Figure 3.1 for air pollution.

3.3.1 Sources and pathways

There are many different pathways and each of them may require a different exposure assessment approach. Furthermore, for certain substances, multiple pathways are important. We will now discuss exposure assessment for various pathways.

3.3.1.1 Air

For exposure to *air pollutants*, the relevant time integration period varies from seconds for odorous substances to years or decades for substances having long-term effects, such as carcinogens. Some substances, such as airborne particulate matter, may have short-term as well as long-term effects, and the relevant time integration period then varies with what sort of effect is being investigated. An important consideration for air pollution is that people cannot stop breathing except for a very short time, so in principle, there is exposure whenever there are pollutants in the air people breathe. This is different for all other pathways, as will be discussed later. One of the main sources of air pollution is traffic; other sources are industry, agriculture, gas cookers and tobacco smoking. The amount of air being inhaled during a day varies with body size, metabolic rate and physical activity.

Assessment of exposure to air pollution is complicated for several reasons:

◆ Concentrations in ambient air vary considerably over time, even when emissions into the air are constant. This is due to meteorological factors such as wind speed and direction, turbulence, height of the mixing layer etc. When emissions are well defined in terms of quantity, height and location, dispersion modeling can be used to estimate air pollution concentrations at specific receptor points. Such models tend to become unreliable, however, when the integration time is short, when sources are not well

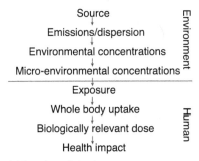

Fig. 3.1 Source receptor model for air pollutants.

defined, and when topography is complicated. Such conditions typically prevail in urban areas where many potentially exposed subjects live.

♦ People spend much of their time indoors, principally in their own homes. In addition, time is spent at work, school, in transit, etc., so that the time spent outdoors is typically only a few hours or less in many countries. The proportion of time spent outdoors may vary considerably with climate and with the proportion of the population living in cities. Most studies on the use of time have been performed in developed countries with moderate or cold climates; there is a lack of data concerning time use in many other countries where climate and the proportion of subjects working in agriculture may be such that a much higher proportion of time is spent outdoors. Indoors, the concentration of air pollutants may be considerably different from the concentration in ambient air. This is because pollutants may be filtered when passing through the building envelope, or because pollutants may react with indoor surfaces, or because there may be indoor sources contributing pollution to the indoor air. Suspended particulate matter is an example of a form of air pollution that is being filtered out to some extent when moving from outdoors to indoors. The extent of filtration depends on the particle size, large particles penetrating less, in general, than small particles. Gaseous pollutants may have very different chemical reactivities. Ozone, for example, is very reactive, and indoor concentrations are usually much lower than outdoor concentrations for this reason. Carbon monoxide (CO), on the other hand, is quite inert, and concentrations indoors will not be very different from those outdoors in the absence of indoor CO sources.

♦ Especially in homes, many sources of air pollution may exist, contributing to the pollution load of indoor air. Unvented or inadequately vented combustion appliances for space or water heating or for cooking are a major source of indoor air pollution. In many developing countries, the burning of coal or biomass fuels indoors leads to concentrations of particles, sulphur oxides, nitrogen oxides and carbon monoxide which can be much higher than concentrations encountered outdoors. In addition, many other sources have been identified, such as soil and building materials (radon), particle board and certain forms of cavity wall insulation (formaldehyde), tobacco smoking (environmental tobacco smoke), pets, fungi and dust mites (allergens).

♦ Ventilation habits and possibilities vary within and between countries, and the concentration of a pollutant indoors is to a large extent determined by the ventilation rate. When there are no indoor sources, a low ventilation rate will generally lead to lower concentrations indoors, because there is more time for decay of pollution. When there are indoor sources, however, the concentration goes up with a low ventilation rate, because there is less removal of pollution from the indoors.

♦ Air pollution tends to occur as a mixture and at often low concentrations. Particles for example are complex mixtures and we tend often only to focus on physical properties such as size. Polycyclic aromatic hydrocarbons (PAHs) are a mixture of many different substances but investigators only tend to measure one or two.

Despite these complications, exposure assessment methods have been developed and used successfully for outdoor air pollution studies. The most commonly applied designs have utilized exposure contrasts over *time* or exposure contrasts in *space* as a starting point. The focus of many of these studies has been on so-called 'community air pollution', a term which usually refers to air pollution components that occur widespread because they have many sources that are more or less evenly dispersed. Well-known components are sulphur dioxide (SO_2), nitrogen oxides (NO_x), carbon monoxide (CO), ozone (O_3), polycyclic aromatic hydrocarbons (PAH), airborne particulate matter (APM) of various sizes such as Total Suspended Particulate matter (TSP) with no specific upper size cut, PM_{10} and $PM_{2.5}$. Often, there are health–based guidelines or standards for these components that mandate that they be measured routinely in ambient air with a certain density in time and space. Historically, many epidemiological studies on the potential effects of air pollution on health have relied on such routine measurements for exposure assessment. The many recent time-series studies relating the day-to-day variation in time of air pollution to the day-to-day variations in health end points such as total and cause specific mortality, respiratory or cardiovascular hospital admissions, etc. would not have been possible without the existence of large, routinely collected databases on air pollution levels in many areas of the world. The advantage of this approach is that one does not have conduct often costly air pollution measurements for the sole purpose of epidemiological studies. There are also disadvantages, including:

- the choice of components that are measured usually reflects yesterday's legislation, which in turn usually reflects scientific knowledge of the day before yesterday;

- the location of measurements may be focused on 'hot spots' such as busy roads rather than on sites representative of average population exposure; and

- the frequency and duration of measurements may be dictated by instrumental characteristics rather than biological insights.

Nevertheless, when due attention is paid to the choice of monitoring sites from which to extract data for epidemiological studies, the existing data have often been used successfully, as the multitude of published time-series studies shows. Because there are limitations to routinely collected data, investigators have set up their own air pollution monitoring in some studies to obtain more accurate or precise measures of human exposure to air pollution, or they have resorted to modeling, which is discussed later.

3.3.1.2 Water

For exposure to drinking water pollutants, the relevant time integration period may be short in case of infectious agents, or long when substances such as carcinogens are involved. One of the archetypical epidemiologic studies was that carried out by John Snow, who demonstrated that the incidence of cholera in some London boroughs was related to the pump or the water company people used to obtain their drinking water (see Chapter 1). Exposure assessment was relatively simple in this case, with many people using the water from just a few pumps. In developed regions, drinking water is piped into most if not all homes nowadays, but this is not so in many less developed regions, where people may still obtain their drinking water from wells or streams. The challenges for assessment of exposure to contaminants in drinking water are obviously different in the respective situations.

The consumption of drinking water varies from person to person, but may be in the order of 1–2 liters per day. This is not necessarily tap water; people may also use bottled water. Tap water, after boiling, is however often used for beverages such as tea and coffee. Furthermore, a proportion of the population may use filters on their taps, or obtain their water from private wells rather than the public drinking water supply. These factors need to be taken into account when assessing exposure to pollutants in drinking water. Drinking water may become polluted in various stages. The raw material may be contaminated, e.g., with arsenic in Bangladesh, and inadequately purified. The purification process itself (e.g., chlorination) may add pollutants such as chloroform to the drinking water. The piping material may add pollutants as well. In many areas, lead was used for making drinking water pipes for a long time, and especially when the drinking water is somewhat acidic, large quantities of lead may be leached from the pipes into the water supply. Various pollutants may get into the water supply when pipes leak or are permeable to certain pollutants. The problem with pollutants added or formed after the water has left the pumping station is that they are more difficult to control and monitor than when the pollutants are already present in the raw material. For exposure assessment, it is then necessary to measure or estimate the pollutant concentration in the water as it leaves the tap in individual homes.

Uptake of water contaminants may not only occur through ingestion but also through inhalation and skin absorption as, for example, with trihalomethanes, by products of chlorination (see section 3.3.2). This is of potential concern, especially when uptake of the contaminant following inhalation is more efficient than uptake through the gut.

3.3.1.3 Soil and dust

Direct exposure to *soil pollution* occurs when soil particles are ingested or inhaled. Ingestion may occur when soil particles adhering to food crops are insufficiently removed through washing, or through the normal 'hand to mouth' behavior children exhibit when they are between one and three or four years old. In normal children, the amount of soil or dust particles ingested this way is in the range of 50 to 100 mg per day.

Polluted soil may lead to indirect exposure when contaminants are released into the air, are taken up by food crops and livestock, or are leached into the drinking water supply or into surface waters. Prediction of the environmental fate of pollutants in soil is complex, and often, measurements in relevant pathways will be needed to estimate indirect human exposure to soil pollutants with some accuracy.

However, not many environmental epidemiological studies examine the relationship between soil contaminants and adverse health effects. This may be partly due to the relatively low uptake of soil contaminants. For example, mining and smelting have left certain areas of south-west England with high arsenic levels in soil. There has been considerable concern about these high soils levels, although it was unclear how much was taken up by the residents. Kavanagh *et al.* [3] measured arsenic levels in soil, house dust and urine of residents in three areas: two exposed areas (Gunnislake and Devon Great Consols)

Table 3.1 Arsenic (As) in soil, house dust and urine in the south-west of England

	Cargreen	Gunnislake	Devon GC	Ratios between sites
Soil (μg/g)	37	365	4500	1: 10: 122
House dust (μg/g)	49	217	1167	1: 4: 24
Urine (μg/g creatine)				
Total As	4.7	9.2	10.0	1: 2: 2
Arsenite (As III)	<LOD	1.7	0.9	
Arsenate (As V)	<LOD	0.9	1.3	
DMA	4.7	5.6	8.5	
MMA	<LOD	0.3	0.7	

<LOD = below limit of detection.

GC = Great Consols.

DMA = Dimethylarsinic acid.

MMA = Monomethylarsonic acid.

Adapted from [3]. Reproduced with permission from Kavanagh P, Farago ME, Thornton I, Goessler W, Kuehnelt D, Schlagenhaufen C, et al. Urinary arsenic species in Devon and Cornwall residents, UK. A pilot study. Analyst. 1998 123(1):27–9. Reproduced by permission of The Royal Society of Chemistry.

and one unexposed area (Cargreen) (Table 3.1). High levels of arsenic were found in the soil and, to a lesser extent, in house dust. Marked variations were evident, however, between the different areas. Concentrations of arsenic in the soil were up to 122 times greater in areas with high exposure compared to nonexposed areas. For house dust, concentrations were up to 24 times higher. In urine, there was only a twofold difference in arsenic levels between the areas. This suggests that the actual uptake of arsenic from soil and house dust is relatively low, particularly if people do not eat home-grown vegetables.

3.3.1.4 Food

Exposure to contaminants through the food chain is one more important pathway to consider. Many contaminants may be present in food, and exposure may vary considerably with dietary habits. When a population depends primarily on home or locally grown food, local contamination may lead to high exposures. Some of the classical and tragic examples of environmental epidemiology include methylmercury poisoning of Japanese fishermen and their families, who were dependent on fish caught from a bay that was heavily contaminated with effluents from the Chisso factory that produced (among other substances) acetaldehyde which involved use of mercury. The mercury was transformed by microorganisms into methylmercury, a highly neurotoxic component. In the 1950s, exposed nearby residents were found to suffer from serious neurological disorders, and although corrective measures were taken at the factory many years ago, ongoing studies still show long-term consequences of this exposure. A National Institute for Minamata Disease was founded and is still following exposed subjects and conducting studies on the toxicology of methylmercury poisoning (http://www.nimd.go.jp). A description of the case can be found at http://www.american.edu/ted/minamata.htm.

Another example, also from Japan, is cadmium poisoning in older rural women living in the Toyama prefecture, whose diet depended heavily on locally grown rice. The cadmium pollution came from waste water from the Kamioka mining plant that was used for irrigating the rice fields. Exposed persons suffered from renal disease, and also from a bone disorder called osteomalacia which causes bones to fracture easily with intense pain as a result ('*itai itai*' is Japanese for 'ouch ouch'). The reason why older women suffered most was that they were more likely to have weaker bones after having borne a number of children, and after developing degrees of osteoporosis with age. The importance of dependence on locally grown food in this case can be illustrated by comparing the fate of the affected Japanese with that of the inhabitants of Shipham, a village in the UK located in an area where the soil cadmium levels were even higher than in the affected Japanese areas. The difference was likely one of exposure, related to the much smaller dependence of the Shipham population on locally grown food [4].

3.3.2 Exposure routes

There are three possible exposure routes for substances:

* inhalation through the respiratory system;
* ingestion through the gastrointestinal system; and
* absorption through the skin.

The exposure route(s) of a substance depends on the biological, chemical and physical characteristics of the substances, location and activity of the person, and the persons themselves. Inhalation of particles through the respiratory system depends on the particle size diameter. Smaller particles penetrate more deeply into the lungs. The thoracic fraction (particles with a 50 percent cut off diameter of 10 μm) is the fraction that enters the thorax and is deposited within the lung airways and the gas exchange region, and is generally referred to as PM_{10}. $PM_{2.5}$ (particles with a 50 percent cut off diameter of 2.5 μm) are deposited in the gas-exchange region (the alveoli). Furthermore, inhalation depends on the breathing rate of the subject, where those carrying out heavy work may breath in much more air and more deeply (20 L/min for light work versus 60 L/min for heavy work). People also move through different microenvironments with different particle concentrations.

Skin absorption can play an important role for uptake of substances such as solvents, pesticides and trihalomethanes. Trihalomethanes are volatile compounds that are formed when water is chlorinated and the chlorine reacts with organic matter in the water. In this context there are a number of possible exposure pathways and routes (Figure 3.2). The main pathway of ingestion is generally drinking tap water or tap water-based drinks (e.g., tea, coffee and squash). Swimming, showering, bathing, and dish washing may all result in considerable uptake through inhalation and skin absorption and, for the first three, ingestion to minor extent. Water standing or flushing in the toilet may lead to uptake through inhalation through volatilization of the chloroform.

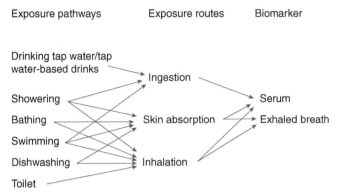

Fig. 3.2 Examples of exposure pathways, routes and biomarkers for trihalomethanes.

The total uptake of trihalomethanes may be assessed using the concentration measured in exhaled breath or serum.

In the human body, the uptake, distribution, transformation and excretion of a substance such as trihalomethanes can be modeled using physiologically based pharmicokinetic (PBPK) models [1]. These models are becoming more sophisticated, although they are still rarely used in environmental epidemiology. They can be used to estimate the contribution of various exposure pathways and routes to the total uptake and model the dose of a specific target organ. For example, where trihalomethanes through ingestion may mostly be metabolized rapidly in the liver and not appear in blood, uptake through inhalation and skin increases the blood levels substantially. Furthermore, metabolic polymorphisms may lead to different dose estimates under the similar exposure conditions.

3.4 **Exposure parameters**

Respiratory and dermal exposures to substances generally have three dimensions:

- duration (e.g., in hours or days);
- concentration (e.g., in mg/m^3 in air or mg/L in water); and
- frequency (e.g., times per week).

In case of ingestion, the dimensions of exposure are concentration, amount (e.g., liters) and frequency. Any of these can be used as an exposure index in an epidemiological study, but they can also be combined to obtain a new exposure index, for example by multiplying duration and concentration to obtain an index of cumulative exposure. The choice of index depends on the health effect of interest. For substances that cause acute effects such as ammonia, the short-term concentration is generally the most relevant exposure index, while for substances that cause chronic effects, such as asbestos, long-term exposure indices such as cumulative exposure may be a more appropriate index.

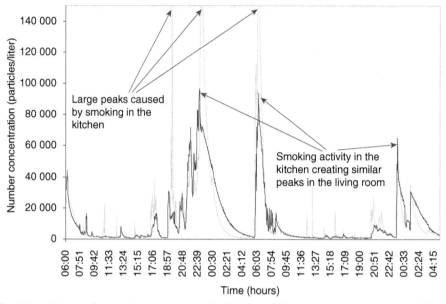

Fig. 3.3 Variation in fine particulate levels in the kitchen and living room over a day. From [5]. Reproduced with permission from Wigzell E, Kendall M, and Nieuwenhuijsen MJ. (2000) The spatial and temporal variability of particulates in the home. *J Expos Anal Environ Epidemiol* **10**:307–314.

3.5 **Exposure level and variability**

The concentration of exposure generally varies temporally and spatially. Figure 3.3 provides the exposure levels of $PM_{2.5}$, expressed as the number of particles in a house over a day [5]. Peak exposure levels, i.e., exposure levels considerably higher than the overall average, are caused by someone smoking in the house. Furthermore, the measurements show that although there appears to be a very good correlation between the $PM_{2.5}$ levels in the kitchen and the living room, the actual levels differ. Spatial variations also exist over much larger areas, for instance in air pollution levels between large cities and rural areas, in exposure to ultraviolet radiation between areas at different latitude, in selenium intake between areas with high and low background selenium concentrations in agricultural soils, etc.

Exposure data often show a log normal distribution i.e., the distribution of the measured or model data is skewed to the right. Figure 3.4 provides an example of the distribution of approximately 50 personal exposure measurements of $PM_{2.5}$. The y axis shows the number of measurements, the x axis the $PM_{2.5}$ concentration. As can be seen, the distribution is skewed to the right; some persons were exposed to much higher levels than the average. Statistical tests can be carried out to assess if this is a lognormal distribution (e.g., Kolmogorov–Smirnov or Shapiro–Wilk tests).

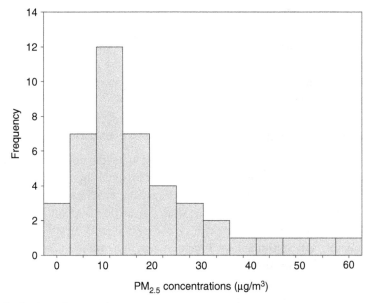

Fig. 3.4 Distribution of personal exposure measurements of PM$_{2.5}$.

The central tendency (i.e., the peak of the distribution) of a lognormal distribution is generally described by the Geometric Mean (GM), while the variability is described by the Geometric Standard Deviation (GSD). They can be calculated as follows:

$$\mu = \frac{\sum \ln x}{n}$$

$$\sigma^2 = \frac{\sum (\ln x - \overline{\ln x})^2}{n-1}$$

Geometric mean (GM) = exp μ
Geometric Standard Deviation (GSD) = exp σ
Arithmetic mean = $\frac{\sum x}{n}$

X = concentration of the substance in a sample, n = number of samples
Σ = sum, in =natural logarithm
μ = average of log transformed measurements
σ^2 = variance of log transformed measurements

The arithmetic mean (AM) provides the average of the exposure measurement and is generally used to calculate cumulative exposure rather than the geometric mean. Besides the AM, GM and GSD the range, minimum, maximum or 95 percent confidence intervals are often reported.

Exposure generally varies from day to day for any given person and from person to person, often referred to as the within and between subject exposure variability, respectively. The within and between subject variability can be estimated when repeated exposure measurements have been obtained using analysis of variance models [1]. Besides variability caused by persons, there may be other determinants of exposure such as source strength or ventilation, and these need to be identified to get a better understanding of what is causing the variability in exposure to make use of this in the exposure assessment.

3.6 Ecological versus individual exposure estimates

To obtain exposure estimate(s) for a population in an epidemiological study, two main approaches are available: (a) the individual and/or personal approach and (b) the group or area approach. In the individual approach, exposure estimates are obtained at the individual level, e.g., every member of the study population is monitored either once or repeatedly, or estimates are modeled at an individual level. In the group approach, the group is first split into smaller subpopulations, more often referred to as exposure groups, based on specific determinants of exposure, and group or ecological exposure estimates are obtained for each exposure group. In environmental epidemiological studies, exposure groups may be defined, for example, on the basis of presence or absence of an exposure source (a gas cooker or smoker in the house), distance from an exposure source (roads or factories), or activity (playing sport or not). The underlying assumption is that subjects within each exposure group experience similar exposure characteristics, including exposure levels and variation. A representative sample of members from each exposure group can be personally monitored, either once or repeatedly, or the exposure for the group or area can be modeled. For the former, if the aim is to estimate mean exposure, the average of the exposure measurements is then assigned to all the members in that particular exposure group. Alternatively, other exposure estimates can be assigned to the groups, e.g., data from ambient air pollution monitors in the area where the subjects live. Ecological and individual estimates can be combined, e.g., in the case of chlorination by-products where routinely collected trihalomethane measurements providing ecological estimates, at times are combined with individual estimates on actual ingestion, showering and bathing [6].

Intuitively, it is expected that the individual estimates provide the best exposure estimates for an epidemiological study. This may not be true, however, particularly when taking measurements, because of variability in exposure and the limited number of samples obtained for each individual. In this case, personal estimates lead to attenuated, though more precise, health risk estimates than ecological estimates. Modeled individual estimates and ecological estimates, in contrast, result in less attenuation of the risk estimates, albeit less precise [7–9]. These differences can be explained by Classical- and Berkson-type error models (see Chapter 5). Between-group, between-subject and within-subject variance can be estimated using analysis of variance models and this information can be used to optimize the exposure–response relationship, for example, by changing the distribution of exposure groups [10, 11]. In the case of the group approach, the aim is to increase the contrast of exposure between exposure groups, expressed as the ratio between the between group variance and the sum of the between and within group variance, while maintaining a reasonable precision of the exposure estimates of the exposure groups.

3.7 **Exposure classification, measurement or modeling**

Exposure can be classified, measured or modeled and different tools are available such as questionnaires, air pollution monitors and statistical techniques respectively. The methods are often divided into direct and indirect methods (Figure 3.5).

3.7.1 **Classification**

Subjects in an epidemiological study can be classified to a particular substance on an ordinal scale, for example as exposed:

♦ no, yes; or

♦ no, low, medium, high.

This can be achieved by, for example, expert asessment or self-assesment questionnaire:

♦ *Expert assessment*, e.g., a member of the research team decides based on prior knowledge whether the study subject is exposed or unexposed, e.g., using distance from a point source such as a factory [12], radio and TV transmitters [13], incinerators [14], emissions from roads [15–17], landfill [18]; or categorization by industrial sources, land use or urban zone [19]. Many of the studies using these simple surrogates or proxies for exposure have reported positive associations with health outcomes. How to interpret these reports, however, is wrought with challenges. The relationship between the proxy

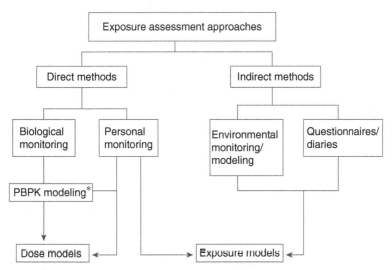

*PBPK modeling = physiologically pharmacokinetic modeling.

Fig. 3.5 Different approaches to human exposure assessment.

measures used and actual exposure is certainly not simple. This is further compounded because concentrations away from source, for example, do not decline linearly, but typically fall sharply in the first few tens of meters before gradually declining to background levels, and also depend on meteorological conditions.

◆ *Self-assessment by questionnaire* i.e., the study subject is asked to fill out a questionnaire where they are asked about a particular substance, for example pesticides. Questionnaires are often used to ask a subject if they are exposed to a particular substance and also for the estimation of the duration of exposure [1, 20, 21].

Questionnaires can be used not only to ask the subjects to estimate their exposure but also obtain information related to the exposure such as where people spent their time (time microenvironment diaries), work history including the jobs and task they carried out, what they eat and drink, and residential history. These variables could be used as exposure indices in the epidemiological studies or translated into a new exposure index, for example by multiplying the amount of tap water people drink and the contaminant level in the tap water to obtain the total ingested amount of the substance. When used on their own they are often referred to as exposure surrogates.

Expert and self-assessment methods are generally the easiest and cheapest, but can suffer from a lack of objectivity and knowledge and may therefore bias the exposure assessment. Both experts and study subjects may not know exactly what the subjects are exposed to or at what level and therefore misclassify the exposure, while diseased subjects may recall certain substances better than subjects without disease (recall bias) and cause differential misclassification, leading to biased health risk estimates.

3.7.2 Measurement

A more objective way to assess the exposure, particularly the concentration of exposure, is by measuring the exposure. Some examples:

◆ Levels of outdoor air pollution can be measured by ambient air monitors (i.e., ambient air monitoring). These monitors are placed in an area and measure the particular substance of interest in this area. Subjects living within this area are considered to be exposed to the concentrations measured by the monitoring station. This may or may not be true depending on for example where the person lives, works, or travels. The advantage of this method is that it could provide a range of exposure estimates for a large population. Nowadays there are many monitors that routinely monitor air pollutants for regulatory purposes, particularly in cities in the developed world. For example, epidemiological study designs for outdoor air pollution such as the time series studies have related day-to-day variation in air pollution to day-to-day variability in morbidity and mortality [22, 23]. Others such as the Harvard Six Cities study have used the spatial differences in air pollution to define the exposure index [23, 24]. The environmental measurements for most of these studies were obtained from stationary ambient monitoring stations that routinely measured the air pollution levels at one or more points in the area where the subjects lived. Specific monitoring campaigns can be conducted to measure environmental exposure levels, but only for current exposure, and these are often thought to be too expensive.

◆ Levels of air pollution can be measured by personal exposure monitors. These monitors are lightweight devices that are worn by the study subjects [1, 25–27]. They are often used in occupational studies and are being used more frequently in environmental studies. The advantage of this method is that it is likely to estimate the subject's exposure better than ambient air monitoring. The disadvantage is that it is often labor-intensive and expensive and can often only be used for relatively small populations. They are however ideal for validation studies of modeled exposure estimates.

◆ Levels of water pollutants and soil contaminants can be estimated by taking water samples and soil samples respectively, and analyzing these sample for substances of interest in the laboratory. Often these need to be combined with assessment of behavioral factors such as water intake, contaminated food intake or hand-to-month contact to obtain a level of exposure. Epidemiological studies of chlorination disinfection by-products have used routinely collected trihalomethane concentrations in a water zone or distribution network as their exposure index. Occasionally these environmental measurements have been combined with personal data on ingestion, showering or swimming obtained by questionnaire to obtain more specific individual exposure indices [6].

◆ Levels of uptake of the substance into the body can be estimated by biomonitoring. Biomonitoring consists of taking biological samples such as urine, exhaled breath, hair, adipose tissue or nails, e.g., the measurement of lead in serum. Biomonitoring is expected to estimate the actual uptake (dose) of the substance of interest rather than the exposure. Biomonitoring can be very informative, particularly for substances that have multiple pathways and routes. A major drawback is often the fairly short biological half life of many substances which makes it only useful for estimating current exposures or doses. Biomonitoring (e.g., blood lead) has also been used frequently in studies on the effects of exposure to lead [28].

The measurement of exposure is generally expensive, particularly for large populations, and, as mentioned above, can be restricted due to inaccessibility to subjects or the need for a historical assessment of exposure rather than assessment of current exposure. It may be very useful for validation purposes. For example, epidemiological studies of the effects of environmental tobacco smoke have often used questionnaires (e.g., whether spouse is smoking or not) or biomonitoring (e.g., serum or salivary cotinine) to obtain exposure estimates. The latter only indicates recent exposure, but can be used to validate questionnaire data [29, 30]. Furthermore, methods can be combined. Studies on radon and electromagnetic fields have relied on a mixture of questionnaire data, expert knowledge, environmental measurements and modeling of determinants [31, 32].

3.7.1.2 Modeling

Modeling of exposure can be carried out preferably in conjunction with exposure measurements either to help to build a model or to validate a model. It is particularly important that model estimates are validated.

Modeling can be divided into two categories: deterministic and stochastic.

3.7.3.1 Deterministic modeling

In deterministic modeling (i.e., physical) the models describe the relationship between variables mathematically on the basis of knowledge of the physical, chemical and biological mechanisms governing these relationships [33].

For example, Hodgson *et al.* [34] used the Atmospheric Dispersion Modeling System (ADMS) to assess mercury dispersion in Runcorn in the north-west of England. ADMS uses algorithms that take account of stack height and diameter, volume flow rate, temperature and emission rates of pollutants, as well as meteorology, local geography, atmospheric boundary layer and deposition parameters, to calculate concentrations of pollutants at ground level. Three authorized processes were included in the model, a chlor alkali plant, an associated multi-fuel power station, and a coal-fired power station. Compared to using distance as a proxy for exposure, the model identified a much smaller exposed population (Figure 3.6). The correlation between modeled and measured mercury levels was high (r =0.9) (Figure 3.7).

3.7.3.2 Stochastic modeling

In stochastic modeling (i.e., statistical) the statistical relationships are modeled between variables. These models do not necessarily require fundamental knowledge of the underlying physical, chemical and/or biological relationships between the variables.

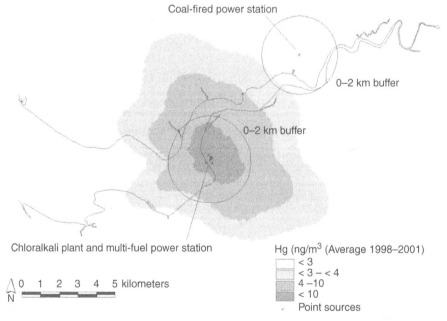

Fig. 3.6 Comparison of modeled exposure output (average 1998–2001) to exposure analysis based on distance as a proxy for exposure for a study of mercury in the north-west of England. From [34]. Reproduced with permission from Hodgson S, Nieuwenhuijsen MJ, Colvile R, Jarup L. Assessment of exposure to mercury from industrial emissions: comparing 'distance as a proxy' and dispersion modeling approaches. *Occupational and Environmental Medicine*. 2007 64(6):380–8.

Monitored versus modeled mercury levels at nine monitoring sites over 14 consecutive weeks.

Graph shows the weekly average (mean) monitored value plotted against the weekly average (mean) modeled value.

Although the model underestimates the measured values, there is a good correlation between the values (Pearson's correlation coefficient = 0.90, p = <0.00)

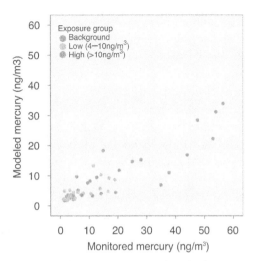

Fig. 3.7 Correlation between modeled and measured mercury concentrations in the north-west of England. Hodgson S. *Renal effects in a population exposed to chloralkali plant emissions*. (PhD thesis). London, United Kingdom: Imperial College London, University of London, 2005.

Examples are regression and Bayesian modeling. For regression modeling, a statistical regression model can be expressed in the form:

$$Ln(C_{ij}) = \beta_0 + \beta_1 var_i + \beta_2 var_j + E$$

whereby $ln(C_{ij})$ denotes the log transformed exposure concentration, β_0 the background level, var_x the potential determinant of exposure, β_x the regression coefficient of var_x providing the magnitude of the effect, and E a random variable with mean 0, often called the error term.

This technique was applied in a study of pesticides. Harris *et al.* [35] measured 2,4 D [2,4-dichlorophenoxyacetic acid], mecopop [2-(4-chloro-2 methylphenoxy) propionic acid, MCPP] and dicamba [3,6-dichloro-*o*-anisic acid] in urine for two consecutive 24 hour periods collected from a group of 98 professional turf applicators from 20 companies across south-western Ontario. The group also filled out questionnaires to acquire information on all known variables that could potentially increase or decrease pesticide exposure to the amount handled. They used linear regression to assess the relationship between the concentrations of the substances in urine and the questionnaire data. They found that the volume of pesticide applied was only weakly related to the total dose of 2,4 D absorbed (R^2 = 0.21). Two additional factors explained a large proportion of the variation in measured pesticide exposure: the type of spray nozzle used and the use of gloves while spraying. Individuals who used a fan-type nozzle had significantly higher doses than those who used a gun-type nozzle. Glove use was associated with significantly lower doses. Job satisfaction and current smoking influenced the dose, but were not highly predictive. In the final multiple regression model it was concluded that approximately 64 percent of the variation in doses could be explained by the small number of variables identified (Table 3.2). Biological monitoring in this case was important in order to be able to determine the true effect of wearing protective equipment such as gloves. This study provided extremely useful information for epidemiological and health risk assessment studies, which could focus on obtaining information on these particular variables in a larger population.

A problem in exposure assessment is that often few routinely collected measurements are available to model exposure estimates and therefore more sophisticated statistical techniques need to be used, as was demonstrated in a study of chlorination by-products. Trihalomethane (THM) concentrations were used as the marker for chlorination by-products in a study of chlorination by-products and birth outcomes. In the UK, where the study was conducted, water samples are routinely collected and analyzed from each water zone (population up to 50 000 people) using random samples at the tap (an average of four measurements per zone). Because the small number of THM measurements in some water zones did not meet the need for quarterly estimates (to allow for trimester-weighted exposure estimates), it was necessary to model the raw THM data to obtain more robust estimates of the mean THM concentration in each zone. This was done using a *hierarchical mixture model* in the software WinBUGS (Bayesian inference using Gibbs sampling) [36], as described in detail elsewhere [37]. A three-component mixture model was fitted in which zones were assumed to belong to one or some mixture of three components which were labeled 'ground', 'lowland surface' and 'upland surface' waters (Figure 3.8). The hierarchical model was assigned over the zone-specific mean individual THM concentrations, enabling zones to 'borrow' information from other zones with the same water source type. This resulted in more stable estimates for zones where few samples were taken. Seasonal variation was taken into account by estimating a quarterly effect common to all zones supplied by the same source type. These quarterly zone mean THM estimates were then back-transformed onto the original scale and summed to give THM levels for various seasons (Figure 3.9).

Table 3.2 Regression models predicting the log of total dose of 2,4 D in 94 volunteers ($R^2 = 0.64$)

Variable	Estimate	SE	*p*- value	Partial R^2
Intercept	−1.09	0.01	0.29	
Log spray	0.96	0.12	0.001	0.44
Nozzle	1.37	0.23	0.001	0.29
Glove wear	−1.50	0.25	0.001	0.29
Satisfaction	−0.39	0.17	0.021	0.06
Smoke	0.51	0.22	0.02	0.06

Adapted from [35]. Reproduced with permission from Harris SA, Sass-Kortsak AM, Corey PN, Purdham JT. Development of models to predict dose of pesticides in professional turf applicators. *Journal of Exposure Analysis and Environmental Epidemiology*. 2002 12(2):130–44. Reprinted by permission from Macmillan Publishers Ltd.

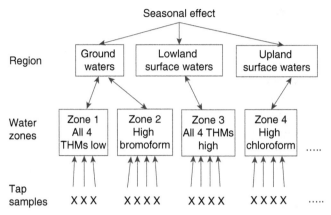

Fig. 3.8 Hierarchical mixture model to estimate the water zone means of THMs by water source using tap water samples and applying a common seasonal effect. From [37]. Reproduced with permission from Whitaker H, Best N, Nieuwenhuijsen MJ, Wakefield J, Fawell J, Elliott P. Modeling exposure to disinfection by-products in drinking water for an epidemiological study of adverse birth outcomes. *Journal of Exposure Analysis and Environmental Epidemiology.* 2005 15(2):138–46.

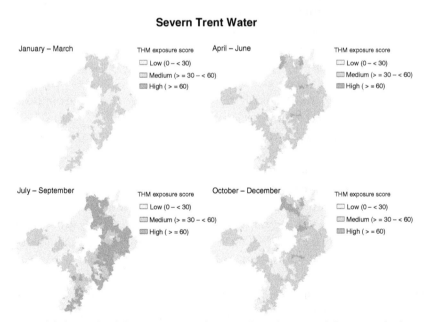

Fig. 3.9 Modeled THM levels by water zone using Bayesian mixture modeling. From [37]. Reproduced with permission from Whitaker H, Best N, Nieuwenhuijsen MJ, Wakefield J, Fawell J, Elliott P. Modeling exposure to disinfection by-products in drinking water for an epidemiological study of adverse birth outcomes. *Journal of Exposure Analysis and Environmental Epidemiology.* 2005 15(2):138–46.

The modeled exposure estimates provided a better exposure relationship than when using estimates based on the mean of the raw THM concentrations for each zone.

A further problem is that pollutants such as outdoor air pollution and chlorination by-products in water often occur as mixtures. Statistical techniques such as *principle component analysis* have recently been used to identify sources of the pollutants and use this type of information to further refine the exposure estimates in epidemiological studies [38, 39]. Laden *et al.* [38] used the elemental composition of size fractionated particles to identify several distinct source-related fractions of fine particles and examined the associations of these fractions with daily mortality in six cities. Using specific rotation factor analysis for each city, they identified a silicon factor classified as soil and crustal material, a lead factor classified as motor exhaust, a selenium factor representing coal combustion and up to two additional factors. Motor exhaust and coal combustion, but not crustal particles, were associated with mortality.

3.8 Geographical information systems

In recent years, many of the exposure assessments have been greatly strengthened by the use of geographical information system (GIS) techniques [40, 41]. Looked at simply, GIS techniques are computerized mapping systems. As such, they comprise a computer, software, data and whatever other devices are needed to capture and display the data (e.g., scanner, plotter, printer). GIS, however, can do more than simply map data. It also provides the capability to integrate the data into a common spatial form, include or link to stochastic or deterministic models, and to analyze the data geographically. It is these capabilities that give GIS its special power in relation to exposure assessment. However, there are often problems in acquiring the data needed to carry out geographic methods of exposure assessment, and regarding the resolution that is required. Another issue is that all the data used in GIS models must be *georeferenced*. Given the importance of GIS methods, some specific examples are discussed below.

Various GIS and geostatistical techniques have been used to assign geographical locations, e.g., distance from a road or modeling local pollution patterns, on the basis of the monitored data—for example, using inverse distance weighting, (co)kriging or regression methods (Table 3.3). These essentially fit a surface through the available monitored data, in order to predict pollutant concentrations at unmeasured sites. The approach appears to work well in areas where there is relatively gentle variation in air pollution or where the density of the monitoring network is high; conditions that are often not fulfilled. Co-kriging with roads as the covariate seems to be a major improvement in most models. In other situations, it is helpful to supplement the available monitoring data through the use of covariates: variables that correlate with monitored concentrations, but for which data are available at a higher density of locations [42]. Both co-kriging and regression methods enable this. A few examples follow.

3.8.1 GIS-based interpolation modeling

Jerret *et al.* [43] interpolated $PM_{2.5}$ data from 23 state and local district monitoring stations in the Los Angeles, US, basin for the year 2000 using five interpolation

Table 3.3 GIS-based modeling methods

Indicators
Distance, traffic volume
Kriging
Uses only monitoring data, interpolates local surface
Co-kriging
Kriging with covariates
Regression modeling
Regression model for covariates (e.g. land cover, road), trained on monitoring sites
Focal sum
Kernel function of emissions, trained on monitoring sites
Dispersion modeling
Physical model of dispersion processes
Time-space modeling
Any of above, linked to time-activity data

methods: bicubic splines, two ordinary kriging models, universal kriging with a quadratic drift, and a radial basis function multiquadric interpolator. They emphasized kriging interpolation because this stochastic method produces the best linear unbiased estimate of the pollution surface. After cross-validation, they used a combination of universal kriging and multiquadric models. This approach takes advantage of the local detail in the multiquadric surface and the ability to handle trends in the universal surface. They averaged estimated surfaces based on 25 m grid cells. They conducted sensitivity analysis using only the universal estimate and found the results to be similar; therefore, only the findings from the combined model were used. Sensitivity analyses were also implemented with the kriging variance. Exposure assignments were down weighted with larger errors in exposure estimates in these analyses (i.e., weight equal to the inverse of the standard error in the universal kriging estimate). Finally, they assessed the impact of traffic by assigning buffers that included zip code-area centroids within either 500 or 1000 meters of a freeway. This distance from the zip code-area centroid to the freeway approximates exposure to traffic pollution, which may exert independent effects in addition to pollutants such as $PM_{2.5}$ and O_3 that vary over larger areas.

3.8.2 GIS-based regression modeling

Regression techniques were used as part of the SAVIAH study to model exposures to NO_2 (as a marker for traffic-related air pollution) in four study cities [44]. Data from 80 monitoring sites were used to construct a regression equation using information on road traffic (e.g., road network, road type, traffic volume), land cover and use, altitude and monitored NO_2 data. The results showed that the maps produced extremely good predictions of monitored pollution levels, both for individual and for the mean annual concentrations, with $r^2 \sim 0.79$–0.87 across 8–10 reference points, although the accuracy of the predictions for individual periods was more variable. Subsequently it was shown that regression models developed in one location could successfully be applied, with local calibration using only a small number of sites, to other study areas or periods [45]. The same approach was further developed to assess exposures to particles in a number of different cities as part of the TRAPCA study [46] and to model traffic-related air pollution in Munich [47]. Brauer *et al.* [46] did the modeling in three locations, and in each location, 40–42 measurement sites were selected to represent rural, urban background and urban traffic locations. At each site, fine particles and filter absorbance (a marker for diesel exhaust particles) were measured for four two-week periods distributed over approximately one-year periods between February 1999 and July 2000. They used these measurements to calculate annual average concentrations after adjustment for temporal variation. Traffic-related variables (e.g., population density and traffic intensity) were collected using GIS and used in regression models to predict annual average concentrations. From these models, the investigators estimated ambient air concentrations at the home addresses of the cohort members. Regression models using traffic-related variables explained 73, 56 and 50 percent of the variability in annual average fine particle concentrations for the Netherlands, Munich and Stockholm County, respectively. For filter absorbance, the regression models explained 81, 67 and 66 percent of the variability in the annual average concentrations. Cross-validation to estimate the model prediction errors indicated root mean squared errors of 1.1–1.6 µg/m for $PM_{2.5}$ and 0.22–0.31*10 m^{-5} for absorbance. The work showed that different input variables of the models can be used, but that each location needs its own model construction and validation, because regression equations can be different.

3.8.3 GIS-based air dispersion modeling

A case-control study of air pollution and lung cancer in Stockholm used emission data, dispersion models and GIS to assess historical exposure to several components of ambient air pollution and compared estimates with actual measurements [48, 49]. For NO_2, the investigators used information from a detailed regional database which included information on approximately 4300 line sources related to traffic, 500 point sources, including major industries and energy plants as well as small industry and ferries in ports. Limited diffuse emission sources, e.g., air traffic and merchant vessels in commercial route were treated as area sources, and several population-density-related sources such as local heating were mapped as grid sources, as were work machine emissions. They collected information on the growth of urban areas, the development of district heating, and the growth and distribution of the road traffic over time. They used the Airviro model, together with population data, to derive population-weighted average exposures from 1955 to 1990. In the case of traffic-related NO_2, exposures were seen to increase over this period, from about 15 µg/m^3 in 1955 to about 24 µg/m^3 in 1990, showing the effect of increasing traffic volumes. Modeled SO_2 exposures, in contrast, fell from above 90 µg/m^3 to less than 20 µg/m^3, as a result of improvements in fuel technology, emission controls and a shift to district heating.

3.8.4 **Comparison of methods**

Cyrys *et al.* [50] compared the measured NO_2 and $PM_{2.5}$ levels with the levels predicted by the two modeling approaches (for 40 measurement sites), stochastic and dispersion modeling. NO_2 and $PM_{2.5}$ concentrations obtained by the stochastic models were in the same range as the measured concentrations, whereas the NO_2 and TSP levels estimated by dispersion modeling were higher than the measured values. However, the correlation between stochastic- and dispersion-modeled concentrations was strong for both pollutants: at the 40 measurement sites, for NO_2, $r = 0.83$, and for PM, $r = 0.79$; and identically at the 1669 cohort member sites, for NO_2, $r = 0.83$ and for PM, $r = 0.79$. Both models yielded similar results regarding exposure estimate of the study cohort to traffic-related air pollution.

Figure 3.10 provides an example of the different NO_2 concentration patterns one can get using different techniques such as distance from road, traffic density, dispersion modeling and regression modeling from a study in Sheffield. It shows that there could be considerable differences depending on which method is used.

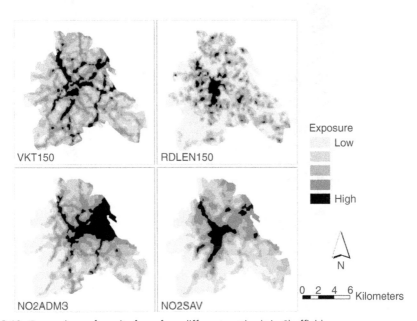

Fig. 3.10 Comparison of results from four different methods in Sheffield.

3.8.5 **People movement and remote sensing**

People, of course, do not only move in the longer term; they also move around during the day. These behavior patterns can greatly affect exposure. The importance of this was clearly shown by a study in Helsinki [51], which used dispersion modeling to predict nitrogen dioxide concentrations across the city at different times of the day. These models were then overlaid onto data showing where people were at different periods in order to build up a picture of exposure variations throughout the day. An interesting development in this area is that it is possible to track people through their environment using global positioning systems (GPS) with enough resolution to make it useful for

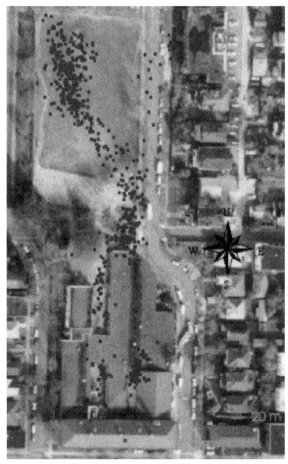

Fig. 3.11 Path traveled by one child on a week day during school hours. The playing field is located near the top of the picture, the school building near the bottom, and the main entrance is located at the center. There is a street along the right side of the school grounds. From [53]. Reproduced with permission from Elgethun K, Fenske RA, Yost MG, Palcisko GJ. Time-location analysis for exposure assessment studies of children using a novel global positioning system instrument. *Environmental Health Perspectives*. 2003 111(1):115–22.

this type of studies (Figure 3.11) [52, 53]. There are some restrictions as a result of the limitations in the technology, e.g., the reception of the satellite signals can be adversely impacted by the shielding from buildings of certain material (concrete, steel), electrical power stations, and to some extent vehicle body panels. However, combining pollution maps with information on where people spend their time may greatly improve exposure estimates if further improvements to the technology can be made.

A further promising development is the use of remote sensing to obtain information on ground levels of pollutants, which could be used for large-scale epidemiological studies and has the advantage that data are available in electronic format. However, it has had only limited use so far in epidemiological studies, e.g., in the identification of land use to predict pesticides use [54].

Table 3.4 provides an overview of the various approaches. These different approaches are not exclusive and often are combined to obtain the best exposure index. It is often difficult or impossible to measure the exposure to the actual substance of interest and therefore exposure to an 'exposure surrogate' is estimated. The National Research Council (NRC) in the US came up with a ranking of exposure data and surrogate measures around point sources such as landfill sites (Table 3.5) [55].

The data at the top of this hierarchy will provide some fairly good information on the exposure of the subjects, while at the bottom the exposure estimates are the worst and they may not be helpful in the interpretation of an epidemiological study. Of course there are still other issues that are important in the ranking, for example many quantified area measurements may still be better than a few quantified personal exposure measurements.

3.9 Validation studies

In epidemiological studies it is often not possible to obtain detailed exposure information on each subject in the study. For example, in a large cohort study it is generally not feasible to take measurements on each subject and administer a detailed exposure questionnaire. In this case it is desirable to carry out a small validation study on a subset of the population that is representative for the larger population. Ideally this will be carried out before the main study starts and can make use of information from the literature. Questions in the questionnaire could be validated with measurements and exposure models could be constructed. The exposure assessment in the whole population could focus on key questions that have a large influence on the exposure estimates and thereby reduce the length of the questionnaire. Information on key determinants will also provide a better understanding of the exposure and how it may affect exposure–response relationships in epidemiological studies. Besides the validity, the reproducibility of various tools can be evaluated in a sub sample.

3.10 Conclusion

This chapter provided an overview of various issues and methods that are common to exposure assessment for environmental epidemiological study, and a number of

Table 3.4 Input and strength and limitations of various methods

Method	Input/requirements	Strength	Limitations
City/monitoring station	Monitoring stations	Relatively easy to place monitoring in community of interest	Does not reflect within community variability Placement may affect results Provides concentration estimates but not necessarily exposure estimates
Distance from the road/source	GIS Road network Road network attributed with traffic composition	Relatively easy to obtain Reflects 'all' exposures from traffic	Emissions from roads may not be easily characterized and be the same Not directly giving concentrations—only a proxy for various traffic-related pollutants
GIS-based interpolation modeling e.g. (co) kriging	Locations of monitoring sites attributed with pollutant concentrations For co-kriging, covariates might include road geography and altitude	A further refinement of the distance from the road measure Fairly straightforward to do nowadays Provides concentration estimates Validation studies show good correlations with actual measurements	It requires a dense monitoring network and good input data such as land use, traffic volume for co-kriging
GIS-based regression modeling	Locations of monitoring sites attributed with pollutant concentrations Covariates might include road geography and altitude	A further refinement the distance from the above measures Fairly straightforward to do nowadays Provides concentration estimates Validation studies show fairly good correlations with actual measurements	It requires good input data such as land use, traffic volume, and monitoring data It requires a specific model for each location
GIS and air dispersion modeling	Road geography Point or area sources for non-traffic emissions Hourly or daily wind speed and direction, plus temperature and cloud cover or sensible surface heat flux	A further refinement of above methods Specific emissions can be modeled It can be used to model past exposures, although certain assumptions have to be made Provides concentration estimates	Need to include all the relevant input parameters in the model It is quite time-consuming

Table 3.4 (continued) Input and strength and limitations of various methods

Method	Input/requirements	Strength	Limitations
Personal exposure monitoring	Contact with subjects Personal monitoring equipment	It reflects personal exposure Incorporates exposure from different sources	Very time-consuming and expensive Can only be used for validation purposes in large studies
Biological monitoring	Contact with individuals Biomonitoring methods	It reflects actual uptake	Very few good biomarkers Often only reflects recent exposure Need contact and consent of individuals May only be used for validation purposes

examples. The exposure assessment that is possible very much depends on the epidemiological study design and resources available. The methods outlined in this chapter often appear straightforward and easily achievable—in reality this of course is not the case, and considerable effort and resources are needed. The variability in exposure is often complex due, e.g., to spatial and temporal variability in environmental levels of pollutants, behavior of subjects and the presence of mixture. The main challenge is

Table 3.5 Hierarchy of exposure data and surrogates for fixed source contaminants

Type of data	Approximation to actual exposure
1 Quantified personal measurement	Best
2 Quantified area measurements in the vicinity of the residence or sites of activity	↑
3 Quantified surrogates of exposure (e.g. estimates of drinking water use)	
4 Distance from the site and duration of exposure	
5 Distance or duration of residence	
6 Residence or employment in the geographical area in reasonable proximity to the site where exposure can be assumed	
7 Residence or employment in a defined geographical area (e.g. a county) of the site	Worst

Adapted from [55]. Reproduced with permission from National Research Council (U.S.). Board on Environmental Studies and Toxicology. Committee on Advances in Assessing Human Exposure to Airborne Pollutants. Human exposure assessment for airborne pollutants: advances and opportunities. Washington, DC: National Academy of Sciences 1991.

how to get to grips with this and produce robust and meaningful estimates of exposure for the epidemiological study. The interpretation of the epidemiological study depends on the extent to which we succeed. Much work lies ahead of us.

3.11 **References**

[1] **Nieuwenhuijsen MJ.** *Exposure assessment in occupational and environmental epidemiology.* Oxford and New York: Oxford University Press 2003.

[2] **Armstrong BG.** Optimizing power in allocating resources to exposure assessment in an epidemiologic study. *Am J Epidemiol.* 1996 **144**(2):192–7.

[3] **Kavanagh P, Farago ME, Thornton I, Goessler W, Kuehnelt D, Schlagenhaufen C, *et al*.** Urinary arsenic species in Devon and Cornwall residents, UK. A pilot study. *Analyst.* 1998 **123**(1):27–9.

[4] **Elliott P, Wakefield J, Best N, Briggs D.** *Spatial epidemiology: methods and applications.* Oxford: Oxford University Press 2000.

[5] **Wigzell E, Kendall M, Nieuwenhuijsen MJ.** The spatial and temporal variation of particulate matter within the home. *Journal of Exposure Analysis and Environmental Epidemiology.* 2000 **10**(3):307–14.

[6] **Nieuwenhuijsen MJ, Toledano MB, Elliott P.** Uptake of chlorination disinfection by-products; a review and a discussion of its implications for exposure assessment in epidemiological studies. *Journal of Exposure Analysis and Environmental Epidemiology.* 2000 **10**(6 Pt 1):586–99.

[7] **Kromhout H, Tielemans ELP, Heedrik D.** Estimates of individual dose from current measurements of exposure. *Occupational Hygiene.* 1996 **3**:23–9.

[8] **Seixas NS, Sheppard L.** Maximizing accuracy and precision using individual and grouped exposure assessments. *Scand J Work Environ Health.* 1996 **22**(2):94–101.

[9] **Heederik D, Kromhout H, Braun W.** The influence of random exposure estimation error on the exposure–response relationship when grouping into homogenous exposure categories. *Occupational Hygiene.* 1996 **3**:229–41.

[10] **Kromhout H, Heederik D.** Occupational epidemiology in the rubber industry: implications of exposure variability. *Am J Ind Med.* 1995 **27**(2):171–85.

[11] **van Tongeren M, Gardiner K, Calvert I, Kromhout H, Harrington JM.** Efficiency of different grouping schemes for dust exposure in the European carbon black respiratory morbidity study. *Occupational and Environmental Medicine.* 1997 **54**(10):714–9.

[12] **Dolk H, Thakrar B, Walls P, Landon M, Grundy C, Saez Lloret I, *et al*.** Mortality among residents near cokeworks in Great Britain. *Occupational and Environmental Medicine.* 1999 **56**(1):34–40.

[13] **Dolk H, Elliott P, Shaddick G, Walls P, Thakrar B.** Cancer incidence near radio and television transmitters in Great Britain. II. All high power transmitters. *Am J Epidemiol.* 1997 **145**(1):10–7.

[14] **Elliott P, Shaddick G, Kleinschmidt I, Jolley D, Walls P, Beresford J, *et al*.** Cancer incidence near municipal solid waste incinerators in Great Britain. *British Journal of Cancer.* 1996 **73**(5):702–10.

[15] **Livingstone AE, Shaddick G, Grundy C, Elliott P.** Do people living near inner city main roads have more asthma needing treatment? Case control study. *BMJ (Clinical Research edn).* 1996 **312**(7032):676–7.

[16] **English P, Neutra R, Scalf R, Sullivan M, Waller L, Zhu L.** Examining associations between childhood asthma and traffic flow using a geographic information system. *Environmental Health Perspectives.* 1999 **107**(9):761–7.

[17] **Hoek G, Brunekreef B, Goldbohm S, Fischer P, van den Brandt PA.** Association between mortality and indicators of traffic-related air pollution in the Netherlands: a cohort study. *Lancet.* 2002 **360**(9341):1203–9.

[18] **Elliott P, Briggs D, Morris S, de Hoogh C, Hurt C, Jensen TK, et al**. Risk of adverse birth outcomes in populations living near landfill sites. *BMJ (Clinical research edn)*. 2001 **323**(7309):363–8.

[19] **Barbone F, Bovenzi M, Cavallieri F, Stanta G**. Air pollution and lung cancer in Trieste, Italy. *Am J Epidemiol*. 1995 **141**(12):1161–9.

[20] **Cooney MA, Daniels JL, Ross JA, Breslow NE, Pollock BH, Olshani AF**. Household pesticides and the risk of Wilms tumor. *Environmental Health Perspectives*. 2007 **115**(1):134–7.

[21] **Teitelbaum SL, Gammon MD, Britton JA, Neugut AI, Levin B, Stellman SD**. Reported residential pesticide use and breast cancer risk on Long Island, New York. *Am J Epidemiol*. 2007 **165**(6):643–51.

[22] **Katsouyanni K, Zmirou D, Spix C, Sunyer J, Schouten J, Pönkä A, et al**. Short-term effects of air pollution on health: a European approach using epidemiological time-series data. The APHEA project: background, objectives, design. *Eur Respir J*. 1995 **8**:1030–8.

[23] **Dockery D, Pope C**. Outdoor air I: particulates. In: Steenland K, Savitz D, eds. *Topics in environmental epidemiology*. New York: Oxford University Press 1997: 119–66.

[24] **Dockery DW, Pope CA, 3rd, Xu X, Spengler JD, Ware JH, Fay ME, et al**. An association between air pollution and mortality in six U.S. cities. *The New England Journal of Medicine*. 1993 **329**(24):1753–9.

[25] **Kramer U, Koch T, Ranft U, Ring J, Behrendt H**. Traffic-related air pollution is associated with atopy in children living in urban areas. *Epidemiology (Cambridge, MA)*. 2000 **11**(1):64–70.

[26] **Magari SR, Schwartz J, Williams PL, Hauser R, Smith TJ, Christiani DC**. The association between personal measurements of environmental exposure to particulates and heart rate variability. *Epidemiology (Cambridge, MA)*. 2002 **13**(3):305–10.

[27] **Magnus P, Nafstad P, Oie L, Carlsen KC, Becher G, Kongerud J, et al**. Exposure to nitrogen dioxide and the occurrence of bronchial obstruction in children below 2 years. *Int J Epidemiol*. 1998 **27**(6):995–9.

[28] **Bellinger D, Schwartz J, eds**. *Effects of lead in children and adults*. New York: Oxford University Press 1997.

[29] **Etzel RA**. Environmental tobacco smoke I: childhood diseases. In: Steenland K, Savitz DA, eds. *Topics in environmental epidemiology*. New York: Oxford University Press 1997: 227–53.

[30] **Wu A**. Environmental tobacco smoke II: lung cancer. In: Steenland K, Savitz D, eds. *Topics in environmental epidemiology*. New York: Oxford University Press 1997: 227–53.

[31] **Brownson R, Alavanja M, eds**. *Radiation I. Radon*. New York: Oxford University Press 1997.

[32] **Savitz D**. Radiation II: elecromagnetic fields. In: Steenland K, Savitz D, eds. *Topics in environmental epidemiology*. New York: Oxford University Press 1997: 295–313.

[33] **Brunekreef B**. Exposure assessment. In: Baker D, Kjellström T, Calderon RHP, eds. *Environmental epidemiology: a textbook on study methods and public health applications*. Geneva: World Health Organization 1999: 65–102.

[34] **Hodgson S, Nieuwenhuijsen MJ, Colvile R, Jarup L**. Assessment of exposure to mercury from industrial emissions: comparing 'distance as a proxy' and dispersion modeling approaches. *Occupational and Environmental Medicine*. 2007 **64**(6):380–8.

[35] **Harris SA, Sass-Kortsak AM, Corey PN, Purdham JT**. Development of models to predict dose of pesticides in professional turf applicators. *Journal of Exposure Analysis and Environmental Epidemiology*. 2002 **12**(2):130–44.

[36] **Spiegelhalter D, Thomas A, Best N, Gilks W**. *The BUGS Project 0.5 – Bayesian inference using gibbs sampling manual (Version ii)*. 1996 cited; Available from: http://www. mrc-bsu.cam.ac.uk/bugs/.

[37] **Whitaker H, Best N, Nieuwenhuijsen MJ, Wakefield J, Fawell J, Elliott P**. Modeling exposure to disinfection by-products in drinking water for an epidemiological study of adverse birth outcomes. *Journal of Exposure Analysis and Environmental Epidemiology*. 2005 **15**(2):138–46.

[38] **Laden F, Neas LM, Dockery DW, Schwartz J**. Association of fine particulate matter from different sources with daily mortality in six U.S. cities. *Environmental Health Perspectives*. 2000 **108**(10):941–7.

[39] **Vallius M, Janssen NA, Heinrich J, Hoek G, Ruuskanen J, Cyrys J, et al**. Sources and elemental composition of ambient PM(2.5) in three European cities. *Sci Total Environ*. 2005 Jan **337**(1–3):147–62.

[40] **Nuckols JR, Ward MH, Jarup L**. Using geographic information systems for exposure assessment in environmental epidemiology studies. *Environmental Health Perspectives*. 2004 **112**(9):1007–15.

[41] **Briggs D**. The role of GIS: coping with space (and time) in air pollution exposure assessment. *J Toxicol Environ Health A*. 2005 **68**(13–14):1243–61.

[42] **Bayer-Oglesby L, Grize L, Gassner M, Takken-Sahli K, Sennhauser F, Neu U, et al**. Decline of ambient air pollution levels and improved respiratory health in Swiss children. *Env Health Perspect*. 2005 **113**(11):1632–7.

[43] **Jerrett M, Arain A, Kanaroglou P, Beckerman B, Potoglou D, Sahsuvaroglu T, et al**. A review and evaluation of intraurban air pollution exposure models. *Journal of Exposure Analysis and Environmental Epidemiology*. 2005 **15**(2):185–204.

[44] **Veen AVD, Briggs DJ, Collins S, Elliott P, Fischer, P, Kingham S, et al**. Mapping urban air pollution using GIS: a regression-based approach. *International Journal of Geographical Information Science*. 1997 **11**(11):699–718.

[45] **Briggs DJ, de Hoogh C, Gulliver J, Wills J, Elliott P, Kingham S, et al**. A regression-based method for mapping traffic-related air pollution: application and testing in four contrasting urban environments. *The Science of The Total Environment*. 2000 **253**(1–3):151–67.

[46] **Brauer M, Hoek G, van Vliet P, Meliefste K, Fischer P, Gehring U, et al**. Estimating long-term average particulate air pollution concentrations: application of traffic indicators and geographic information systems. *Epidemiology (Cambridge, MA)*. 2003 **14**(2):228–39.

[47] **Carr D, von Ehrenstein O, Weiland S, Wagner C, Wellie O, Nicolai T, et al**. Modeling annual benzene, toluene, NO2, and soot concentrations on the basis of road traffic characteristics. *Environ Res*. 2002 **90**(2):111–18.

[48] **Nyberg F, Gustavsson P, Jarup L, Bellander T, Berglind N, Jakobsson R, et al**. Urban air pollution and lung cancer in Stockholm. *Epidemiology (Cambridge, MA)*. 2000 **11**(5):487–95.

[49] **Bellander T, Berglind N, Gustavsson P, Jonson T, Nyberg F, Pershagen G, et al**. Using geographic information systems to assess individual historical exposure to air pollution from traffic and house heating in Stockholm. *Environmental Health Perspectives*. 2001 **109**(6):633–9.

[50] **Cyrys J, Hochadel M, Gehring U, Hoek G, Diegmann V, Brunekreef B, et al**. GIS-based estimation of exposure to particulate matter and NO2 in an urban area: stochastic versus dispersion modeling. *Environmental Health Perspectives*. 2005 **113**(8):987–92.

[51] **Kousa A, Monn C, Rotko T, Alm S, Oglesby L, Jantunen MJ**. Personal exposures to NO2 in the EXPOLIS-study: relation to residential indoor, outdoor and workplace concentrations in Basel, Helsinki and Prague. *Atmospheric Environment*. 2001 **35**(20):3405–12.

[52] **Phillips ML, Hall TA, Esmen NA, Lynch R, Johnson DL**. Use of global positioning system technology to track subject's location during environmental exposure sampling. *Journal of Exposure Analysis and Environmental Epidemiology*. 2001 **11**(3):207–15.

[53] **Elgethun K, Fenske RA, Yost MG, Palcisko GJ**. Time-location analysis for exposure assessment studies of children using a novel global positioning system instrument. *Environmental Health Perspectives*. 2003 **111**(1):115–22.

[54] **Ward MH, Nuckols JR, Weigel SJ, Maxwell SK, Cantor KP, Miller RS**. Identifying populations potentially exposed to agricultural pesticides using remote sensing and a geographic information system. *Environmental Health Perspectives*. 2000 **108**(1):5–12.

[55] **National Research Council (U.S.). Board on Environmental Studies and Toxicology. Committee on Advances in Assessing Human Exposure to Airborne Pollutants.** *Human exposure assessment for airborne pollutants: advances and opportunities*. Washington, DC: National Academy of Sciences 1991.

Chapter 4

Health effects assessment

Dean Baker

4.1 Concepts of health effects measurement

All organs and systems of the body can be affected adversely by exposures to environmental hazards. Adverse effects range from subtle physiological and biochemical changes that may be asymptomatic, to individual perceptions or symptoms of illness, to clinically diagnosed disease, and finally, to death (see Figure 2.1 in Chapter 2). In general, toxic agents have specific molecular and cellular components which they target, so many toxic agents cause specific effects in particular target organs while other agents impact on multiple tissues and organs of the body.

Toxicity is the capacity of a toxic agent to produce injury in an organism. Severity of toxicity depends on the route and magnitude of exposure and on the dose received by the target organ system. The extent and pattern of injury at a given dose is modified by route of absorption and, in the case of chemicals, by the distribution and metabolism in the body, and the rate of excretion. The severity of toxicity is also affected by the extent to which the person is susceptible to the hazard. Consequently, even with a similar dose, toxic effects can vary between humans and other organisms, among human subpopulations such as adults compared to children, and among individuals within the same subpopulation.

Lead is an example of an environmental hazard that produces a wide range of adverse effects at different doses, including both clinical and subclinical toxicity, and produces different effects at different concentrations in children compared to adults. (See Figure 2.2 in Chapter 2.) *Sub-clinical toxicity* refers to harmful health effects that may have been caused by an environmental exposure to a toxic agent but are not clinically recognizable. For example, anemia, encephalopathy, wrist drop and renal failure are among the clinically obvious manifestations observable at the upper end of the range of lead toxicity. Slowed nerve conduction, impaired biosynthesis of heme, and altered excretion of uric acid are some subclinical effects. It is important to note that these subclinical changes represent adverse reactions to lead and are not merely physiological adjustments to its presence.

Exposure to organophosphate pesticides (OPs) provides another example of the range of clinical manifestations of toxicity. In acute OP poisoning, symptoms and signs of poisoning can vary from respiratory distress to diarrhea, nausea and vomiting; all of which could be confused with an acute infectious disease process. However, the presence of blurred vision, slowing of the heart rate, pinpoint pupils, and muscle fasciculation point to a chemical etiology. These findings in association with a history of recent pesticide exposure lead to a tentative clinical diagnosis of OP toxicity. Laboratory measures of cholinesterase activity (red blood cell or plasma cholinesterase depression) may be used to verify the diagnosis and monitor recovery from the poisoning.

The concepts of health effects caused by environmental hazards were introduced in Section 2.1.2. When developing strategies to measure health effects in an epidemiological study, it is relevant to understand the concepts discussed in the Chapter 2—such as local and systematic effects, reversible and irreversible effects, acute and chronic effects, and immediate and delayed (latent) effects.

4.1.1 Acute and chronic effects

Damage to human health by chemical or biological hazards is generally related to the dose. In the short term, *acute toxicity* may be defined as hazard dose associated with an adverse health effect occurring in a timeframe of minutes, hours or days. With exposure to some hazards, adverse health effects are delayed. Mechanistically, *delayed toxicity* can be related to a wide variety of factors. Neural tissue damage and behavioral sequelae arising from acute carbon monoxide intoxication may be expressed several weeks after the initial insult. Effects of repeated exposure to asbestos such as development of lung cancer or lung disease (asbestosis) may take many years, even decades, before becoming clinically apparent.

The delay before appearance of disease is generally called the induction or latent period, although these terms have different precise meanings. The *induction period* is the time interval from the causal exposure to initiation of disease, while the *latent period* is the time interval from disease initiation to the clinical manifestation of disease (Figure 4.1). Because the exact causal exposure cannot be determined, the induction period is generally considered the time interval beginning with onset of exposure. Furthermore, because it is difficult to determine exactly the time of disease initiation for most chronic diseases, it may be difficult to distinguish in practical terms between the induction and latent periods. In actuality, epidemiologists tend to use the terms—induction period and latent period—interchangeably to mean the time interval between onset of exposure and clinical manifestation of disease.

For biological agents, the incubation period represents the period of time between exposure and the manifestation of disease. During the incubation period, the bacteria,

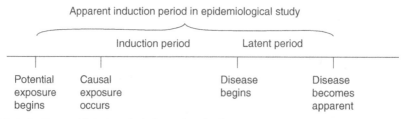

Fig. 4.1 Induction and latent periods for a chronic disease.

viruses or parasites grow in number and are transported to the target organ, in which the disease will develop. This period may be hours, days, weeks, or decades in length. For some bacteria, the damage to the target organ is due to the production of chemical toxins by the bacteria. The incubation period for a biological agent has a different technical definition than the latency period for a chemically induced disease, but in epidemiological studies these terms have the same operational definitions (time between exposure and manifestation of disease) and represent the same concept.

4.1.2 Specific and non-specific effects

Exposure to some toxic agents such as asbestos are linked with specific effects, in this case mesothelioma, while other exposures, such as traffic related air pollution, may cause a number of adverse effects including, e.g., respiratory and cardiovascular disease and adverse reproductive outcomes. Environmental epidemiology studies can be designed to measure a specific outcome related to an identified exposure, or the design can encompass an array of health outcomes within a more general study. The degree of specificity in the health effects assessment will generally depend on existing knowledge about the epidemiological and biological processes, and the quality of the exposure monitoring information for the putative environmental hazard. Studies may focus on one primary effect, but collect information on other secondary or nonspecific effects as well. For example, large population-based studies designed to evaluate the effects of chemical air pollutants on respiratory lung disease may also be designed to observe the effects on cardiovascular disease in the study population.

4.1.3 Variation and susceptibility

The likelihood of developing an adverse health effect following exposure to an environmental hazard is often affected by characteristics of the individuals in the exposed population. The most fundamental consideration is whether the individuals are 'at risk' of developing a health outcome due to an environmental hazard. Individuals may not be at risk of developing a health outcome for gender-specific diseases depending on their gender (e.g., prostate cancer can only affect males), if they already have a health outcome, or if they had a disease and cannot develop the disease again (e.g., immunity following some infections). Even among the at-risk population, there is usually variation in the degree of risk depending on characteristics of the persons. General host factors that should be taken into consideration include age, ethnicity, behavior (such as smoking and amount of physical exercise), hygiene, diet, and coexisting health conditions.

Traditionally investigators have distinguished between 'genetic' and 'environmental' causes of health effects; however, this distinction is not appropriate because of the close interaction between genetic and environmental factors. Environmental hazards can cause genetic damage, which includes chromosomal aberrations as well as alterations in specific genes. Genetic damage to somatic and germ cells may be the underlying mechanism responsible for many types of health effects, including reproductive failure and cancer. Many chemicals can induce chromosome aberrations in somatic cells [1]. These include benzene, pesticides, nitrosamines, vinyl chloride monomer and a number of other industrial chemicals and drugs. Therefore, substantial effort has been made to quantify genetic damage in humans as a health outcome in itself.

Furthermore, some people may have a genetic predisposition to increased susceptibility to specific environmental hazards. For example, the nevoid basal cell carcinoma syndrome predisposes to radiation-induced skin cancer. In people with this syndrome, the development of basal cell carcinoma is accentuated, occurring only months after even very low dose X-ray exposure. Similar genetic susceptibility is suspected for some chemicals due to individual variation in metabolic pathways or enzyme systems (e.g., aromatic hydrocarbons). An example of susceptibility is the enzyme, glutathione-S-transferase (GST), which functions in metabolism to detoxify absorbed chemicals. This family of isoenzymes catalyses the conjugation of reactive intermediates, such as epoxides formed during early stage metabolism with glutathione scavengers occurring naturally in the body. Those individuals with a low capacity for producing the enzyme have a reduced capacity for conjugating electrophiles, and are more at risk for a mutational event that could be associated with cancer, as was found in a study of bladder cancer and GSTM1 [2]. Another example is N-acetyltransferase (NAT), a non-inducible enzyme that functions in detoxifying aromatic amines such as benzidine and 4-amino biphenyl by acetylation. Two phenotypes are in human populations, one with low acetyltransferase activity (slow acetylators), and one with high enzyme activity (fast acetylators). Those individuals who are NAT2 slow acetylators are at increased risk of bladder cancer because they can not detoxify aromatic amines as quickly as fast acetylators [2].

Susceptibility is a particularly important factor to be aware of in environmental epidemiology because the relationships between exposure and biological effect or disease can be modified in that portion of a population that is susceptible, and the association between exposure and disease for the susceptible subpopulation can be masked or weakened in any study that does not consider variation in individual susceptibilities. Use of susceptibility biomarkers could improve the precision and strength of putative exposure–disease associations by avoiding the dilution effect that occurs in populations with a large proportion of nonsusceptible people. Consequently, susceptibility biomarkers should be used in stratifying the study populations, so a more accurate estimate of disease risk can be made. An increasing proportion of environmental epidemiological research studies now include genetic measurements in order to examine the interaction between gene and environment. More information on methods to study gene-environment interactions is presented in Chapter 8, Section 8.5.

4.1.4 **Hyperreactivity and hypersensitivity**

Hyperreactivity and hypersensitivity are similar terms which are also used to identify highly sensitive individuals in the population, but they have different meanings than 'susceptibility'. In *hyperreactive* persons, the effects of the agent are qualitatively the same as expected, but quantitatively increased. 'Normal' effects occur, but at a lower dose than in the majority of the population. It is possible that the variation in susceptibility is due to the interaction of genetic and other host factors, but in practice, it is not possible to determine exactly why hyperreactive persons are more sensitive than other members of the population.

Hypersensitivity refers to when persons react with 'allergic' effects following exposure to a certain substance (allergen). The allergic reaction involves a person's immune system after it has become sensitized to the substance. These allergic reactions include skin conditions such as eczema and contact dermatitis, as well as respiratory conditions such as asthma and hypersensitivity pneumonitis.

4.2 Assessment of health effects

4.2.1 Strategy of what to measure

What health outcome to assess depends on the study question, hypothesis and design and available resources. It is also generally based on what is known from the toxicological literature or from previous epidemiological studies for the exposure of interest itself or similar substances. For example, air pollution research started off by examining respiratory morbidity and mortality effects, but has now progressed and includes cardiovascular and reproductive effects. It follows a trend that was seen in tobacco research, which involves similar pollutants albeit at a higher level. The particle sizes of interest have also been expanded from PM_{10}, to $PM_{2.5}$, to ultrafine. This was partly based on observed effects in animal studies. Whereas some environmental epidemiologists focus on one particular outcome, others study the whole range of health effects associated with air pollution.

Assuming that the health outcome of interest is known (e.g., respiratory), the potential outcomes to assess range from biomarkers of lung permeability (e.g., surfactant A and B); pro-inflammatory cytokines and chemokines (e.g., interleukin-8); inflammation (e.g., intracellular adhesion molecule, increased sputum neutrophil and esinophilic cationic protein levels); oxidative stress (e.g., the production of nitrogen oxide and carbon monoxide, thiobarbituric acid reactive substances, 8-isoprostane, and myeloperoxidase); physiological changes (e.g., FEV_1); self-reported disease; doctor-diagnosed respiratory disease; and respiratory morbidity and mortality data from hospital and death registries. Some health outcome data from hospital records needs to be collected on individuals (e.g., surfactant A and B, FEV_1), while others may be obtained from routine sources (e.g., hospital and death records). The research question, sample size, logistics of collecting new health outcome data, and availability of existing medical records determine to a large extent what will be studied.

A principal reason to study sub-clinical changes is that such changes may occur earlier than and be predictive of the future development of clinical disease, leading to strategies for surveillance and prevention of the disease. Sub-clinical changes are also studied because these changes may provide insight about the mechanisms by which the environmental hazard causes the disease. Finally, at any specific dosage level, sub-clinical changes may occur in a larger proportion of the population than overt clinical disease, so epidemiological studies of sub-clinical effects may have greater statistical power.

On the other hand, registry data of clinical effects may be used to evaluate long-term trends and spatial distribution of a disease.

4.2.2 Case definition

An initial step in many environmental epidemiological studies is to describe the problem by defining the case. A *case definition* is a set of criteria for deciding whether an individual should be classified as having the condition of interest. It includes clinical criteria as well as criteria relating to place and time, and type of individual. Within the framework of developing a case definition, several questions must be addressed:

- How does the disease present clinically?
- How does one define a case in terms of clinical observations and laboratory tests?
- In what particular population is the disease occurring and is there truly an excess?
- What etiological possibilities immediately present themselves in terms of clinical and population observations?

Whenever possible, a case should be defined on the basis of data derived from clinical and laboratory findings, rather than on the basis of symptoms reported by participants or their families. Ideally, the clinical criteria should be objectively measurable (e.g., fever >38°C, FEV_1 lower than 80 percent predicted, elevated antibody titers, three or more loose bowel movements per day). However, when clinical evidence is not available or is inappropriate, then it may be necessary to use other means of establishing a case definition. For example, following the contamination of flour with polybrominated biphenyl (PBB) in Michigan, US, a 'PBB syndrome' was defined through the use of questionnaire data (consisting largely of symptoms such as fatigue, sleep disturbance, joint pain, and headache).

Questionnaire data may also be combined with clinical data to establish the case definition. For example, in a historical cohort study of uterine leiomyoma (fibroids) among women potentially exposed to dioxin from the Seveso, Italy, chemical plant explosion in 1976, Eskenazi *et al.* [3] used a combination of interview responses and medical records to categorize women as 'cases' with uterine leiomyoma. First the research staff asked the women whether they had been diagnosed with fibroids. If the woman responded 'yes', the investigators requested past medical records for confirmation. These women were considered cases if the medical records did not contradict the self-reported historical diagnosis. In addition, among women who answered 'no' to the question about fibroids, the investigators obtained medical records (generally requested for other diseases) and examined whether the medical records documented a diagnosis of fibroids. If the medical record showed such a diagnosis, these women were also considered to be 'cases' even though they did not report this diagnosis during their interview. Therefore, the investigators categorized cases based on a combination of the best information available from the interview and the medical records.

Case definitions for cancer, respiratory, or cardiovascular disease, are generally well understood by health practitioners. However, for diseases with unknown etiologies, often involving either subtle immunologic or neurological responses that may be related to environmental exposures, case definitions are not as well defined. Furthermore, outcomes that consist of a blend of subtle and non-specific conditions may be difficult to define. For example, it may be difficult to establish a precise case definition when studying the impact of heavy metal exposure on postnatal development in children. Investigators typically measure several indicators of development, such as gestational age at birth; birth weight; postnatal changes in weight and length; the child's ability to roll over, sit up, and walk at appropriate stages of development; and neurobehavioral function at different ages. Analysis of these variables taken together (e.g., factor analysis or other multivariate analysis techniques) can help to develop a case definition to be used in further studies.

Whenever possible, it is advisable to use standard definitions of clinical outcomes, so the findings of one study may be compared to those of other studies. This approach is especially important for epidemiological studies that use disease information reported to registries, since the investigators do not personally conduct the health outcome assessment. A widely used coding scheme for this purpose is the International Statistical Classification of Diseases and Related Health Problems. Currently in its 10th Revision (ICD-10), it is a coding of diseases and signs, symptoms, abnormal findings, complaints, social circumstances and external causes of injury or diseases, as classified by the World Health Organization (WHO) (Table 4.1). The version for 2007 is available at http://www.who.int/classifications/apps/icd/icd10online. Most registries follow the ICD classification, which provides a standardized approach to ascertainment. An issue with long-term studies is how to bridge from previous ICD codes (e.g., ICD-8 to ICD-9 to ICD-10) because disease categories have been changed. The WHO provides some guidelines. Furthermore, it is important to remember that the actual classification may differ between different registries because it is dependent upon who does the classification. In cases like congenital anomalies, this may not be straightforward, and considerable differences in case ascertainment between registries have been observed [4]. Congenital anomalies such as gastroschisis are easy to detect at birth and are generally well recorded, but others such as certain congenital anomalies of the heart are more difficult to detect and ascertainment rates differ between registries. In addition, some registries may record many minor anomalies, while others record only the major anomalies, which is important to consider when classifying anomalies as single or part of a syndrome. Furthermore, congenital malformations are often categorized as main categories, e.g., neural tube defects and heart defects while generally they are heterogeneous with respect to both phenotype and etiology. It may therefore be necessary to identify subsets of the main categories for analyses (see, for example, Table 4.2) [5].

Although it is essential for many environmental epidemiological studies to establish a case definition so there is a clear understanding of the health outcome, it is not always necessary to treat health outcomes as being dichotomous, i.e., either a case or not a case. Indeed it may be appropriate in many epidemiological studies to evaluate health effects as continuous variables to evaluate gradations of effects, even within the clinically normal ranges. For example, some investigators may examine respiratory health

Table 4.1 International Statistical Classification of Diseases and Related Health Problems 10th Revision. Version for 2007.

Chapter	Blocks	Title
I	A00–B99	Certain infectious and parasitic diseases
II	C00–D48	Neoplasms
III	D50–D89	Diseases of the blood and blood-forming organs and certain disorders involving the immune mechanism
IV	E00–E90	Endocrine, nutritional and metabolic diseases
V	F00–F99	Mental and behavioral disorders
VI	G00–G99	Diseases of the nervous system
VII	H00–H59	Diseases of the eye and adnexa
VIII	H60–H95	Diseases of the ear and mastoid process
IX	I00–I99	Diseases of the circulatory system
X	J00–J99	Diseases of the respiratory system
XI	K00–K93	Diseases of the digestive system
XII	L00–L99	Diseases of the skin and subcutaneous tissue
XIII	M00–M99	Diseases of the musculoskeletal system and connective tissue
XIV	N00–N99	Diseases of the genitourinary system
XV	O00–O99	Pregnancy, childbirth and the puerperium
XVI	P00–P96	Certain conditions originating in the perinatal period
XVII	Q00–Q99	Congenital malformations, deformations and chromosomal abnormalities
XVIII	R00–R99	Symptoms, signs and abnormal clinical and laboratory findings, not elsewhere classified
XIX	S00–T98	Injury, poisoning and certain other consequences of external causes
XX	V01–Y98	External causes of morbidity and mortality
XXI	Z00–Z99	Factors influencing health status and contact with health services
XXII	U00–U99	Codes for special purposes

outcomes by defining a 'case' of chronic obstructive pulmonary disease (COPD) as a person having a FEV_1/FVC ratio <0.70 (the volume of air exhaled in the first second divided by the total volume of air that can be exhaled during a forced expiratory maneuver). For these studies, the health outcome would be the proportion of COPD 'cases' in a population. On the other hand, some investigators may evaluate the effect of an environmental hazard on respiratory function by examining the FEV_1/FVC ratio as a continuous proportion. In this latter situation, it would not be necessary to define a specific cut-point that constituted a 'case' of COPD. Both of these approaches are acceptable and

Table 4.2 Selection of a subset of congenital anomalies from the major congenital anomalies grouping for a study on the relationship between chlorination by-products and congenital anomalies.

Birth defect	ICD 10 codes (with BPA extension) for 'broad' category	Subset for inclusion in 'narrow' category	Subset for exclusion in 'narrow' category	Comment
Cleft lip/palate	Q35–Q37	Q35.* Q36.* Q37.*		Analysis should be split into: (a) Q35: cleft palate (b) Q36–Q37.99: cleft lip and cleft palate with cleft lip
Abdominal wall defects	Q79	Q79.0 (congenital diaphragmatic hernia) Q79.1 (absence of diaphragm, CM of diaphragm NOS, eventration of diaphragm) Q79.2 (exomphalos) Q79.3 (gastroschisis)		Analysis should be split into: Exomphalos (older women, part of chromosomal anomaly) Gastroschisis (younger women, not part of a chromosomal anomaly)
Major cardiac defects	Q20–Q28	Q20.*, Q21.2 (atrioventricular septal defect), Q21.3 (tetralogy of Fallot), Q22.*, Q23.*, Q25.1, Q25.2, Q25.3 Q25.4, Q25.5, Q25.6, Q25.7, Q25.8. Q25.9 Q26.*	Q21.0, Q21.1, Q21.4, Q21.8, Q21.9, Q24.*, Q25.0, Q27.*, Q28.*	Q21.8: possibly include this if, after sensitivity check on text field they are not atrial septal defects or ventricular septal defects but are tetralogy of Fallot Q23.4: useful for sensitivity check as should have a high ascertainment
Respiratory defects	Q30–Q34	Q33.*	Q30.*, Q31.*, Q32.*, Q34.*	
Urinary tract defects	Q60–Q64, except for Q64.0 (epispadias)	Q60.* Q61.* Q62.* (but see exclusion) Q64.* (but see exclusion)	Q62.0 Q63. * Q64.0 Q64.8 Q64.9	Analysis should be split into: (a) All renal disease (Q60 and Q61) (b) Obstructive disease (Q62 and Q64)

*All codes within the subset.

From [5]. Nieuwenhuijsen MJ, Toledano MB, Bennett J, Best N, Konstantinou K, Hambly P, et al. The relationship between disinfection byproducts in drinking water and congenital anomalies in England and Wales. *Environmental Health Perspectives*. 2008; 116: 216–22.

widely used. The differences in how the health outcomes are conceived and defined by investigators will depend largely on the study objectives and whether it is relevant to define a specific clinical outcome (i.e., mortality or morbidity event) to be studied.

4.2.3 Data sources

Health effects data may be classified as either primary or secondary depending on the reasons why the data were first recorded. Primary data are data that have been collected specifically for a particular study, such as by questionnaires or medical examinations. Secondary data (often referred to as routinely collected or registry data) are data that have been collected for purposes other than for a particular study and generally must be abstracted from existing records. The completeness of registration and accuracy of the information that the records contain can vary widely. Therefore, it is important to be aware of the quality of existing records.

Existing data sources for epidemiological studies include birth and death registries, cancer registries, hospital records, chronic and infectious disease registries, birth defects registries, hospital admissions, outpatient visits, well child clinics, and environmental monitoring programs. Data gathered from well-managed sources are useful because they are collected in a reasonably standardized fashion. Data collection for existing data may also be divided into direct (also called primary by some investigators) and indirect techniques. Direct data collection is when an investigator records data on study participants, expressly for the purpose of study (e.g., abstracting information on the study participant from a medical record). An indirect approach may be used if cases of a disease to be studied can be identified through an existing data system. The use of death certificate data is an example of such an indirect, secondary data source.

In many countries laws exists which expressly require reporting of morbidity and mortality data relating to specific chronic or infectious diseases. Such laws compel institutions and healthcare professionals to report cases of selected diseases or mortality to a central agency or registry.

4.2.3.1 Mortality data

Mortality data are used commonly in environmental epidemiology, especially in ecological studies and in case-control studies (see Chapter 6). An example of an ecological study based on mortality is the study by Chen and Wang [6] in which the investigators examined the association between arsenic concentration measured in water wells and cancer mortality data reported by administrative district in Taiwan. They found that administrative districts that had higher concentrations of arsenic in well water had elevated rates of cancers of the liver, nasal cavity, lung, skin, bladder and kidney. The 'Harvard Six Cities' study is an example of a cohort study that examined the effects of air pollution on mortality by following more than 8000 adults who were randomly recruited from six US cities with different levels of air pollution [7]. Mortality was assessed by sending informational letters to the subjects annually. The vital status of subjects who did not respond was determined by questioning family members, friends, or neighbors. In addition, the investigators searched the US National Death Index for the follow-up years.

For each person in the cohort who died, the investigators obtained death certificates and coded the causes of death according to the International Classification of Diseases. They found that fine-particulate air pollution was associated with excess mortality from lung cancer and cardiopulmonary disease in the study cohort.

Mortality data can be quite useful for epidemiological studies, but one must be aware of the strengths and limitations of these data sources. Mortality data are influenced by factors that affect disease duration and survival, such as detection and treatment, as well as incidence. Death certificates are based on the concept of the underlying cause of death, defined as 'the disease or injury which initiated the train of morbid events leading directly to death, or the circumstances of the accident which produced the fatal injury' [8]. The completeness and reliability of information on mortality varies widely throughout countries. In North America and Europe, for instance, death registration is virtually complete and death certificates generally contain reliable information regarding mortality. In some other countries and regions of the world, less than 50 percent of deaths are registered.

The basis for a mortality records system is that all deaths are medically certified by cause and recorded on a registry that is accessible to appropriate parties. For example, in the US, researchers can submit names and other identifying information to the National Death Index to determine an individual's vital status and place of death. The appropriate state's Office of Vital Statistics is then contacted for a copy of the death certificate, as was done in the Harvard Six Cities study. Other sources of information regarding the occurrence of death include records relating to employment, tax, military service, driver's licence, electoral status and insurance. Professional, union or alumni societies may also yield useful information.

Without accurate clinical data, the cause of death may be incorrectly recorded on the registry. Co-morbidity data are rarely available, unless all causes mentioned on the certificate have been coded (immediate and contributory, as well as underlying). Furthermore, in the absence of coding for multiple causes of death, or information collected at autopsy, the cause of death information that is coded from the death certificate may be misleading. Also death certificates generally do not contain information on other risk factors (e.g., tobacco smoking, occupational exposures). Consequently, it is difficult to use mortality data generated from a registry without supplementing those records with other data sources.

4.2.3.2 Morbidity data

Morbidity is defined as an incidence of ill health or disease, so morbidity data are those records of diseases or ill-health events that are the health outcomes of the epidemiological studies. Morbidity data may be gathered from health surveys, medical records (including those kept by hospitals, emergency rooms, clinics and physician's records) and disease registries such as cancer and congenital anomalies registries. Abstracting information of interest from paper records can be time-consuming, but fortunately that is generally not necessary for more recent years since the data is often available in digital (computer) form.

Hospital records

Hospital records can provide useful information on morbidity and mortality, although the investigators must be careful in using such records because of factors associated with admission practices of the hospital (hospital records are not always complete; physicians do not hospitalize all their patients with a particular disease; some patients die before admission); or because the study participants do not accurately reflect the catchment area for all hospital admissions. For example, if an appreciable proportion of patients admitted to the hospital are from areas outside the community of interest, that hospital's morbidity or mortality statistics will not be reliable as measures of disease prevalence within that community. Clearly, socioeconomic status as well as medical insurance policies may play a role in the hospital admissions process, as well as in the mode of treatment. One should be aware of such issues in deciding whether hospital records are reliable to use for study data.

Employment and school records

Records from work or school may be used to estimate morbidity within selected populations. There are two main limitations in these records. First, they are applicable only to generally unrepresentative source populations. Second, medical information in the records may not be accurate. In some instances, 'sick leave' may be reported for reasons other than sickness. For example, school absenteeism is known to relate to the day of the week, season of the year, and to social events or behavioral factors influencing the student population.

Registries of reportable diseases

When healthcare providers are legally required to report the occurrence of specific disease conditions, such as tuberculosis, congenital malformations, stillbirth or cancer to a centralized system, the accumulated datasets are known as registries (e.g., cancer registries). Environmentally related disease incidence data may also be reported to registries (e.g., pesticide poisonings to Poison Control Center data banks) in some governmental jurisdictions. However, the completeness of reporting is determined by the willingness of the providers to report the cases in a timely and reliable fashion. The validity of such reports can be assessed through the use of community surveys and by checking medical records.

Data generated from birth and birth defects registries are useful for evaluating effects (e.g., stillbirth, reduced birthweight) related to environmental exposures within communities. However, birth certificates contain only limited information regarding adverse health outcome measures (e.g., the birth record will only record the most severe structural or functional abnormality noted at birth, and not late developing abnormalities) and must be evaluated with care. Furthermore, as for a lot of the registry data, there is often only limited data on potential confounders.

4.2.3.3 Health interview and examination surveys

In *health interview surveys*, a sample of individuals is questioned about their social setting, their recognition of signs and symptoms of disease, their attitude towards sickness and health, and contact they have had with health services. The population sample may be representative of the total population, or selected subpopulations chosen by geographic distribution, or other characteristics. Such a survey can be a cost-effective means of obtaining data from a large sample of respondents. Data can be obtained from subjects by a variety of methods, including self-completion questionnaires, telephone interviews, direct interviews, group interviews, or diaries. The disadvantages of health interview surveys are that answers tend to be subjective and that no objective measures of disease may be available.

In *health examination surveys*, information is collected by interview and by physical examination. An example is the US National Health and Nutrition Examination Survey (NHANES), which is an ongoing survey of a representative sample of the US population conducted by the government to determine the prevalence of risk factors, health behaviors, sub-clinical conditions (e.g., elevated blood pressure), and clinical conditions. Data from the NHANES survey was used, for example, to examine the association between exposure to volatile organic compounds measured by passive personal monitoring and the prevalence of doctor-diagnosed asthma and wheezing [9]. Problems that may be encountered with this type of survey include the magnitude of resources required to collect the sample and to examine the study population. It can be expensive to conduct the physical examinations, combined with the costs of the collection of human tissue and fluid samples, and the analysis of samples. However, the benefit of health examination survey is that health outcome assessments can be based on physiological, neurological and psychological parameters, so that studies are not limited to examining only death or recorded diseases, or relying solely on self-reported health status.

4.2.3.4 Primary health outcome assessment

For many epidemiological studies, existing data on mortality and morbidity will not be sufficient for the health outcome assessment. In these situations, investigators will need to collect health outcome data specifically for the study. The major methods to collect such data are questionnaires, physical examinations, clinical testing (e.g., spirometry to evaluate lung function), and collection of biological specimens for laboratory analysis.

Questionnaires

Questionnaires are a major tool by which epidemiologists gather data on the characteristics of a study population. Through questionnaires, epidemiologists can gather information on the demographics associated with the study population (e.g., age, sex, race, ethnic group); social factors (e.g., occupation, education, socioeconomic status); personal habits (e.g., smoking, medications, drug use); genetic characteristics (e.g., familial health conditions); and individual and family health histories (e.g., hypertension, diabetes, heart disease, cancer, reproductive effects). As discussed in Chapter 3, questionnaires are also used to collect information on a person's time, activity, and location – which is useful for estimating exposures. An example of questions concerning hypertension is shown in Table 4.3. A disadvantage of questionnaires

Table 4.3 Questions about hypertension in a study population

1. I have some questions about hypertension (high blood pressure):
a. Have you ever been told by a doctor that you had high blood pressure? Yes ( ) No ( )
b. Another name for high blood pressure is hypertension. Have you ever been told by a doctor that you had hypertension?   Yes ( )   No ( )
c. If you have been told by a doctor that you have high blood pressure (hypertension), how long ago were you told? (specify number) ____ months ____ years
d. Was it in the past year?   Yes ( )   No ( )

is that the information is subjective and may lead to misclassification of disease. Therefore, validation and standardization of the questions is important. Whenever possible, questionnaires should be based upon previously used and tested questionnaires. This is especially useful if data are to be compared with those from previous surveys.

Some specific issues related to questionnaire design and administration are given in Table 4.4. In conducting a survey, the investigators must decide whether to use a self-administered questionnaire or to use interviewers to elicit information from the respondents. Although self-administered questionnaires are less costly, the response rate is frequently better with interviewer-administered questionnaires. Interviewers are also able to communicate with the participant, both to allay concerns, and to elicit difficult to derive information. With an interviewer, the respondent can also seek and receive clarification of a question, or help in completing the form. Thus, with an interviewer,

Table 4.4 Issues in questionnaire design

When designing questionnaires the investigator should ensure that:

- Adequate demographic information on study participants is requested
- Questions are properly grouped and are answered so as to reduce the likelihood of misinformation, bias, or non-response
- Skip patterns are clearly stated and easily identified
- Directions for recording answers are clear, space is adequate, and there is a mechanism to separate missing data (non-response) from 'zero' data
- The questions are understandable by the study population; questions should be kept as simple and to the point as possible
- Questions should be expressed in simple, unambiguous language so that they are readily understood by all members of the study population
- Only necessary questions are asked of the respondents
- The 'did a doctor tell you' approach is used, which reduces the opportunity for misinformation through improved recall. People are more likely to recall a health event correctly when there has been a physician's diagnosis
- Validity and reliability of questions is ensured
- The questionnaire is properly coded and machine readable, if possible

there is a better opportunity for reducing bias arising from failure of the respondent to respond entirely or to provide an incomplete response. On the other hand, the study participant may feel more comfortable using a self-administered questionnaire format to answer sensitive questions about issues such as sexual activity or use of illicit drugs. The person can record their answers privately without having to discuss these issues with the interviewer.

As the cost of mobile or notebook computers has decreased and they have become more available, it has become more common for investigators to have research staff administer questionnaires with the assistance of computers to enter the responses during the interview. This technique is referred to as computer-assisted interviews (CAI) or similar terms. Tablet notebook computers (i.e, mobile computers that allow direct entry of information by tapping or writing on the computer screen) can be used, so the interviewer can easily complete the interview responses without having to type the answers to each question. An advantage of this approach is that the questionnaires can have more structured branches in which answers to one question can determine the subsequent series of questions. Also the responses are directly entered into a database, so this approach reduces paperwork and the separate effort needed by office staff to enter the data from a hard copy of the questionnaire. It is likely that this approach will become increasingly common as the cost of mobile computers continues to decrease worldwide.

Physical examinations

It can be challenging to obtain high-quality data based on physical examinations, even when collaborating with highly qualified clinical examiners. Physicians and other health practitioners are not generally accustomed to performing and interpreting physical examinations in a highly uniform manner, which is essential for quality assurance in an epidemiological study. Interpretation of routine clinical findings, qualitative (e.g., skin pallor) and quantitative (e.g., respiratory rate), are variable between clinical specialists. Measures should be taken to minimize variability between clinical observers by establishing uniform clinical criteria and review procedures and by providing sufficient training in the examination protocol.

Prior to beginning a study, the investigators should establish detailed guidelines for examination and interpretation of the physical findings. The examination procedures should be reviewed with the clinician observers in a random sample of the study population prior to the definitive study. For quality control purposes, one clinician or an appropriate clinical panel should periodically review the clinical data for final interpretation.

Where possible, quantitative clinical measures of pathophysiological effects should be employed. Blood pressure, pulse, respiratory rate, and temperature are examples of routine clinical measures which can be most efficiently quantified and calibrated through instrumentation. Less efficient, semi-quantitative measures include pupil diameter, extremity reflexes, joint range of motion, gait, liver and spleen size. These semi-quantitative measures depend almost entirely on consensus among participating clinicians. Careful coordination among the investigators and the clinical observers is essential to ensure accuracy and consistency. As discussed in Chapter 11, training even of qualified clinicians and quality assurance review of physical examination procedures are necessary in every study.

Physiological measures

Measurement of physiological effects offers another means of assessing adverse health outcomes. However, because of considerable intra- and intervariability encountered between individuals, and equipment, investigators need to ensure that standardized procedures are used. For example, in measuring lung function following exposure to airborne pollutants, one sees daily and seasonal variability with specific lung function parameters such as forced expiratory volume in one second (FEV_1).

Lung function tests (e.g., spirometry) are often used to determine the respiratory health status of subjects participating in air pollution epidemiologic studies. When using spirometry to measure lung functions such as forced volume capacity (FVC), FEV_1, etc., the comparability of the equipment used and of the operators will determine whether results from separate studies can be compared. Guidelines have been published to standardize the performance of pulmonary function tests so that findings of epidemiological studies are comparable [8, 10].

The advantages or disadvantages of physiological measurement techniques or instruments have to be judged on the basis of:

- acceptability to the study population;
- the accuracy and reliability of the results obtained using them;
- their ease of use and the availability of technicians who know how to use them.

The sensitivity and specificity of the test must be determined. The determination of what constitutes a true or false positive or negative will depend on the standards employed.

Laboratory testing

Each laboratory test has three properties: sensitivity, specificity and predictive value. Sensitivity refers to the ability of the test to identify or detect a biologic or analytic end point at some concentration. Specificity refers to the ability of the test to identify an effect with minimal interference from competing reactions or biologic effects. Predictive value refers to the ability of the test to determine a relationship to a specific health effect.

Analytic chemical techniques in general are highly sensitive methods designed to quantify concentrations of a given chemical, element or biologic (protein, DNA, lipid). Current analytic technologies are highly specific, although they lack predictive value. For example, knowledge of the concentration of dioxin in tissue alone does not identify whether a subject has or will have an immunodeficiency condition. On the other hand, laboratory assays that detect a specific infectious agent in consistent association with disease outcome have specificity and predictive value with variable sensitivity. For example, use of western blot technology, an immunoassay, to detect AIDS is highly sensitive, relatively specific and is predictive of a long-term health consequence of infection. Detection of *Yersinia pestis* by culture of lung fluid at autopsy in association with multiple cases of unexplained lethal pulmonary edema is highly specific with relatively low sensitivity and good predictive value.

Biological markers or *biomarkers* can be considered a special type of laboratory test that is being increasingly used in epidemiological studies. The basic principles concerning biomarkers are described in Chapter 2. Biomarkers have been identified for many different types of outcomes. For example, biomarkers of reproductive effects are reduced sperm count, altered sperm morphology, mutagens in body fluids, micronuclei, and somatic cell mutation. Biomarkers of neurological effect include depressed acetyl-cholinesterase in serum and plasma, and slowed nerve conduction in peripheral neuropathy. Biomarkers of early kidney disease include, e.g., N-Acetyl-β-D-glucosaminidase (NAG) and β-2-microglobulin. Biomarkers of lung permeability include Surfactant A and B, and Clara-16 cells. Biomarkers of pro-inflammatory cytokines and chemokines include interleukin-8; for inflammation they include intracellular adhesion molecule (ICAM), sputum neutrophil and esinophilic cationic protein (ECP) levels; for oxidative stress they include, e.g., the production of nitrogen oxide and carbon monoxide, thiobar-bituric acid-reactive substances, 8-isoprostane, and myeloperoxidase. Sister chromatid exchange (SCE), a cellular measure of chromosome damage and repair, is a sensitive semi-quantitative measure of extent of damage by some genotoxic agents (ethylene oxide, styrene) but is an insensitive marker for a number of other genotoxic agents including benzene. Biomarkers of susceptibility involve genetic or environmentally derived metabolic reactions and variability in response to stimuli that potentially influence the response of the target organ to environmental exposure (e.g GST, NAT).

4.3 **Data linkage**

It is beneficial to develop capabilities for linking data sources to provide the best infor-mation possible for epidemiological studies. Clearly, the linkage of disease registry data with environmental databases would facilitate such research. A passive system involving linkage of databases with information on persons with the disease of interest is frequently used. Although a passive approach is less expensive, it is subject to whatever ascertain-ment limitations were present in the original databases. Alternatively, an active approach is used. The active approach to the data collection process involves two steps. First, an emphasis is placed on case finding. Then, a more detailed data set may be collected for a subset of persons (i.e., those suspected of being exposed or at risk). This approach is often used in case-control studies in which case ascertainment is done through cancer registries, but then cases and a population-based sample of controls are recruited as the study population for more detailed data collection.

One of the main problems with data linkage in many countries is getting permission to link the data, which is particularly relevant when information on individuals is required. A way to get around this is to not use information that can identify individuals but infor-mation based on a small geographical unit such as city or postcode, something that has successfully been done by the Small Area Health Statistics Unit (SAHSU) in the United Kingdom. For some countries, such as the Scandinavian countries, this is less of a prob-lem, and individuals can be tracked through life and linked to environmental databases.

4.4 Methodological issues in health effects assessment

4.4.1 Validity and reliability of health outcome measurements

Interpretation of findings from epidemiological studies depends upon the validity and reliability of the measurements undertaken. These issues are discussed in Chapter 2 and the reader should refer to that section for more information. For a health outcome, validity is characterized by sensitivity (i.e., the probability that a sick person will be classified as sick) and specificity (i.e., the probability that a healthy person will be classified as healthy).

To ensure the validity of symptom questionnaires, the diseases that are being assessed must be defined accurately; and the symptoms described should be manifestations of these disease entities. The use of stricter diagnostic criteria can be problematic in that improvements in specificity may reduce sensitivity. If the amounts of disease in different populations are to be compared, it is essential that the levels of sensitivity and specificity do not vary between populations. The International Study of Asthma and Allergies in Childhood (ISAAC) is an example of a large international study that was designed to develop and evaluate standardized methods and criteria to diagnose asthma in children [11, 12]. The goal of this project was to compare the prevalence of asthma among children in different countries, but to do so, the investigators had to ensure that the questionnaires and examinations methods performed consistently across the research centers.

The validity of a measurement recorded by an instrument is determined by the accuracy with which it quantifies the effect that it is intended to measure. The reliability of an instrument can be determined by frequent tests in which everything is the same except the time (test–retest). Some instruments are or can be set up to obtain measurements of duplicate samples and results at the same time (split-half testing). This method is often used in conjunction with questionnaires in which 'identical' questions are repeated in several sections.

4.4.2 Intra-individual variability in effects

Humans display distinct variation in personal physiological functions that can be identified and measured (e.g., personal cholinesterase values will vary from hour to hour or day to day, or even from month to month depending on the degree of exposure to either exogenous or endogenous agents). Lung function shows a diurnal rhythm, and blood pressure can also be highly variable. It is therefore important to pick the right time for measurements or take multiple measurements. Standardization of protocols is very important in order to be able to compare results.

4.4.3 Inter-individual variation

Variation in biological response measured in one individual and compared with another individual is known as interindividual variation. Inter-individual variation must be taken into account when recording biological measurements.

4.4 **References**

[1] Rosenkranz H. Experimental and computational strategies for the rapid identification of environmental carcinogens In: Rom WN, ed. *Environmental and occupational medicine*, 3rd edn. Philadelphia, PA: Lippincott-Raven Publishers 1998:197–207.

[2] Garcia-Closas M, Malats N, Silverman D, Dosemeci M, Kogevinas M, Hein DW, et al. NAT2 slow acetylation, GSTM1 null genotype, and risk of bladder cancer: results from the Spanish Bladder Cancer Study and meta-analyses. **Lancet.** 2005 **366**(9486):649–59.

[3] Eskenazi B, Warner M, Samuels S, Young J, Gerthoux PM, Needham L, et al. Serum dioxin concentrations and risk of uterine leiomyoma in the Seveso Women's Health Study. *American Journal of Epidemiology*. 2007 **166**(1):79–87.

[4] Boyd PA, Armstrong B, Dolk H, Botting B, Pattenden S, Abramsky L, et al. Congenital anomaly surveillance in England–ascertainment deficiencies in the national system. *BMJ (Clinical Research edn)*. 2005 **330**(7481):27.

[5] Nieuwenhuijsen MJ, Toledano MB, Bennett J, Best N, Konstantinou K, Hambly P, et al. The relationship between disinfection byproducts in drinking water and congential anomalies in England and Wales. *Environmental Health Perspectives*. 2008; **116**: 216–22.

[6] Chen CJ, Wang CJ. Ecological correlation between arsenic level in well water and age-adjusted mortality from malignant neoplasms. *Cancer Res*. 1990 **50**(17):5470–4.

[7] Dockery DW, Pope CA, 3rd, Xu X, Spengler JD, Ware JH, Fay ME, et al. An association between air pollution and mortality in six U.S. cities. *The New England Journal of Medicine*. 1993 **329**(24):1753–9.

[8] World Health Organization. *World health statistics annual*. 2001 0250–3794 [cited; Available from: http://www.who.int/whosis/en].

[9] Arif AA, Shah SM. Association between personal exposure to volatile organic compounds and asthma among US adult population. *International Archives of Occupational and Environmental Health*. 2007 **80**(8):711–19.

[10] ATS. Standardization of Spirometry, 1994 Update. American Thoracic Society. *Am J Respir Crit Care Med*. 1995 >152(3):1107–36.

[11] Behrens T, Maziak W, Weiland SK, Rzehak P, Siebert E, Keil U. Symptoms of asthma and the home environment. The ISAAC I and III cross-sectional surveys in Munster, Germany. *International Archives of Allergy and Immunology*. 2005 **37**(1):53–61.

[12] Asher MI, Weiland SK. The International Study of Asthma and Allergies in Childhood (ISAAC). ISAAC Steering Committee. *Clin Exp Allergy*. 1998 **28**(Suppl 5):52–66; discussion 90–1.

Chapter 5

Measurement error

Consequences and design issues

Ben Armstrong

5.1 Introduction

This chapter is concerned with the effects that inaccuracy in data, particularly exposure data (including misclassification of exposure) has on results of epidemiological studies. Readers may be aware that such error impacts adversely on studies, but may not be aware just in what way. Does it add to uncertainty in estimates of measures of effect? If so, is this extra uncertainty reflected in the usual statements of uncertainty, such as confidence intervals? Under what circumstances does it cause bias in a result, and can the direction and extent of bias be known, or even corrected for? Does it compromise the power of the study?

The chapter will summarize, in a manner as accessible to the non-statistician as possible, what is known about the effects of measurement error on the results of a study. The chapter is organized in three sections. The first covers the types and contexts of measurement error and how to describe them formally. The second describes the effects of error according to its type, first qualitatively and then where possible quantitatively; it also includes an introductory discussion of methods of correcting for these effects. Finally, the chapter addresses issues of designing epidemiological studies in the presence of measurement error—what resources to put to exposure measurement, and how large should validity or reliability studies be?

5.1.1 Terms and notation

The term relative risk (RR) is used here in the statistical tradition, generically to include rate ratios, odds ratios, prevalence ratios, etc. The term effect measure is used to denote a summary of the association between exposure and outcome, for example relative risk or regression coefficient. The true exposure is denoted T, the approximate measure X, and the error E, with

$$X = T + E.$$

The standard deviation of T, X, and E are written σ_T, σ_X, and σ_E, respectively.

5.2 **Describing measurement error**

The effects of measurement error depend critically on its context and type. There are three categories of explanatory variables which may be measured with error: a variable of interest (environmental or occupational exposure), a potential confounder (active smoking, socioeconomic status), and a potential effect-modifier (markers of vulnerability to the effects of the variable of interest, for example, age). As described earlier in Chapter 2, the error is called differential if it varies according to the health outcome. The classic example of this is recall bias in case-control studies, in which cases may recall exposure with different error than controls. Non-differential error does not depend on health outcome. This can usually be assumed if the exposure is measured before the outcome is known, or deduced from written records, for example, using work or residential histories. The scale of the variables could be categorical (qualitative), comprising dichotomous ('exposed' vs 'not exposed') and polytomous ('high', 'medium', 'low') categories, or numerical (concentration of particles in air in mg/m^3, number of cigarettes smoked per day). When occurring in categorical variables, measurement error is termed misclassification, i.e., study subjects may be classified incorrectly. Numerical variables can be made into groups, and thus become categorical variables. Conversely, ordered polytomous variables can sometimes be treated as numerical.

Two further distinctions apply to error in numerical variables: systematic—for example, all exposures overestimated by two units or by 20 percent or random—some exposures overestimated, some underestimated (the mean error is zero), and Classical or Berkson. Error often has some systematic and some random component. This chapter concentrates on the random component because effects of systematic error are easier to work out by common sense reasoning. Furthermore, if measurement is known to be subject to systematic error, it can be corrected to remove this. The Classical or Berkson distinction is not well known and a little tricky to understand, but it has major implications for the effects of the error. Classical error occurs where the average of many replicate measurements of the same true exposure would equal the true exposure. Berkson error occurs where the same approximate exposure ('proxy') is used for many subjects; the true exposures vary randomly about this proxy, with mean equal to it.

> Example:
> A study investigates the relationship of average lead exposure up to age 10 with IQ in 10-year-old children living in the vicinity of a lead smelter. IQ is measured by a test administered at age 10. Consider two study designs for assessing exposure:
> **Design 1:** Each child has one measurement made of blood lead, at a random time during his or her life. The blood lead measurement will be an approximate measure of average blood lead over life. However, if the investigators were able to make many replicate measurements (at different random time-points), the average would be a good indicator of lifetime exposure. This measurement error is thus classical.
> **Design 2:** The children's places of residence at age 10 (assumed known exactly) are classified into three groups by proximity to the smelter—CLOSE, MEDIUM, FAR. Random blood leads, collected as described in Design 1, are averaged for each group, and this group average is used as a proxy for lifetime exposure for each child in the group. Here the same approximate exposure ('proxy') is used for all subjects in the same group, and true exposures, though unknown, may be assumed to vary randomly about the proxy. This measurement error is thus Berkson type error.

Often, error has both Classical and Berkson components, although one usually predominates. Exposures estimated from observed determinants using an exposure prediction model have predominantly Berkson error. Indeed, if the determinants are measured without error, the error is entirely of Berkson type.

The two types of error are defined statistically as:

Classical: $X = T + E$, with E independent of T and mean $(E) = 0$;

Berkson: $T = X + E$, with E independent of X and mean $(E) = 0$;

Effects of measurement error usually depend on its magnitude. With random error this will vary from measurement to measurement, so more properly one says that the effect of measurement error depends on its distribution. Error distributions are important conceptually, even if there are no data from which to infer them. However, it makes this section less abstract if data from a validity study are assumed to be available. A validity study is a study in which for a sample of subjects, exposure is measured accurately as well as by the approximate method to be used in the main study. Alternatively, but less usefully, investigators may have data from a reliability study, in which for a sample of subjects exposure is measured two or more times, each time independently. If the same method is used each time, this is called an intra-method reliability study. Otherwise it is an inter-method reliability study. There is more about estimation of magnitude of error from validity and reliability studies later in the chapter, but summaries of error magnitude are introduced here.

The likely extent of misclassification of categorical variables is usually specified as probabilities of misclassification. For dichotomous variables, it is conventional to express these through the sensitivity (the probability of correctly classifying a truly exposed subject as exposed), and the specificity (the probability of correctly classifying a non-exposed subject as non-exposed) of the classification. In the exposure classification illustrated in Table 5.1, sensitivity is 80 percent (0.8) and specificity is 60 percent (0.6); so the probability of misclassifying an exposed subject as nonexposed is $1–0.8 = 0.2$, and the probability of misclassifying a nonexposed subject as exposed is $1–0.6 = 0.4$.

Sensitivity and specificity cannot easily be estimated from a reliability study, although construction of a table of agreement similar to Table 5.1 is often useful. For these studies, there are various ways of summarizing agreement between the measurement, the most

Table 5.1 Describing misclassification of a dichotomous exposure variable

		According to true variable	
		Unexposed n (%)	Exposed n (%)
According to	Unexposed	30 (60)	10 (20)
misclassified	Exposed	20 (40)	40 (80)
variable	Total	50 (100)	50 (100)

popular being the kappa (κ) statistic, which takes the value 1 if there is complete agreement, and 0 if there is no more agreement than can be explained by chance [1]. Although for validity study data sensitivity and specificity is usually a more useful summary than kappa, the calculation of kappa from the data in Table 5.1 is illustrated below. If the four cell counts are labeled clockwise from top left as n_{00}, n_{01}, n_{11}, and n_{10}, the row totals $n_{0.}$ and $n_{1.}$ and the column totals $n_{.0}$ and $n_{.1}$, then

$$\hat{\kappa} = \frac{2(n_0 n_{11} - n_{01} n_{10})}{n_{0.} n_{.1} + n_{1.} n_{.0}} = \frac{2(40 \times 30 - 20 \times 10)}{60 \times 50 + 40 \times 50} = 0.4$$

For categorical variables of more than two levels, many different sorts of misclassification can occur. They can be specified in a matrix of misclassification probabilities, which take the same form as Table 5.1, but with more than two columns and rows. An example is shown in Table 5.2, showing three groups according to proximity of residence to a smelter. Here the only misclassification is from the 'very near' to 'quite near' group. The example will be referred to later. Similar tables of agreement can be assembled from reliability studies, but column percentages can no longer be described as misclassification probabilities, because column classification is not by true level. Summaries (such as a kappa statistic) are possible but often are more complex when there are more than two levels, because some types of disagreement are usually more important than others. For example, misclassification into adjacent categories is usually less important than other misclassification. This can be reflected in summaries if different degrees of misclassification are weighted.

Important aspects of the distribution of random errors (Classical or Berkson) in numerical variables are their standard deviation (σ_E) or variance (σ_E^2). These can be estimated directly from a validity study as the sample standard deviation and sample variance of the observed values of X-T. However, other summaries are often used, sometimes because they are more easily obtained, and sometimes because they are more convenient in deducing consequences of error, or correcting epidemiological results for error (see below). Classical error is generally described by its *coefficient of reliability*, which can be defined as the correlation of independent repeated measurements of exposure (ρ_{XX}), such as might be estimated from a reliability study. In theory (in large samples) this may be shown to be equal to the square of the coefficient of validity, which is the correlation between the true and approximate measurements (ρ_{XT}), such as might be estimated from

Table 5.2 Describing misclassification of a polytomous exposure variable

		According to true variable		
		Very near n (%)	Quite near n (%)	Far n (%)
According to	Very near	80 (80)	0 (0)	0 (0)
misclassified	Quite near	20 (20)	100 (100)	0 (0)
variable	Far	0 (0)	0 (0)	200 (100)
	Total	100	100	200

a validity study. The coefficient of reliability is also theoretically equal to several expressions involving standard deviation of errors (σ_E), true exposures (σ_T), and observed approximate exposures (σ_X) as follows:

$$\rho_{XX} = \rho_{XT}^2$$
$$= \sigma_T^2/\sigma_X^2$$
$$= (\sigma_X^2 - \sigma_E^2)/\sigma_X^2$$
$$= \sigma_T^2/(\sigma_T^2 + \sigma_E^2)$$
$$= 1/(1+\sigma_E^2/\sigma_T^2)$$
$$= 1/[1+(\sigma_E/\sigma_T)^2]$$

These values are only theoretically equal (i.e., in large samples, when the Classical error model is correct). When they are estimated from validity or reliability data, exact values will differ. Choice of which expression to use is discussed further below, after a discussion of which are important in describing consequences of error.

5.3 The consequences of measurement error in exposure

This section begins with and focuses mainly on the effects of non-differential error or misclassification in the exposure of interest, first on effect measures, then on the results of significance tests. Briefer discussion follows on effects of errors on confounder control and the investigation of interaction, and finally on effects of non-differential errors.

5.3.1 Consequences of error in the exposure of interest for effect measures

In general, random measurement error or misclassification leads to bias in effect measures (relative risks, regression coefficients, differences in means). This bias is usually downwards (towards the null), but there are important exceptions. With information on the magnitude of measurement error and exposure variability (or prevalence), the extent of bias can be estimated.

For exposure measured on a dichotomous scale, non-differential error always biases the effect measure toward the null value (there is a technical but unrealistic exception when the sum of sensitivity and specificity of exposure classification is less than 1, implying measurement that tends to reverse exposed and unexposed categories!)

> Example:
> A study of lung cancer in relation to proximity of residence to a coke oven classifies subjects (cases and populations) by distance of residence from the oven at the time of follow-up—NEAR = <4 km from oven; FAR = 4–10 km. The incidence rate is compared in the two groups. Here there is misclassification due to migration—not all persons living NEAR the oven at time of follow-up will have lived there at the etiologically relevant time. Thus if the true relative risk for subjects living in these areas throughout their lives were 1.5, the observed relative risk would tend to be less.

The extent of bias depends upon, and may be calculated from, the sensitivity and specificity of the classification as well as the proportion of truly exposed in the non-diseased. This calculation may be by first principles, calculating number of cases and non-cases expected to move between cells of a two × two table, or by a formula:

$$OR_{Obs} = [pD \times (1 - pN)] / [pN \times (1 - pD)]$$

where

pD = sensitivity × PD + (1 – specificity) × (1 – PD),

pN = sensitivity × PN + (1 – specificity) × (1 – PN)

and 'P' = true proportion exposed, 'p' = observed population exposed
'D' = Diseased, 'N' = Non-diseased.

Suppose misclassification (migration) in the above example was such that 10 percent of the NEAR group was in fact FAR at the time of relevant exposure, and vice-versa (i.e., sensitivity = specificity = 0.9), and that 50 percent of the population overall lived in the NEAR area. The observed relative risk would then be 1.38.

Further examples are given in Table 5.3. Notice that where exposure is less common than not (<50 percent) poor specificity biases the odds ratio much more than poor sensitivity.

There is also an approximate formula using the kappa (κ) statistic for agreement between two independent classifications with the same instrument to link the observed naïve and the true odds ratio [1]:

$$OR_{Obs} \approx (OR_{True}-1) \times \kappa+1$$

For example, if a repeat classification gave
κ: = 0.7, and OR_{True} = 1.5, then $OR_{Obs} \approx (1.5–1) \times 0.7+1 = 1.35$

Table 5.3 The effect of non-differential misclassification on relative risks in two groups

Exposure sensitivity	Exposure specificity	Proportion of exposed in the population	Observed relative risk
1.00	1.00	Any	2.00
0.90	0.90	0.01	1.08
0.90	0.90	0.50	1.72
0.90	0.99	0.01	1.47
0.90	0.99	0.50	1.82
0.99	0.90	0.01	1.09
0.99	0.90	0.50	1.89
0.99	0.99	0.01	1.50
0.99	0.99	0.50	1.97

For exposure measured on a polytomous scale, non-differential error biases downwards estimates of trend across ordered groups, but comparisons between specific categories can be biased in either direction.

Assume that in the above example the NEAR group was split into two: VERY NEAR and QUITE NEAR, with true relative risks, relative to FAR, of 2.0 and 1.3. If there is 20 percent migration from VERY NEAR to QUITE NEAR, but not otherwise (as in Table 5.2), observed risks for VERY NEAR group relative to the FAR group is unchanged on average, but that for the QUITE NEAR group is increased by contamination by the VERY NEAR migrants. The specific value of the misclassified RR was calculated assuming that the NEAR group divided into two equal-sized groups (25 percent of total population each), so the misclassified RR is a weighted mean of 1.3 and 2, with weights $w_1 = 25$ and $w_2 = 0.2*25 = 5$ (the migrants from VERY NEAR). Thus RR = $(1.3*25 + 2*5)/(25 + 5) = 1.42$. The relative risk is increased by misclassification (Table 5.4).

For exposure measured on a numerical scale, classical errors bias regression coefficients (relative risks per unit exposure) towards zero. The association is described as attenuated. In fact, for linear regression the bias factor is equal to the coefficient of reliability (ρXX); with the observed regression coefficient. Thus if

$$Y = \alpha_{TRUE} + \beta_{TRUE} \times T; \text{ then}$$

$$Y = \alpha_{OBSERVED} + \beta_{OBSERVED} \times X, \text{ with } \beta_{OBSERVED} = \rho_{XX} \times \beta_{TRUE}$$

The parameter $\beta_{OBSERVED}$ is sometimes called the 'naive' regression coefficient.

Lead-IQ example – design 1. Suppose that a regression of IQ on true lifetime average blood lead has a regression with coefficient –2 (IQ reduces by 2 points per μg/dl blood lead). With classical measurement error with coefficient of reliability 0.5, this would be attenuated, on average, to $(0.5)(-2) = -1$.

From the alternative expressions for the coefficient of reliability given above ($\rho_{XX}=1/[1+(\sigma_E/\sigma_T)^2]$) bias in β is seen to depend on the average magnitude of measurement error relative to the average magnitude of the true exposure (σ_E/σ_X). This implies that measurement error will have less effect if the true exposures are more spread out (σ_X is greater). Table 5.5 gives attenuation bias as a function of the ratio of the standard deviation of errors to that of true exposures (σ_E/σ_X). This is quite reassuring—error has to be relatively big to give serious bias.

For logistic and log-linear (Poisson) regression coefficients, the same qualitative result is true, and the quantitative one approximately so, with the approximation good except

Table 5.4 The effect on non-differential misclassification on relative risks in three exposure groups – example

	Relative risk		
	VERY NEAR	QUITE NEAR	FAR
True	2.0	1.3	1.0
Misclassified	2.0	1.42	1.0

Table 5.5 The attenuation bias due to exposure measurement error in linear regression

Error σ_E/σ_X	0.0	0.1	0.2	0.3	0.4	0.5	0.75	1.0	1.5	2.0
Attenuation*	1.0	0.99	0.96	0.92	0.86	0.80	0.64	0.50	0.31	0.20

*Attenuation is the factor by which the naive regression slope will underestimate the true slope.

for large error and large relative risks. For logistic and log-linear regression, relative risk is linked to the regression coefficient by the formula RR=exp(β), thus

$$RR_{OBSERVED} = (RR_{TRUE}) \cdot \rho^{xx}$$

If, in the children exposed to blood lead, investigators were to use as an outcome a child having IQ below 80, and if the relative risk (odds ratio) increment per 10 µg/dl true blood lead (from logistic regression) was 1.5, then the observed RR is given by:

$$RR_{OBSERVED} = 1.5^{0.5} = 1.22$$

Berkson errors, however, lead to no bias in linear regression coefficients, and little or no bias in logistic or log-linear regression coefficients. The distinction between classical and Berkson error is thus important.

Lead-IQ example—design 2. In this grouped design the error is of Berkson type, so there is no bias in the regression coefficient. However, precision would be lost (width of confidence interval would be wider), and power would not be as great as without measurement error, or as in the biased design 1.

5.3.2 Consequences for significance tests and power

All types of non-differential random measurement error or misclassification reduce study power—the chance that a study will find a statistically significant association if one is truly present. This is true for Berkson as well as Classical error, and for misclassification. The extent of power loss can be quantified if magnitude of measurement error and exposure variability (or for a dichotomous measure prevalence) are known.

A cohort study is designed to have 80 percent power to detect a relative risk of 2.0 between truly exposed and truly unexposed persons (80 percent of similar-sized studies would find the association), by inclusion of sufficient subjects (equal numbers exposed and unexposed) to expect 20 cases in each group under the null hypothesis [2]. If approximate measurements were used, the power would be less. If the measure of exposure has sensitivity = specificity = 0.9 and 10 percent of the population are exposed, then a true relative risk of 2.0 would be attenuated, on average, to 1.48. Power to detect this reduced RR is only 30 percent [2]. To restore 80 percent power would require a study about four times bigger.

According to Lagakos [3], for numerical exposure variables (and approximately for dichotomous exposures if coded 0 and 1), power loss is based on the result that the effective loss in sample size is equal to the coefficient of reliability of the measure.

A study with exposure measured with a coefficient of reliability of 0.5 will have similar power to one with accurate exposure assessment and half the number of subjects.

Despite the bias and power loss noted above, the p-values obtained by using the usual methods on data subject to random error or misclassification are valid. Spurious 'significant' results (where there is in fact no association) are no more likely with than without measurement error.

> A study finds an association between dust and loss of lung function, with $p = 0.02$, but dust measurements were known to be subject to error. Providing that the error is non-differential, the low p-value cannot be attributed to the measurement error.

5.3.3 Confounders

The general rule is that errors in confounders compromise our ability to control for their effect, leaving 'residual' confounding. The effect measure adjusted using the approximate confounder will on average lie between the crude, unadjusted effect measure and the effect measure adjusted using the true (unknown) confounder. The validity of significance tests on the effect of exposure is compromised.

> A study of the relationship of lung cancer to air pollution adjusts for smoking using a crude estimate of pack-years for each subject. Any confounding of the relative risk for lung cancer vs air pollution will be only partially controlled. For example, if $RR_{(crude)} = 1.50$ (95% CI 1.20, 1.88; $p<0.001$), and RR $_{(adjusted\ for\ true\ pack-years)} = 1.04$ (95% CI 0.86, 1.24; $p = 0.67$), then the partially adjusted RR $_{(adjusted\ for\ approximate\ pack-years)}$ will in general lie between 1.50 and 1.04, and the partially adjusted p-value will lie between 0.001 and 0.67.

The degree of residual confounding depends on the coefficient of reliability of the measure of the confounder. A coefficient of reliability of 0.5 will imply that about half the confounding present will be controlled, in the sense that the observed log (RR) (more generally the regression coefficient) will on average lie about halfway between the crude unadjusted log (RR) and the fully adjusted log (RR).

> Continuing the same example, if the coefficient of reliability of measured pack-years is 0.5, then log (RR $_{(adjusted\ for\ approximate\ pack-years)}$) will lie about half way between log (RR$_{(crude)}$) and log (RR $_{(adjusted\ for\ true\ pack-years)}$), which gives RR $_{(adjusted\ for\ approximate\ pack-years)} = 1.25$(95% CI 1.03, 1.52; $p = 0.03$).

There are a few exceptions. Entirely systematic error (everyone underreporting their smoking by 20 percent) will not usually compromise control of confounding. In special situations (when the effects of the confounder and the exposure of interest are strictly additive) Berkson error (for example, use of group mean rather than individual pack-years of smoking) also leaves no residual confounding. Most importantly, if the variable suspected of confounding is in fact not associated with the exposure of interest (smoking is not associated with air pollution) then there is no confounding or residual confounding, however strongly the variable is associated with the outcome (however bad the smoking data, the observed association of lung cancer with air pollution is not biased). Correlation between errors in measuring confounders with errors in measuring the exposure of interest or with exposure itself further complicates the situation, although the same broad conclusion – that error compromises control of confounding, remains.

Having to control for confounders, whether measured with error or not, increases somewhat the effect of error in the variable of interest on the relative risk of interest. The formulae above for the simple situation without confounders can be extended to cover this situation by replacing each of the coefficients with their value conditional on the presence of the confounder [4, 5]. For example, the reliability coefficient of an exposure measure conditional on age is the partial correlation between independent repeat measures after control for age, which is typically lower.

5.3.4 **Effect modifiers**

An effect modifier is a variable that modifies the effect of the exposure of interest (for example identifying subgroups vulnerable or resistant to the exposure). In statistical terms, this is described as an interaction between the effect modifier and the exposure. Error in measuring effect-modifiers tends to diminish apparent effect modification. Vulnerable subgroups are thus made harder to identify.

> Lead-IQ example. Suppose diet modified the effect of lead on IQ, children with vitamin-deficient diets having a regression slope of –3, and others a slope of –1. If diet is measured with error (misclassified), the apparent modification will tend to be less, for example the slope in vitamin-deficient children might be –2.5, and that in others –1.5.

Even if the putative effect-modifier is measured without error, error in the variable of interest can distort effect-modification, and even create spurious modification. This may happen because the magnitude of error, and hence bias due to it, depends on the putative modifier. Even if this is not the case, the variation of exposure may depend on the putative modifier, in which case the bias due to measurement error will again depend on the putative modifier.

Suppose now that the interest is in modification of the effect of lead on IQ by sex, which is measured without error, but lead is again measured with (Classical) error. Suppose also that although the average error was the same for boys and girls, boys had more varied lead exposures than girls (σ_T is higher in boys than girls). In this case, if the true regression slope of IQ on lead is –2 for both boys and girls, the estimated slope will tend to be more attenuated for girls (say to –0.5) than for boys (say to –1.5). (For girls the standard deviation σ_T is lower, and hence the attenuation bias σ_E^2/σ_T^2 is greater.) Thus sex appears to modify the effect of lead on IQ, but does not in fact do so.

5.3.5 **Differential error**

Differential error can cause bias in the effect measure either upwards or downwards, depending on whether adverse outcomes are associated with over or underestimation of exposure. Significance tests are not valid in the presence of differential error. For dichotomous exposure, the bias can be quantified if the sensitivity and specificity of the approximate classification are known.

> The association of exposure to video display units (VDU) use with spontaneous abortion is investigated by means of a case-control study in which women are interviewed after a live birth or abortion, and asked about the number of hours per week that they spent using a VDU. The relative risk of spontaneous abortion in women using VDUs for 15 or more hours per week was 1.20 (95% CI 1.06–1.34). Due to media attention to the hypothesized association, women who had experienced spontaneous abortions may have been more likely to recall their VDU use fully. In this case, some or all of the excess of VDU users in the cases relative to the controls would be spurious, so that the true relative risk would be more than 1.20.

5.3.6 **Correcting for measurement error**

If there is information on the magnitude and type of error, it is possible (but not always easy) to allow for it in estimating the effect measure, at least for reasonably simple forms of measurement error. Sometimes, it is sufficient to invert the formulae shown above for deriving the effects of measurement error. For example with dichotomous exposure subject to non-differential misclassification:

$$OR_{True} \approx (OR_{Obs}-1)/\kappa+1$$

More exact '*matrix inversion*' methods are also available; details are discussed by Kuha [6]. Similarly for numerical exposures and outcomes:

$$\beta_{TRUE} = \beta_{OBSERVED}/\rho_{xx}, RR_{TRUE} = (RR_{OBSERVED})^{(1/\rho_{xx})}$$

In the Lead-IQ study, if investigators had observed a regression coefficient ($\beta_{OBSERVED}$) of -1 and known that the coefficient of reliability of measurement (ρ_{xx}) was 0.5, then they could estimate

$$\beta_{TRUE} = -1/0.5 = -2$$

Similarly, if investigators observed an increment in relative risk of low IQ per 10 µg/dl observed blood lead: $RR_{OBSERVED} = 1.22$, then approximately

$$RR_{TRUE} = 1.22^{(1/0.5)} = 1.5$$

Corrections will not, in general, affect the *p*-value of a test of the null hypothesis of no association, nor will the power of the test be improved. However, confidence intervals will normally get wider.

In the Lead-IQ study mentioned above, suppose the regression coefficient of -1 had a 95% CI $(-1.8, -0.2)$, with $p = 0.01$. Assuming a coefficient of reliability of 0.5, the corrected coefficient is -2, the 95% CI $(-3.6, -0.4)$, and $p = 0.01$, as before. If there were uncertainty in the coefficient of reliability, then a more sophisticated approach that reflected this would give a wider confidence interval, but its lower limit would remain below zero, consistent with the *p*-value, for which a correction is not required.

Other methods are available which refine and generalize this approach. The aim of these more sophisticated methods is usually to use other sorts of information on measurement error, to more exactly eradicate bias, or to reflect in the estimate and confidence intervals uncertainty as to the magnitude of the error. A review is given by Carroll [5].

Probably the most popular group of methods is called '*regression calibration.*' In general, these seek to correct an observed effect measure by applying to it a calibration factor, typically obtained from a validity or reliability study. For example, from validity study data one can estimate the calibration factor λ as the regression coefficient of true accurate exposure (Y variable) on approximate exposure (X variable)—this estimates the average change in the accurate exposure corresponding to unit change in the approximate variable. Observed regression coefficients from the main study are divided by λ to obtain an unbiased estimate of the true coefficient: $\beta_{TRUE} = \beta_{OBSERVED}/\lambda$. Using the formulae given above with ρ_{XX} or ρ_{XY} estimated from reliability of validity studies are also examples of regression calibration.

Zeger *et al.* [7] applied the regression calibration method when correcting estimates of increased mortality per $\mu g/m^3$ PM_{10} from a time series mortality study in Riverside, California, which used a central site monitor to estimate exposure. The study found mortality to increase by 0.84% per 10 $\mu g/m^3$ PM_{10} (95% CI 0.06, 1.76). A validity study had been carried out in which 49 people from Riverside had worn personal monitors for a total of 178 sampling days. Regressing ambient measure (Y variable) on personal exposure (X variable) gave a regression calibration slope of 0.60 (se 0.08). (Thus each 1 $\mu g/m^3$ change in PM_{10} in personal exposures was on average reflected in a 0.6 $\mu g/m^3$ change in ambient levels.) This allowed the observed regression slope of 0.84 to be corrected by dividing by 0.60: True regression slope = 0.84/0.60 = 1.40. Confidence limits were obtained by applying the same correction to the naïve limits, thus (−0.11, 2.95). These confidence limits are slightly too narrow, because they do not reflect uncertainty in the calibration factor. As Zeger discusses, the measurement error in this situation is a mixture of Berkson and Classical type. Regression calibration making direct use of the calibration slope provided a way of quantifying the correcting for bias without having to assume either all-Berkson or all-Classical error.

The '*method of moments*' estimator is an alternative correction procedure. For this, one estimates just the variance of the error distribution $-(\sigma_E^2)$ from a reliability study (half the variance of differences in measurements) or validity study. This estimate can be transported to the main study with fewer assumptions than needed for λ, ρ_{XX}, or ρ_{XY} (see below). The variance of observed exposures (σ_X^2) is then estimated from the main study and correct the naïve regression slope using the expression $\rho_{XX} = (\sigma_X^2 - \sigma_E^2)/\sigma_X^2$.

For an example showing two methods of correction for measurement error applied to occupational epidemiology, see Spiegelmann and Valanis [8].

An intriguing method that can be used only for hierarchical studies which combine regression coefficients across many centers has been proposed and applied to multi-city time series studies of air pollution and mortality [9]. This exploits the within-city associations of the pollutant of interest with other pollutants, which are used as 'instruments' from which to extract an overall coefficient that is bias-free under some assumptions, though there is a precision cost.

5.3.7 Limitations of corrections for measurement error

To obtain information on measurement error, the magnitude is needed. This requires reliability studies (a sample of repeated independent measurements) or validity studies (a sample of gold standard measurements in parallel with the approximate measurements). These are not often available, and even if they are, much uncertainty remains unless they are large. If corrections are carried out on the basis of incorrect information on error magnitude, bias may be increased, rather than decreased. 'Corrections' for attenuation can also magnify confounding or other information bias, rather than a true association. Researchers should give the naïve effect measure (using the approximate exposure in a regular analysis), even if including effect measures corrected for measurement error. Also worth considering is calculating corrections under a variety of assumptions, in the spirit of a sensitivity analysis.

5.4 **Design issues**

5.4.1 **What resources should be put into estimating exposure?**

Random exposure measurement error reduces power of a study and, except Berkson error, biases affect measures. To avoid these problems it is desirable to design studies with minimum measurement error. However, making exposure measurement more accurate may be costly and must be considered against alternative uses for the resources. Thus the practical question is usually 'What proportion of resources should be put into exposure measurement in order to improve accuracy?'

Where a study aims to add to evidence as to whether an exposure causes an outcome, study power is the main consideration. For these studies, Lagakos' result [3], cited above, can be used to address this question by justifying the principle:

> To maximize study power, resources should be spent on improving accuracy until the proportional increase in the square of the validity coefficient (ρ_{XT}^2) is less than the proportional increase in total study cost per subject that is required to achieve it.

For example, if it is possible to increase ρ_{XT}^2 from 0.6 to 0.9 (i.e., by a factor of 1.5) by spending 30 percent more per subject, it is worth doing. If it cost 100 percent more, it is not—the money would be better spent recruiting more subjects. As usual in such design decisions, input information (ρ_{XT}^2 or equivalent) may have to be obtained from pilot studies if it is not available from prior studies or the literature. More details and examples are given by Armstrong [10].

5.4.2 **Deciding on the number of repeat exposure measurements**

A special case of this problem occurs where increase in precision is possible by making independent repeat measurements of exposure for each study subject, and the question is 'How many replicates?' With costs of each exposure measurement C_Z, other marginal study costs per subject (e.g., outcome measurement) C_I, and the reliability of the measurement ρ_{XX}, the principle cited above yields the optimal number of n replicates:

$$n = \frac{C_I(1-\rho_{XX})}{C_Z\rho_{XX})}$$

For example, if ρ_{XX} is 0.6, C_Z is $20, and C_I is $100, then $n = 100(1–0.6)/(20 \times 0.6) = 40/12 = 3.3$; i.e., about three repeat exposure measurements per subject. The square of the validity coefficient, or another of the equivalent expressions noted above can be substituted for reliability coefficient in this expression.

5.4.3 **Limitations to designing for maximum power**

Where a study aims not only to add evidence as to whether an exposure causes an outcome, but also to quantify how much risk is consequent to a measured level of exposure (the absolute dose–response relationship), then the bias in effect measure assumes an added importance, and power is an inadequate criterion for choice of resources to go into exposure measurement. Increasing the sample size does not reduce measurement error bias—although it does increase power. Formal approaches to this problem require more assumptions. Less formal trade-offs between bias and power, perhaps informed by the power criterion, are likely to be necessary. The sections below address this situation.

5.4.4 Designing for Berkson rather than Classical error

If bias in effect measure is the major consideration (rather than study power), there is sometimes scope to design exposure measurement to utilise the fact that Berkson error causes little bias. There are two main ways to do this:

- **By using mean exposure over groups of subjects.** The Lead-IQ study can provide an example. Using each child's blood lead measurement gives rise to classical error, biasing the regression coefficient, but if investigators group children according to proximity to smelter, this error is changed to mainly Berkson type, not biasing the coefficient. ('Mainly' rather than 'entirely' Berkson, because any error in the mean as an estimate of true group mean remains classical, but this will be small unless the number of measurements per group is small.) Using the group mean thus eliminates or greatly reduces bias. Remaining bias can be reduced by making groups larger. However, this procedure does not improve power. In fact, using group means in this way usually reduces power. Thus, there is a choice between retaining power and reducing bias.

- **By using a prediction model.** This is a generalization of the grouping method. Individual measures are used to estimate coefficients of a model for predicting exposure given some easily measured predictor variables. Then, predicted values from the prediction model are used in place of the individual measures when investigating the association of exposure with outcome. The resulting error is again of mainly Berkson type. Some Classical error will remain if the sample on which the prediction model is based is small, as when using group means, and also if the predictor variables are measured with error. Again, bias will be reduced, but usually at the cost of lost power.

In fact, both grouping and prediction models are more usually used when not all subjects in the study have individual exposure measures, so their use is forced rather than a choice. Nevertheless it may be useful when deciding between strategies to be aware that the resulting primarily Berkson type error will bias effect measures little if at all, but will reduce power. The use of grouping methods for this purpose is discussed further by Tielemans [11].

5.4.5 Validity, reliability, and two-stage studies

As an alternative to or in addition to improving exposure assessment for every study subject, investigators can use a less costly approximate method for the main study, and supplement this by a smaller validity study (a sample of gold standard measurements in parallel with the approximate measurements) or reliability sub-study (a sample of repeated independent measurements). In this section we discuss analysis of such sub-studies, and how parameters estimated from the sub-study can be used to inform interpretation of the main study, and sometimes to correct the effect measure in the main study for measurement error. It is usually best if the validity or reliability study samples can be drawn from among the main study subjects. This is partly to improve portability of error parameters (see Section 5.4.7 on portability), and partly so that the additional information on exposure in the sub-sample can be used to improve the power of the main study (see Section 5.4.9 on two-stage studies).

5.4.6 Analysis of validity and reliability studies

Data from a validity or reliability sub-study should be analyzed first to describe agreement rather generally, rather than immediately focusing on estimation of parameters required for correction of attenuation of exposure–response relationships under specific assumptions. A few key features of standard analysis of agreement between two numerical measurements are given here. More complete treatment is available in Shoukri [12] and in Bland [13].

- The mean (and CI) of differences between numerical measurements displays the extent to which one instrument measures consistently higher than another.

- The standard deviation of the differences in measurements displays the extent of variation in agreement (random error). The mean and standard deviation can be brought together to define 'limits to agreement', for example, mean ± 1.96SD estimates the limits within which the difference will lie 95 percent of the time. In a validity study, the standard deviation of differences estimates the standard deviation of measurement error σ_E. In an intra-method reliability study, the standard deviation estimates $(\sqrt{2})\,\sigma_E$. (The variance of differences estimates twice the variance of errors.)

- Various plots can be used to explore whether agreement depends on other factors. For example, plotting differences against the mean or sum of the two measurements identifies whether agreement varies according to the magnitude of exposure, and will suggest departure from additivity if present.

- With data from a validity study, Classical and Berkson error can be distinguished by examining whether differences are correlated with true or approximate measurements, for example by plotting.

The analyses described above allow evaluation of some assumptions of measurement error models and correction techniques (additivity, Berkson or Classical distinction). Also, most investigators will wish to be aware of features of error, for example additive bias, even if it does not affect study power or bias effect measures. Once one has a general description of agreement, it is reasonable to focus on the parameters that determine the extent of attenuation due to measurement error, and hence are needed to correct it. The standard deviation (σ_E) or variance of errors (σ_E^2) may be the most useful parameters for this purpose (see the discussion on portability in Section 5.4.7). However, the parameters most directly related to the attenuation are the validity and reliability coefficients.

If there are two repeats of each measurement the validity or reliability coefficient can be estimated directly as the Pearson correlation coefficient from the paired measurements. However, it is more efficient to estimate them as 'intra-class' correlation coefficients (ICC) or equivalently from variance components, as described below. When there are several repeat measurements, the ICC/variance component method is the only one.

The ICC can be expressed as a function of the ratio of variances within (σ_W^2) to between (σ_B^2) pairs (or triplets, etc.): ICC = $1/[1+ (\sigma_W^2/\sigma_B^2)]$ [1, 12], if these variances are estimated from the measurements in the substudy as variance components. Variance components and ICC are obtainable from most statistical software. Interpretation of the ICC will depend on context. With data from a reliability study, the ICC estimates the reliability coefficient ρ_{xx}, which in simple models is the attenuation factor and loss in effective sample size and hence power. With data from a validity study, the ICC estimates the validity coefficient, which estimates the square root of the reliability coefficient. If the mean for a subject is the true exposure, and repeated measurements are taken on a sample of subjects, the variance components become those between and within subjects. If the main study relating exposure to outcome uses just one exposure measure per subject, the above formula for ICC again estimates reliability coefficient and attenuation. If means of exposures from m repeats are used in the main study, the attenuation reduces to $1/[1+(\sigma_W^2/\sigma_B^2)/m]$ [14].

It is not in general possible to use measures of agreement from inter-method reliability studies to estimate the bias that use of either method might produce in an epidemiological study. The problem is in apportioning the lack of agreement between the two methods. However, the regression calibration method can be used if the errors of the two measures are independent [15].

5.4.7 Portability of coefficients from sub-studies to main studies

Using results from a validity or reliability sub-study to inform a main study requires 'transporting' estimates of agreement, for example a validity coefficient, from one to the other. This should be done cautiously, with a view to possible factors that might make the underlying values of the coefficients different in the two contexts. For example, a reliability coefficient depends not only on the variance of the error distribution, but also on the variance of true exposures. Thus, even if the measurement instrument used in the main and reliability studies are identical, the reliability coefficient is not portable if the distribution of true exposures differ. The same applies to calibration regression coefficients and to kappa statistics.

This problem can be minimized by choosing the reliability or validity sample randomly from the main study subjects. Alternatively, more portable coefficients can be used. For example, the method of moments correction requires only the variance of the error from a validity or reliability study, which is usually more portable than the reliability coefficient.

5.4.8 Sample size of validity and reliability studies

Given that the motivation for conducting validity and reliability studies usually goes beyond their use for correcting exposure–response relationships, it is useful to consider simple general-purpose aids to deciding their sample size. Perhaps most important is the following frequently misunderstood point: sample size determinations for identifying the presence of an association (e.g., by a chi-squared test or test of a correlation being zero) are of no interest when determining sizes of validity or reliability studies. Such tests merely assess evidence for the two measurements being associated at all. This would not advance us much—even very poor measurements are associated somewhat with the true exposure. The requirement is to quantify the strength and features of the association. Depending on the context, the parameter or parameters of interest may be any of those mentioned above, for example, sensitivity and specificity (proportions), validity of reliability coefficients (correlation coefficients), a regression coefficient, a mean difference, or a kappa coefficient. Usually, the most straightforward and generally adequate approach is to show how the precision of an estimate to be made from the proposed study depends on the sample size and to choose a sample size that reflects the trade-off between the advantages of a precise estimate and the cost of obtaining it.

For example, a validity coefficient of 0.5 estimated from a validity study would have confidence intervals depending on sample size as displayed in Table 5.6. The method of estimating confidence intervals is given in most intermediate-level statistical methods textbooks, and they may be obtained from many statistical software. The results are quite sobering, suggesting that with less than say 100 pairs of measurements the validity coefficient would be rather imprecisely estimated. Of course, investigators do not know that the correlation coefficient will be 0.5, but the pattern of widths of confidence intervals does not usually depend very strongly on such guessed values. To check, the calculations can always be repeated using a range of values for them.

5.4.9 **Two-stage studies**

Epidemiological studies with more accurate exposure assessment on a sub-sample are sometimes called 'two-stage' studies. Careful choice of which subjects to include in the sub-sample can improve precision and power, although analysis to achieve this becomes more complicated [16]. The optimal design of two-stage and other studies with validation sub-studies has been discussed by Greenland [17], who concludes that unless the cost of the better measurement is many times that of the approximate one, a 'fully validated' study using the better measure or replicate measures on all subjects is frequently the optimal one. Where differential error is a concern, validation studies must be particularly large.

Table 5.6 Effect of reliability study sample size on estimate of reliability coefficient

Sample size (pairs)	10	25	50	100	250	500
Confidence interval	−0.19, 0.86	0.13, 0.75	0.26, 0.69	0.34, 0.63	0.40, 0.59	0.43, 0.56

5.5 **Error in outcomes**

Along with many authors on the subject of measurement error, we have concentrated on error in measuring exposure. This is partly because in much environmental epidemiology exposure measurement has less certainty than outcome measurement, but there is also a statistical reason: random error in measuring a numerical outcome does not cause bias in regression coefficients, although will decrease precision and power. This useful result does not help us, however, when the outcome is dichotomous, as often occurs in epidemiology. Here, there is though another simplification, because the effect of misclassification in outcome is essentially identical to that in a dichotomous exposure variable. In this context 'non-differential' misclassification in outcome means that which does not depend on exposure level. The result we saw for misclassification of exposure then translates to:

◆ Non-differential outcome misclassification biases effect measures toward the null.

◆ Differential outcome misclassification biases effect measures, with no general rule as to direction.

Essentially the same approaches can be used to quantify bias due to outcome misclassification as can be used for dichotomous exposure misclassification. The bias can also be corrected with similar methods if information on misclassification probabilities is available [6]. Simultaneous misclassification in outcome and exposure can be handled by these methods.

5.6 **Issues not covered in this chapter**

For simplicity of presentation some assumptions and points of interpretation have been passed over. The most important of these are:

◆ *Bias*. Many of the results above concern bias in an effect estimate. Bias is an average effect if the study were to be repeated many times. In a large study, the effect of measurement error will be close to this average 'bias'. However, in a single small sample, the effect may differ appreciably from this average [18]. In these cases, random error can sometimes even lead to an effect measure estimated from approximate exposures that is more extreme than that with the true exposure. It remains more likely, however, that if true exposure has an effect, it is stronger than the estimate using the approximate measurement [19].

◆ *Prediction*. It has been assumed in this chapter that it is the relationship between the true exposure and health outcome that is of interest. Sometimes this is not the case. If you wish to use the study to predict risks in subjects using the same approximate measure of exposure and drawn from the same population, then the naïve effect estimate, (e.g., β_{Obs}), is appropriate.

◆ *Multiplicative error* (proportional to the true exposure), with lognormal distribution of true exposures, is common in environmental epidemiology. Here, measurement error changes the shape of the regression—for example, from a quadratic curve to a straight line [20, 21].

- *Ecological studies* (which have groups as the unit of analysis) have some unexpected error effects. Where the exposure is the proportion of individuals in the area with an attribute (e.g., proportion of smokers) and the individual measure is subject to misclassification, then the slope of the regression of outcome against the proportion with the attribute will be greater than the true individual effect of the attribute on the outcome, i.e., bias away from the null [22]. Where the group exposure measure is a good approximation to the mean true exposure across individuals in the group, then error is of Berkson type, as discussed above, and little or no bias results from it.

- *Causality*. The impact of random non-differential exposure measurement error on inference about the size of an effect is fairly clear once a causal relationship is assumed—the true effect of exposure is most likely to be greater than that estimated. The impact of measurement error on the evidence that such a study brings on whether a causal relationship exists is more problematic. The following points should be considered:

  (i) One should usually be more cautious, if there is measurement error, in concluding from a 'negative' study that no causal association exists. The reduced power implies that missing a true underlying association is made more likely.

  (ii) One should not use the uncorrected confidence interval for relative risk (or other measure of effect) to indicate the highest risk that is compatible with the data. For example, an uncorrected confidence interval for a relative risk of (0.80, 1.25) suggests that relative risks in excess of 1.25 can be excluded. With exposure measurement error, however, the true uncertainty is greater, so that a higher relative risk is possible.

  (iii) Random non-differential measurement error should not lead us to discount an observed association of exposure with disease—observing a positive association is no more likely with measurement error. On the other hand, one cannot assume that a small non-significant or even significant estimated effect of exposure would be larger and more significant in the absence of exposure measurement error. Such small associations could be due to chance or to uncontrolled bias or confounding, in which case they would be no larger, on average, in the absence of measurement error.

5.7 **References**

[1] Armstrong BK, White E, Saracci R. *Principles of exposure measurement in epidemiology*. Oxford and New York: Oxford University Press 1992.

[2] Breslow N, Day N. *Statistical methods in cancer research – the design and analysis of cohort studies*. Lyon, France. International Agency for Research on Cancer 1987.

[3] Lagakos SW. Effects of mismodeling and mismeasuring explanatory variables on tests of their association with a response variable. *Statistics in Medicine*. 1988 7(1–2):257–74.

[4] Armstrong B. The effects of measurement errors on relative risk regressions. *Am J Epidemiol*. 1990 132(6):1176–84.

[5] Carroll R. Measurement error in epidemiologic studies. In: Gail MH, Benichou J, eds. *Encyclopedia of epidemiologic methods*. Chichester and New York: Wiley 2000: xxi, 978.

[6] Kuha J, Skinner C, Palmgren J. Misclassification error. In: Gail MH, Benichou J, eds. *Encyclopedia of epidemiologic methods*. Chichester and New York: Wiley 2000: 530–57.

[7] Zeger SL, Thomas D, Dominici F, Samet JM, Schwartz J, Dockery D, *et al.* Exposure measurement error in time-series studies of air pollution: concepts and consequences. *Environmental Health Perspectives*. 2000 **108**(5):419–26.

[8] Spiegelman D, Valanis B. Correcting for bias in relative risk estimates due to exposure measurement error: a case study of occupational exposure to antineoplastics in pharmacists. *Am J Public Health*. 1998 **88**(3):406–12.

[9] Schwartz J, Coull BA. Control for confounding in the presence of measurement error in hierarchical models. *Biostatistics (Oxford, England)*. 2003 **4**(4):539–53.

[10] Armstrong BG. Optimizing power in allocating resources to exposure assessment in an epidemiologic study. *Am J Epidemiol*. 1996 **144**(2):192–7.

[11] Tielemans E, Kupper LL, Kromhout H, Heederik D, Houba R. Individual-based and group-based occupational exposure assessment: some equations to evaluate different strategies. >**Ann Occup Hyg**. 1998 **42**(2):115–9.

[12] Shoukri M. Agreement, measurement of. In: Gail MH, Benichou J, eds. *Encyclopedia of epidemiologic methods*. Chichester and New York: Wiley 2000: 35–48.

[13] Bland J, Altman D. Statistical methods for assessing agreement between two methods of clinical measurement. *Lancet*. 1986 **1**(8476):307–10.

[14] Liu K, Stamler J, Dyer A, McKeever J, McKeever P. Statistical methods to assess and minimize the role of intra-individual variability in obscuring the relationship between dietary lipids and serum cholesterol. *J Chronic Dis*. 1978 **31**(6–7):399–418.

[15] Wacholder S, Armstrong B, Hartge P. Validation studies using an alloyed gold standard. *Am J Epidemiol*. 1993 **137**(11):1251–8.

[16] Zhao LP, Lipsitz S. Designs and analysis of two-stage studies. *Stat Med*. 1992 >**11**(6):769–82.

[17] Greenland S. Statistical uncertainty due to misclassification: implications for validation substudies. *J Clin Epidemiol*. 1988 **41**(12):1167–74.

[18] Sorahan T, Gilthorpe MS. Non-differential misclassification of exposure always leads to an underestimate of risk: an incorrect conclusion. *Occupational and Environmental Medicine*. 1994 **51**(12):839–40.

[19] Wacholder S, Hartge P, Lubin JH, Dosemeci M. Non-differential misclassification and bias towards the null: a clarification. *Occupational and Environmental Medicine*. 1995 **52**(8):557–8.

[20] Doll R, Peto R. Cigarette smoking and bronchial carcinoma: dose and time relationships among regular smokers and lifelong non-smokers. *J Epidemiol Community Health*. 1978 **32**(4):303–13.

[21] Lyles RH, Kupper LL. A detailed evaluation of adjustment methods for multiplicative measurement error in linear regression with applications in occupational epidemiology. *Biometrics*. 1997 **53**(3):1008–25.

[22] Greenland S. Divergent biases in ecologic and individual-level studies. *Stat Med*. 1992 **11**(9):1209–23.

Chapter 6

Study design and methods

Dean Baker

6.1 **Introduction**

Chapter 2 reviewed the principles of epidemiology and defined classical study designs that are used in virtually all fields of epidemiology. This chapter will describe the role of these study designs in environmental epidemiology, provide examples of how these study designs have been used to investigate environmental health issues, and summarize the methods, strengths and limitations of these study designs in environmental epidemiology. Some study designs have played particularly prominent roles in environmental epidemiology, although they are not used as widely in other areas of epidemiology. Examples include the use of time-series studies and panel studies in air pollution research or the use of cluster studies to evaluate spatial patterns of environmentally related diseases. Chapter 8 will discuss the use and analysis of these special study designs.

In the real world of epidemiological research, the structure of epidemiological studies is more complicated than is presented in introductory epidemiological textbooks. For example, the classical taxonomy of epidemiological study designs makes a clear distinction between ecological studies, for which populations are the unit of analysis, and other analytical studies, for which individuals are the unit of analysis. However, in environmental epidemiological studies, a common scenario is that measures of exposure may be available at a group or community level, while measures of outcomes and perhaps confounders may be available at the individual level. Studies based on these types of data have been called '*semi-individual*' study designs because they share features of ecological and individual study designs [1]. It is also possible that some measures of exposure are available at the individual level, while other measures of exposure in the same study are only available at a group level. These '*multilevel*' studies require hierarchical analytical methods to account for the shared exposure experiences of individuals within the study population. There are many possible combinations of individual and ecological variables in conducting epidemiological studies, so there may not be clear distinction between the study designs as is presented in classical textbooks. Nevertheless, it is worthwhile to understand the strengths and limitations of the classical study designs because these issues still apply generally to the modified designs. This chapter will focus on the use of classical study designs, while commenting on variations to these designs that are relevant for environmental epidemiology.

6.2 **Types of study**

Table 6.1 shows the basic study designs used for epidemiological studies [2]. All of these study designs have been used in environmental epidemiology.

6.2.1 **Descriptive studies**

Descriptive studies examine the distribution of disease or possible environmental determinants of disease in defined populations. They are often the first step in broader environmental health investigations because they may identify hypotheses to be evaluated in analytical studies. Descriptive studies do not formally evaluate the association between exposure and health outcome, although they can be helpful in assessing the possibility that an association exists. Furthermore, if a causal association is well-established, descriptive studies can be useful for establishing the presence or absence of an environmental health problem in a local population and quantifying its impact.

Most descriptive studies are based on existing mortality or morbidity statistics, such as hospital discharge data, and examine patterns of health outcome by age, gender or ethnicity, for specified time periods or geographical areas. For example, the cancer mortality map in Figure 6.1 depicts the mortality rate for melanoma of the skin among white males in the United States (US) [3]. The darker colors indicate the population areas with the highest mortality rates. Although the data shown in the cancer map do not test a specific hypothesis, one can recognize that the gradient of melanoma mortality correlates spatially with latitude or intensity of sunshine in the US. Advances in mapping software have made it easy to explore descriptive health outcome data using Internet-based systems. For example, the US National Cancer Institute has a website that allows users to

Table 6.1 Types of epidemiological study design

Type of study	Alternative name	Unit of study
Descriptive studies		Individuals or populations
Analytical studies		
Ecological	Correlational	Populations
Cross-sectional	Prevalence	Individuals
Case-control	Case-referent	Individuals
Cohort	Follow-up	Individuals
Historical cohort	Retrospective cohort	Individuals
Experimental studies	Intervention studies	
Randomized controlled trial	Clinical trials	Individuals
Community trials		Communities

Adapted from [2]. Reproduced with permission from Beaglehole R, Bonita R, Kjellström T. *Basic epidemiology*. Geneva: World Health Organization 1993.

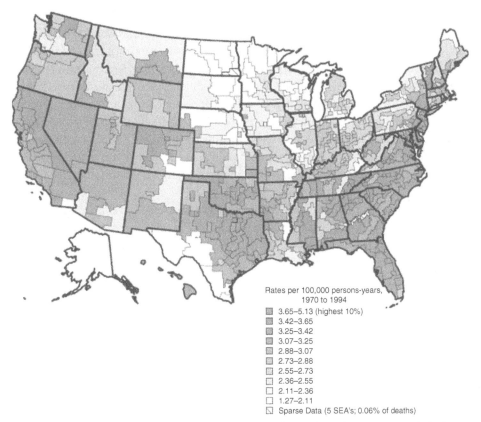

Fig. 6.1 Cancer mortality rates by State Economic Area (Age-adjusted 1970 US population). Melanoma of skin: white males, 1970–1994. From: http://dceg.cancer.gov/atlas/download/ gif-gs/melswm7g.gif [3]. Reproduced with permission from Devesa SS. *Atlas of cancer mortality in the United States, 1950–94*. Bethesda, MD: National Institutes of Health, National Cancer Institute, 1999.

develop cancer mortality maps in the US (http://www3.cancer.gov/atlasplus). Similarly, the International Agency for Research on Cancer (IARC) has developed a program, *Globocan 2000*, that can be downloaded at no cost and used to create cancer maps worldwide (http://www-dep.iarc.fr).

Descriptive data are commonly used to examine patterns of health outcomes by place, time and person. *Geographical comparisons* based on standardized mortality and morbidity rates can be made among countries, or among regions within countries. Variations between countries with respect to rates of mortality attributable to cardiovascular disease and cancers have been the basis of hypotheses regarding the role of environmental factors in these diseases. For example, Forman and Burley [4] examined the global pattern of gastric cancer to evaluate possible environmental risk factors. They observed that gastric cancer incidence and mortality rates were higher in less-developed countries compared to more-developed countries, and that rates were higher in males than females throughout the world. They related these patterns to differences in *Helicobacter pylori* infection, dietary factors, smoking, and other factors. However, international comparisons may be problematic due to differences in diagnostic practices and terminology. For example, the incidence rates of chronic bronchitis and emphysema formerly appeared to be higher in some European countries than in the US, but most of the apparent difference was due to variations in diagnostic practice. In general, geographic contrasts between areas within a single country are likely to be less marked than those between countries, but can be more revealing in relation to environmental factors.

Temporal trends in mortality or morbidity rates can also be of value in indicating the possible effects of environmental factors. Figure 6.2 illustrates changes in male semen density worldwide for the period 1938–1990 [5]. These data suggest environmental factors have a role in the temporal decline in semen quality.

Patterns of disease associated with *personal characteristics* may also provide insight about the effects of environmental factors. Sometimes, differences in exposure patterns between men and women can provide clues about contributory factors, as in the case of lung cancer. The melanoma of the skin mortality in the US, for example, was higher in

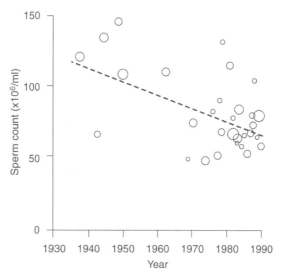

Fig. 6.2 Linear regression of mean sperm density reported in 61 publications, weighted according to the number of participants, 1938–90. From [5]. Reproduced with permission from Carlsen E, Giwercman A, Keiding N, Skakkebaek NE. Evidence for decreasing quality of semen during past 50 years. *BMJ (Clinical Research edn).* 1992 305(6854):609–13.

men compared to women, which was consistent with the greater time men spent working outdoors in the US during 1970–94. The melanoma mortality rates for males and females have become closer over the years as the work patterns and time spent outdoors have become more equal.

Descriptive epidemiological studies of migrant populations, in particular, can provide useful information about the relative roles of environmental and genetic factors [6]. If records on country of origin are available, the health outcomes of migrants can be compared with those of their compatriots in both the country of origin and that of subsequent residence. Cancer morbidity and mortality rates in migrant populations often come to approximate those of the host country, indicating that environmental factors play a role. If genetic factors were the exclusive cause, disease risks would not be influenced within one generation by migration. For example, a descriptive study of cancer risk among migrants and their descendants in Israel found that risks for testis cancer, nasopharyngeal carcinoma and melanoma reflected the father's birthplace even in the second generation; while for ovarian, colorectal, cervical and thyroid cancers, differences in risk between the migrant groups had largely disappeared in the offspring [7]. The investigators concluded that environmental exposures were the major causative factors for the latter group of cancers. There are many examples of cancer studies based on migrants [e.g., 8, 9, 10].

One of the challenges in interpreting descriptive studies of migrants is that the migrants – by virtue of them deciding to migrate and being healthy enough to migrate – may not be like the comparison populations in either their original or new country. Furthermore, people who migrate tend to adopt the customs of their new countries at different rates. A phenomenon called the 'healthy immigrant effect' has been reported, in which many immigrants to developed countries tend initially to be healthier than the populations from their original country, but after a while, these immigrant populations tend to develop worse health status as they adopt habits of their new country [11].

Another type of descriptive study is the *case report* or *case series* in which the investigators report on one or a small number of unusual cases of mortality or disease that might suggest a hypothesis about the causes of the conditions. Often a case report might lead investigators to conduct a descriptive study using existing data to explore the possible causes of the unusual cases, which would be followed by analytical studies to test specific hypotheses. An example of case reports is the series of reports on acute idiopathic pulmonary hemorrhage in infants. This rare condition, in which infants repeatedly cough up fresh blood possibly leading to respiratory failure and death, was reported to occur in a geographical cluster of 10 infants in Cleveland, Ohio, during the early 1990s [12]. This case report lead to a series of case-control studies and surveillance programs, which evaluated the possible role of mold exposure from damp home environments. Although the precise cause of the initial cases events was not determined, additional similar cases continue to be reported from around the world with a continuing focus on factors in the home environment [13].

6.2.2 **Ecological studies**

Ecological studies are studies in which the investigators analyse hypothesized associations between environmental exposures and health outcomes using groups of people, rather than individuals, as the unit of analysis. The numbers of individuals within these populations who have experienced specific combinations of exposure status and health outcome status are not known. Thus an ecological study compares aggregate measures of exposure, such as average exposure or proportion of population exposed, with aggregate measures of health outcome rates, for the same population.

Because descriptive studies also typically examine aggregate measures of exposure or health outcomes, some investigators and textbooks consider ecological studies to be descriptive, rather than analytical studies. Indeed, it is reasonable to think of descriptive and ecological studies as falling along a spectrum, rather than being clearly distinct study designs. In this textbook, we consider ecological studies to be analytical studies because the objectives of these studies are to evaluate specific hypotheses between putative environmental exposures and health outcomes, while descriptive studies examine patterns of exposure or patterns of health outcomes—i.e., characterization of person, place, and time—without formally examining associations between exposures and health outcomes.

The investigation of the association between arsenic and cancer mortality that was conducted in the endemic area of Blackfoot Disease in Taiwan is a classical example of an ecological study [14]. The investigators used data on arsenic concentration measured in over 83 000 wells by the Taiwan Provincial Institute of Environmental Sanitation as a measure of arsenic exposure. These data were used to estimate the average arsenic concentrations in the water supplies of several hundred administrative districts. Cancer mortality data and population size data by administrative district were obtained from the Taiwan Provincial Department of Health. The investigators used correlation and regression analyses to examine the association between arsenic concentration in well-water and age-adjusted mortality for various cancers, controlling for such factors as degree of urbanization and industrialization. Associations were observed between arsenic concentrations in well-water and elevated rates of cancers of the liver, nasal cavity, lung, skin, bladder and kidney.

Traditionally the role of ecological studies has been to perform exploratory analyses using existing population data. However, this study design plays a larger role in environmental epidemiology than in other areas of epidemiology because environmental factors often expose large populations in a similar manner. For example, air pollution in an urban area is likely to cause exposure to most inhabitants and their exposure might be uniformly different from that in a rural area. Similarly, the health effects following exposure to different concentrations of arsenic or chlorination by-products in water supplies might be compared between areas. The potential for misclassification of individual-level exposure is less for these types of exposure. Thus an ecological study of environmental exposures can usually be interpreted with greater accuracy than studies of exposures that are determined by individual behavior, as in the case of cigarette smoking, or an individual exposure that has occurred via food. The distinction between classical (individual-oriented) and Berkson (group-oriented) measurement errors of exposure were discussed in Chapter 5.

6.2.2.1 Design of ecological studies

The strategy for conducting an ecological study is to determine whether those ecological units (i.e., population groups) with a high frequency of exposure also tend to be the groups with a high frequency of health outcome occurrence. Generally, the investigator obtains group rates of the health outcome and a measure of exposure prevalence for the same group. These data are then analyzed statistically to estimate the group-level associations.

In common with the approaches used for descriptive studies, ecological analyses often use *geographical areas*, such as countries or administrative units within countries, as the basis for defining the groups. This was demonstrated by the aforementioned study of arsenic in well-water and cancer mortality [14]. Another example is a study by Lin *et al.* [15] that examined the national mortality rates due to mesothelioma during the period 2000–04 compared to the national asbestos consumption per capita in years 1960–69 for multiple countries. As shown in Figure 6.3, this study found a strong correlation between the aggregate measure of asbestos consumption and the mortality rates due to mesothelioma.

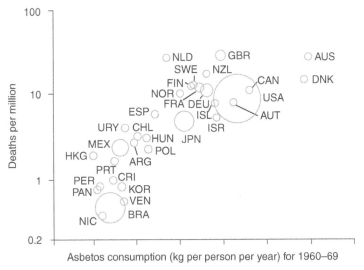

Fig. 6.3 Deaths (per million per year) from mesothelioma in males (2000–04) by country compared to national historical asbestos consumption (kg per person per year) (1960–69). From [15]. Reproduced with permission from Lin RT, Takahashi K, Karjalainen A, Hoshuyama T, Wilson D, Kameda T, et al. Ecological association between asbestos-related diseases and historical asbestos consumption: an international analysis. *Lancet.* 2007 369(9564):844–9, with permission from Elsevier.

Similar geographical ecological studies have been conducted to evaluate the association between radon concentration and childhood leukemia incidence by geographical units in France [8], organochloride pesticide contamination and breast cancer incidence by state in Australia [16], and discharges of chemicals from industrial facilities and breast cancer incidence by county in Texas [17]. The ecological study design has also been used, for example, to compare rates of hospitalizations for diabetes and residential proximity to hazardous waste sites in New York State [18] and the association between the number of indoor chlorinated swimming pools per inhabitant and prevalence of wheezing and asthma in children across Europe [19, 20].

Although comparison of geographical units in an ecological study is conceptually straightforward, determining exposure levels precisely can be difficult if the administrative units providing the health outcome data bear little relation to the occurrence or distribution of the environmental factor being studied. Water monitoring data, for instance, may not be collected specifically for an administrative unit such as a township; yet this may be the unit of analysis for which the health outcome rates are to be estimated. When planning an epidemiological analysis based on geographic areas, an evaluation must be made of how well the available data on exposures and health outcomes match the selected units of analysis.

Controlling for risk factors that may cause bias and confounding in ecological studies needs to be considered because groups of people from different geographic areas often live in different conditions and have different lifestyles. This means that the specific exposure under study, and exposure to other risk factors for the same disease, may vary between groups. Confounding or effect modification cannot be ruled out on the basis of other studies of individuals having demonstrated lack of confounding within each study area [21]. For example, within one area of high air pollution there may be no association between smoking habits and air pollution exposure. The same may also be true of an area of low air pollution. Yet if average air pollution and average smoking habits are correlated, an ecological study of air pollution effects on the lung will suffer from confounding because some of the apparent association between the lung effects and air pollution may actually be due to different rates of cigarette smoking in the groups.

The groups studied in an ecological study also may be defined by *time period*. Temporal comparisons or time-trend studies examine associations between changes in exposure to environmental factors and changes in health outcome rates over time within the same source population. One of the advantages of making a temporal comparison is that population characteristics, such as sociodemographic factors, that could bias group-level associations, may be relatively constant over time in the same geographical area. However, the study of trends over long periods of time may be complicated by substantial changes in demographics. In recent decades such changes have occurred in many developing countries due to increasing population density and industrialization. Furthermore, data on exposure and health outcome rates may not be comparable over time. For example, techniques and instruments to measure air pollution have changed over time. Diagnostic practices and disease coding schemes such as the International

Classification of Diseases have also changed. Investigators should be aware of such changes and develop strategies for rendering data sufficiently comparable.

As mentioned in the introduction, there has been increasing interest among investigators to combine ecological data with individual data in a *semi-individual* study design. This study design has features of both an ecological and individual study design [1]. This design has been used in air pollution epidemiology and to examine spatial patterns of disease (see Chapter 8, Section 8.3 for more information on spatial epidemiology).

6.2.2.2 Strengths and limitations

The principal strength of ecological studies is that they are usually based on existing data and therefore relatively inexpensive to conduct. This study design can be useful for studying rare diseases caused by relatively rare exposures, because the source population for the ecological comparisons can be very large, as when comparisons between countries are made.

However, ecological studies can be difficult to interpret because information about factors that could bias the findings is often limited. An important consideration is the potential for *ecological bias*, in which group-level associations do not accurately reflect individual-level associations [21, 22]. The underlying problem is that the use of aggregate measures of exposure may not reflect individual-level exposure status adequately due to within-group heterogeneity in exposure. This study design must therefore be used with caution because the magnitude of ecological bias is likely to be less predictable than individual bias in estimating the same effect.

Ecological studies have further limitations. For example, nondifferential exposure misclassification can lead to an overestimation of the measure of effect, unlike in individual-level studies; so it cannot be assumed that bias due to inadequate information would result only in underestimation of the exposure effect. Moreover, environmental exposures are often highly correlated, which means that identifying the causal exposure can be difficult. In a study of ambient air pollution, for instance, different regions may have highly correlated concentrations of ozone, acid aerosols and respirable particulates, making separation of the particular effect of each pollutant problematic. Finally, the analysis of ecological data may be limited if the study includes relatively few ecological units of observation, even if the units contain large populations. The statistical precision of ecological studies is based primarily on the number of units and not on the size of the populations that constitute the units.

6.2.3 Cross-sectional studies

Cross-sectional studies examine associations between an environmental exposures and disease prevalence at a particular point in time or during a short period of time. Estimates of exposures and measurements of personal characteristics and health effects are made at the same time. For example, investigators may test lung function in study population and at the same time do personal monitoring or ask questions about exposure to indoor air pollution.

Cross-sectional studies are usually undertaken before cohort or case-control studies because they tend to cost less and take less time to complete. However, cross-sectional studies are not merely quick forms of the latter types of studies since they examine *prevalent* rather than *incident* events. Thus a cross-sectional study design might be used to evaluate the risk of chronic lung disease due to air pollution, but it could not be used to examine respiratory mortality as this is an incident event.

In environmental epidemiology, one of the principal uses of this study design is to assess the role of exposures that result in symptoms and biological changes, such as decreases in lung function or neurological function, but which do not necessarily cause individuals to seek medical care. In many instances, the biological changes are studied because they are early indicators of risk for mortality or the development of disease. Cross-sectional studies have proved effective for the study of chronic conditions such as asthma prevalence, hypertension, chronic obstructive lung disease and arthritis.

Cross-sectional studies are often undertaken in specific communities in response to concern about exposure from a point-source such as an industrial facility or hazardous waste site, or if specific health outcome rates appear to be increasing. This approach is useful if multiple possible exposures and a range of health outcomes must be examined. The findings of the study can then be used to design a more focused cohort or case-control study.

Cross-sectional studies may also be based on national population studies or existing data. For example, Arif and Shah [23] used data from the US National Health and Nutrition Survey to examine the association between exposure to volatile organic compounds measured by passive personal monitoring and the prevalence of doctor-diagnosed asthma and wheezing during the prior 12 months. They found that the risk of having physician-diagnosed asthma was significantly associated with environmental exposures to aromatic compounds, but not to chlorinated hydrocarbons. Table 6.2 shows that the odds ratio (as a measure of relative risk in this cross-sectional study) was 1.63 for each unit increase in a standardized unit of exposure to aromatic compounds, but the odds ratio was less than one for exposure to chlorinated hydrocarbons, suggesting no effect of exposure to the latter compounds.

Wright *et al.* [24] used existing data to conduct a semi-individual study of the effect of trihalomethane (THM) exposure on fetal development using aggregate data on THM concentrations in municipal drinking water and birth records from more than 56 000 singleton infants born in the State of Massachusetts, US. They were able to control for individual potential confounders, such as maternal race, maternal health risk factors and prenatal care, using information from birth records. They found that THM exposure was associated with reductions in birth weight after adjusting for potential confounding variables.

6.2.3.1 Design of cross-sectional studies

The key steps in conducting a cross-sectional study are:

- identify the source population;
- choose a sampling design and sampling frame for selecting the study participants;
- measure the exposure and health outcome status of the study participants.

Table 6.2 Adjusted odds ratios (and 95% confidence intervals [CI]) for physician-diagnosed asthma and exposure to volatile organic compounds in the NHANES cross-sectional study

VOC exposure	Physician-diagnosed asthma	
	Odds ratio[+]	95% CI
Aromatic compounds*	1.63	1.17, 2.27
Benzene	1.33	1.13, 1.56
Ethylbenzene	1.34	1.01, 1.78
Toluene	1.21	0.93, 1.58
o-Xylene	1.32	1.04, 1.67
m,p-Xylene	1.33	1.08, 1.64
Chlorinated hydrocarbons*	0.93	0.66, 1.32
Tetrachloroethene	1.02	0.90, 1.1.5
Trichloroethene	0.94	0.77, 1.14
Chloroform	1.10	0.89, 1.35
1,4-dichlorobenzene	1.16	1.03, 1.30
Methyl tertiary butyl ether	1.19	1.07, 1.32

+ Odds ratio is the increase in the relative risk of reporting physician-diagnosed asthma for each 1 U increase for standardized exposure factor scores.

* The variables "aromatic compounds" and "chlorinated hydrocarbons" were derived by exploratory factor analysis and included loading on the indented individual compounds shown below each factor variable. The analyses for the factor variables and the individual compounds were adjusted for age, sex, race/ethnicity, body mass index, atopy, smoking, environmental tobacco smoke exposure, and poverty level. From [23]. Reproduced with permission from Arif AA, Shah SM. Association between personal exposure to volatile organic compounds and asthma among US adult population. *International Archives of Occupational and Environmental Health*. 2007 80(8):711–19.

Selection of study population

Because cross-sectional studies are generally used to study health outcomes for which identification of a population using mortality or medical records is not possible, the selection of an explicit sampling frame is particularly important. Sampling frames include census lists of all households in a community, population lists based on holders of driver's licenses, voter registration files, medical care registrations, and other public records. If a sampling frame does not already exist, the investigators must create a sampling method that will yield a representative sample of the source population. In many community studies, investigators have found that the most complete coverage and highest participation rates are achieved when study staff go 'door-to-door' to identify subjects and request their participation.

Study populations for cross-sectional studies can be selected using one of three strategies (see Figure 6.4). Perhaps the most common strategy is to obtain a random sample of a population without regard to exposure or health outcome status, i.e., a survey or census

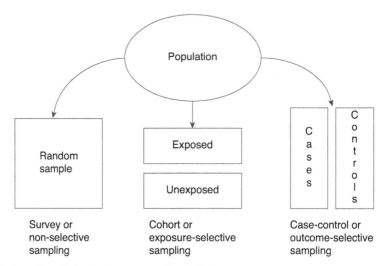

Fig. 6.4 Sampling strategies for cross-sectional study.

sampling strategy. This sampling strategy is feasible when the prevalence of exposure factors and health outcomes are relatively common, as with the aforementioned examples of cross-sectional studies of asthma, hypertension, and arthritis. This approach is suitable for examining multiple exposures and health outcomes. The aforementioned studies based on national examination survey data are examples of the survey approach. In these, the same study population was used to examine a number of exposure and health outcome associations. This sampling strategy is also used when it is not possible to determine exposure or health outcome status before selecting the study population. Investigators may also decide to invite all members of a community to participate in a survey if the community is small or if it would be awkward to include some persons and to exclude others.

A second common strategy is for investigators to select the study population on the basis of *exposure status*. This strategy is used particularly when the study objective is to determine the risk of a specific environmental exposure. Selecting subjects on the basis of exposure status is efficient if exposure prevalence in the source population is relatively low because the statistical analysis of a study with a set study population size is more powerful when the size of the exposed and comparison populations are approximately equal. In order to use this strategy, identification of subjects' exposure status, prior to their being selected for the study, must be possible. This is usually achieved in one of two ways. Investigators may use existing exposure data to identify an exposed community and an unexposed community for an *external* comparison, or to identify various exposure subgroups within a single community for an *internal* comparison. For example, Fujino *et al.* [25] conducted a cross-sectional study of two villages in Inner Mongolia— one with high arsenic levels in the water supply and one with lower arsenic levels—to examine the effect of arsenic exposure on peripheral nerve conduction velocity. People in the village with lower arsenic levels served as an external comparison population for people in the village with higher arsenic levels.

The third strategy for selecting a study population is essentially a case-control design in that participants are identified on the basis of *health outcome status*. Indeed, some textbooks refer to this design as a '*prevalence case-control study*'. This design is an efficient strategy if the proportion of the population with the health outcome is relatively small and participants can be sampled on the basis of health outcome status. For example, medical records in a hospital clinic could be used to identify children with a diagnosis of asthma and a control group of children attending the same clinic who do not have asthma. These children could then be invited to participate in an examination to determine environmental risk factors for asthma. If existing health status records are not available, it still may be efficient to use a two-stage design to first screen the population to determine health outcome status, and then to conduct a more detailed study of cases and controls to determine exposure status. This design would be considered a 'nested case-control analysis' within a cross-sectional study.

Assessment of exposures

Although a primary characteristic of cross-sectional studies is that information on exposures and health outcomes are obtained at the same time, the goal in conducting such studies is to determine the causal relationship between exposure and health status. However, as discussed in Chapter 2, a causal relationship means the causal exposure must precede the development of the health outcome. Therefore, even in cross-sectional studies, investigators must pay careful attention to the temporal relationship between the exposures and health status.

Investigators often conduct cross-sectional studies to assess the effects of past or ongoing exposures on health status. So, for example, investigators might ask about the use of indoor heating sources during the prior month as part of a cross-sectional survey of asthma symptoms [26]. Conceptually, this study design is similar to historical cohort study because the investigators ask about past exposures in relation to current symptoms, but it is still generally considered to be a cross-sectional study because the information on exposures and health status are obtained at the same time, the investigators do not attempt to identify the source population at the time that the exposures occurred, and the outcomes are prevalence rather than incidence measures. These types of cross-sectional studies rely on two assumptions. One, which is similar to the assumption in historical cohort studies and case-control studies, is that accurate information on past exposures can be obtained during the cross-sectional survey. The second assumption is that current exposure status correlates with past exposure status, so that assessment of current exposure is a valid surrogate for measurement of past exposure.

A common strategy to assess past exposures in cross-sectional studies is to use biological indicators of exposure, if they are feasible. For example, von Ehrenstein *et al.* [27] assessed the effect of arsenic exposure on intellectual function tests in 351 children in West Bengal, India, by measuring arsenic concentration in the participants' urine and using parent questionnaire information on lifetime water sources. Similarly,

Carta *et al.* [28] evaluated neurotoxic effects of mercury exposure in 22 fishing-eating males living near the Sardinia Coast of Italy and 22 non-fish eating males by using measures of mercury in urine. Yokoo *et al.* [29] evaluated the effect of methylmercury exposure on neuropsychological function in residents of six villages in Brazil by using questionnaire information on past residences and analysis of mercury in hair. Each of these studies assessed the cross-sectional associations between the biological indicators of exposure and neurological status. The most likely causal exposures occurred before the cross-sectional survey took place, but this past exposure could be assessed using the biological indicators.

Assessment of health effects

The measure of health outcome occurrence in a cross-sectional study is prevalence, that is, the proportion of persons in the group who are affected by the health outcome at a point in time. As a practical matter, many cross-sectional studies examine the *period prevalence* rather than the *point prevalence* for outcomes such as symptoms. The point prevalence is the number of existing cases at a specified point in time, while the period prevalence is the number of cases during a specified interval of time. For example, a questionnaire may ask if the subject has experienced headaches or wheezing during the past month, rather than simply asking the subject if he or she is currently experiencing such symptoms. Although there are subtle differences in interpretation, most investigators analyze and interpret these period prevalence measures as if they were measures of point prevalence.

6.2.3.2 Strengths and limitations

If it is possible to estimate disease risk by studying a prevalent health outcome, a cross-sectional study may be an efficient option since such a study usually costs less and requires less time to conduct than either a cohort or case-control study. Cross-sectional studies can be used effectively to study factors that do not change as a result of disease, such as ethnicity, genetic markers of susceptibility or environmental exposures measured by objective methods. However, exposures measured by questionnaire or biomarkers may be affected by the simultaneous measurement of health outcome. Disease onset may influence subjects' recall of earlier exposures and may affect biological markers of exposure such as pesticide concentration in adipose tissue. Thus cross-sectional measures of exposure can be used effectively only if the investigators can verify that the measures of exposure are not affected by disease onset.

Another limitation of this type of study is that interpretation of cross-sectional associations between exposure and a prevalent health outcome may be subject to selection bias due to 'selective survival'. For example, if persons with lung disease move to areas with low air pollution, a cross-sectional study would underestimate the association between air pollution exposure and lung disease risk. Similarly, if parents of children who had developed asthma reduced their cigarette smoking, a subsequent cross-sectional survey would be less likely to identify an association between the parents' cigarette smoking and their children's asthma.

6.2.4 **Case-control studies**

A case-control study (or case-referent study) examines associations between exposures and a health outcome by comparing *cases*, or individuals who developed the outcome, and *controls* who are a sample of the source population from which the cases were identified. Controls are usually individuals who are similar to the cases in terms of risk characteristics, but who have not developed the health outcome. Having selected cases and controls, the investigators then determine the prior exposure status of the cases and controls by examining existing exposure records and questionnaire information or measuring biomarkers of past exposure.

The efficiency of the case-control study derives from not having to wait for disease occurrence during the induction period of a chronic disease and from limiting the expense of exposure measurement to cases and controls (i.e., exposure is not measured for the entire source population). Case-control studies have been used extensively to study the role of environmental factors in the development of various types of cancer because most types of cancer have long induction periods. Examples include studies of lung cancer and residential exposure to radon [30], brain tumors and exposure to pesticides in France [31], malignant lymphoma and sun exposure in Germany [32], non-melanoma skin cancer and arsenic exposure from power station emissions in Slovakia [33], and mesothelioma risk by residential proximity to deposits of naturally occurring asbestos [34]. Case-control studies have also been used to study noncancer outcomes, such as a study of congenital heart disease and parental exposure to contaminated drinking water [35], and a study of acute myocardial infarction and exposure to traffic [36].

The study of arsenic exposure and non-melanoma skin cancer (NMSC) by Pesch *et al.* [33] is an example of a case-control study that included multimedia exposure assessment for individual and environmental sources. The study included 328 cases of NMSC reported to the Prievidza District reporting center in Slovakia and 286 age- and gender-matched controls who were selected from a mandatory population registry in the same district. The investigators assessed occupational exposures by obtaining personal occupational histories and scoring arsenic exposure using the British job–exposure matrix, they assessed nutritional sources of arsenic exposure by using a food frequency questionnaire combined with data on median arsenic concentrations in the food products, and they assessed environmental arsenic exposure based on the participants' residential histories. Environmental exposure to arsenic was estimated using air dispersion models to calculate arsenic air concentrations over time at the participants' homes. After adjusting for possible selection bias in the control participants, the investigators used logistic regression to calculate the odds ratio for the associations of NMSC with the various sources of arsenic exposure. To express their findings, they divided each of the various exposure measures into three categories based on the percentile distributions in the total study population. Some of the findings are summarized in Table 6.3. The investigators observed increasing risk of NMSC with higher residential exposure and nutritional exposure to arsenic, but no apparent association with occupational exposures. For example, the risk of developing NMSC (odds ratio) was 1.90 times higher or nearly twice as great for people who had higher potential residential exposure to arsenic compared to people with lower residential exposure.

The case-control design has also been used to increase the efficiency of studying cohort populations. If sufficient information is available for identifying a cohort, but the expense of obtaining detailed information on exposure status or confounding factors is prohibitive, the investigator may be able to conduct a case-control analysis within a cohort study population. If so, data on exposure status and other risk factors will be required only for the cases and controls. This design is referred to as a *nested case-control* study.

6.2.4.1 Design of case-control studies

The principal steps in conducting a case-control study are:

- establish a case definition;
- establish criteria for a study population and identify a sampling frame for selecting cases;
- identify an appropriate sampling frame for selecting controls;

Table 6.3 Odds ratio for possible arsenic exposure and non-melanoma skin cancer in Prievidza District, Slovakia, 1999–2000

Source of arsenic exposure	Odds ratio	95% CI
Occupational arsenic exposure		
No	1	–
Low	1.28	0.87, 1.88
High (>90 percentile)	0.75	0.41, 1.37
Residential exposure*		
Low (<30 percentile)	1	–
Medium (30–60 percentile)	1.72	1.42, 20.8
High (>60 percentile)	1.90	1.39, 2.60
Nutritional exposure+		
Low (>30 percentile)	1	–
Medium (30–60 percentile)	1.12	0.77, 1.64
High (>60 percentile)	1.83	0.98, 3.43

* Residential exposure calculated as a function of time and distance from power plants according to an air dispersion model and available emission data.

Nutritional exposure calculated annual arsenic uptake in food from food frequency questionnaire and median concentrations of arsenic in foods, adjusted for consumption of home grown food.

+ From [33]. Reproduced with permission from Pesch B, Ranft U, Jakubis P, Nieuwenhuijsen MJ, Hergemoller A, Unfried K, *et al.* Environmental arsenic exposure from a coal-burning power plant as a potential risk factor for non-melanoma skin carcinoma: results from a case-control study in the district of Prievidza, Slovakia. *Am J Epidemiol.* 2002 155(9):798–809.

- assess prior exposure status and other relevant characteristics of the cases and controls;
- compare the prior exposure experiences of cases and controls in order to estimate the association between the exposures and health outcome.

Case identification

Generally case-control studies are based on officially recorded health outcomes, such as mortality, or conditions requiring hospital admission. Examples include the studies of cancers, birth defects, and myocardial infarctions mentioned previously.

Many case-control studies are based on patients admitted to hospitals or seen for diseases at medical clinics. Such studies have several advantages: the participants and their records are highly accessible, the participants are generally cooperative, and the characteristics of cases and controls can be balanced if both attend the same facility. Howeer, using hospital-based cases is appropriate only if the health outcomes that are being investigated usually result in hospitalization, otherwise cases will be missed. Also if hospital patients are to be used for a study, the investigators should understand the referral patterns to the hospital, so as to be able to identify the true source population and evaluate possible selection bias.

Population-based cases are the principal alternative to hospital-based cases. If a population-based approach is adopted, all incident cases of the outcome in a defined geographical area are included as cases, irrespective of the source or mechanism by which they were identified. A combination of case reporting by all hospitals in a region, as well as other healthcare treatment facilities and offices of medical practitioners, might therefore be used. The advantages of a population-based case approach are that the source population is better defined than for hospital-based cases, and the exposure histories of the cases are more likely to reflect those of persons in the source population who do not have the disease of interest. The disadvantage of this approach is that high costs may be incurred when establishing the network of personnel required for identifying cases, if existing networks such as tumor registries do not already exist in the region of interest.

Selection of controls

Controls should be individuals from the source population who would have been considered cases if they had developed the health outcome. The most commonly used control groups are a random sample of the source population from which the cases were selected or persons seeking medical care at the same institutions as the cases for conditions believed to be unrelated to the health outcome of interest. Less frequently used controls include friends, neighbors, schoolmates, siblings and fellow workers.

Although controls are individuals that could develop the health outcome of interest, they do not have to be disease-free. Indeed, using persons with other diseases as controls may be efficient. The aforementioned study by Pan *et al.* [34] is an example in which persons with pancreatic cancer were used as controls for a study of mesothelioma risk due to asbestos exposure. If this strategy is to be used, the investigators must make sure that the 'control' condition is not causally related to any exposures of interest in the study.

If cases consist of all those individuals within a defined population who develop the disease, the best control group would generally be a sample of individuals from the same source population. However, identifying the control group can be expensive unless the sampling can be based on existing records, such as national security identifications or residents lists. For example, the previously mentioned study of brain tumors in France selected controls from electoral rolls [31], while the study of malignant lymphoma in Germany used lists from a population registration office [32], and the study of acute myocardial infarction in the US used a state resident list [36]. It is more difficult to identify population-based controls when such lists do not exist. Methods have been developed, such as random digit dialing, so the telephone can be used to identify control groups. This approach to control identification has been used extensively in cancer case-control studies, but it is becoming less feasible because of the increasing use of mobile phones and overlapping telephone codes that do not have clear geographical definitions. Also in many countries, intense use of telemarketing has increased the resistance of people to responding to telephone inquires. In some developing countries the proportion of households that have telephones may be low, so this approach would not yield a representative sample of the source population.

During the past few years, the *case-crossover* study design has received increasing use and attention as a variation of the case-control study and alternative to the time-series analysis [37]. In this study design, each case serves as his or her control by comparing exposures near the time of the incident health event with exposures to the same person at another time—either before or after the incident event. As noted by Künzli and Schindler [38], the analysis compares the difference between exposures during the event and control time periods for the same individual, so it is a 'matched' case-control analysis. This study design has been used especially for research on the effects of air pollution on cardiovascular disease events, such as deaths, hospitalizations, ventricular arrhythmias, and intracerebral hemorrhage [e.g., 39, 40, 41]. For example, Peters *et al.* [41] conducted a case-crossover study of 691 persons who had suffered a nonfatal myocardial infarction (MI) in Augsburg, Germany, during 1999 to 2001. The investigators used information on the cases' activities during the day of and the four days preceding the MI, which was collected by nurses using a standardized interview. They used conditional logistic regression to compare the case's exposure to traffic during the six hours prior to the MI with the same person's exposure 24 to 71 hours before the onset of the MI. They found that exposure to traffic was more frequent on the day of the onset of the MI. For example, exposure to any means of transportation was associated with a nearly threefold increased risk of MI within one hour (odds ratio = 2.92). This case crossover study design was used effectively to study transient risk factors, which are factors that may trigger acute events in susceptible persons. Transient risk factors have only short-term effects, whereas chronic risk factors have long-term effects.

Matching

Matching is a strategy for selecting controls so that the distributions of some *a priori* selected risk factors are identical or nearly the same for the controls as for the cases.

Efficiency of the statistical analysis is enhanced because the cases and controls are as comparable as possible in relation to other variables that may confound the association.

In a study of radon exposure and lung cancer, controls could be matched to cases for age, gender and history of cigarette smoking, since each of these could be a risk factor for lung cancer and could also be associated with cumulative exposure to radon. If matching were not performed for such a study, the cases would probably include a much larger proportion of older persons, males, and persons who smoked cigarettes than would the controls randomly selected from the population. Evaluation of the association between radon exposure and lung cancer incidence, while analytically adjusting for these other factors, would be inefficient since it would necessitate use of a larger control group.

6.2.4.2 Strengths and limitations

The case-control study design has several attractive features. It is efficient for studying rare diseases, especially those with a long induction period, and is often less expensive to apply than a prospective cohort study design. Furthermore, by selecting participants on the basis of a health outcome, the investigator can examine the role of multiple environmental factors.

Two of the principal disadvantages of the case-control study design are that identifying an appropriate control population can be difficult, and there can be greater bias in classifying exposure status since this is determined after the outcome has developed. Because of the increasing difficulty of recruiting population-based controls during the past decade, there has been a trend towards investigators again using hospital-based controls or other well-defined sampling frames to identify possible controls. Methods also have been developed to adjust quantitatively for selection bias in case-control studies when some external data are available on the distribution of the exposure variables in the source population. Exposure classification bias may occur in one of several ways. The health outcome itself may affect the exposure measure directly or indirectly. For example, individuals with respiratory symptoms might avoid exposure to tobacco smoke. If they subsequently participated in a case-control study of respiratory disease, the study would probably underestimate the association between respiratory disease and exposure to cigarette smoke. Another problem area concerns individuals' recall of exposure. Many case-control studies rely on subjects to report on earlier exposures, but cases tend to recall exposures more so than controls who have less motivation to recall earlier events.

Another disadvantage of the case-control study design is that the analysis cannot directly yield estimates of health outcome incidence rates, rate differences, or attributable risk.

6.2.5 Cohort studies

In a *cohort study*, the study population consists of individuals who are at risk of developing a particular disease or health outcome. The individuals are divided into groups according to their exposure status. The groups are then followed over time to determine the subsequent incidence of the health outcome within each group. A cohort study enables investigators to measure incidence rates and to estimate all effect measures, such as rate ratios and rate differences, for multiple health outcomes. A cohort study is termed *prospective* if the data are collected as the events unfold and *historical* if it examines past events (using existing records): these terms refer to timing and not to study design.

Cohort studies have been used effectively in environmental epidemiology to assess the long-term health effects of acute exposure to environmental hazards. For example, cohort studies have followed populations exposed acutely to radiation, including populations in Japan who experienced the nuclear bomb explosions during World War II and communities who were affected by the Chernobyl nuclear accident. Cohort studies have also been undertaken to measure chronic effects in populations exposed to environmental releases of toxic chemicals from industrial facilities. An example is the study of communities in the vicinity of the pesticide factory in Bhopal, India, from which methylisocyanate leakage in 1984 killed more than 1700 people and poisoned 200 000 others. Another example is the study of residents in Seveso, Italy, who were potentially exposed to 2,3,7,8-tetrachlorodibenzo-*p*-dioxin following an explosion at a chemical manufacturing plant in 1976 [42, 43]. The role of epidemiology in evaluating the effects of chemical incidents is discussed in Chapter 9.

Cohort studies are also used to evaluate the effects of chronic environmental exposures on health outcomes. For example, a well-known cohort study—the Harvard Six Cities Study— estimated the effects of air pollution on mortality, while controlling for individual risk factors by following a cohort of more than 8000 adults who were randomly recruited from six US cities with different levels of air pollution [44]. The cohort was initially followed for 14 to 16 years with subsequent extended follow-up for 8 years during a period of reduced air pollution concentrations [45]. This study demonstrated that total, cardiovascular, and lung cancer mortality were each associated with exposure to ambient fine particles (aerodynamic diameter smaller than 2.5 µm, or $PM_{2.5}$) in the air of the six cities (see Figure 6.5). The total mortality rate in the most polluted city (Stubenville) was 1.26 times the mortality in the least polluted city (Portage), after controlling for individual risk factors. This cohort study was a semi-individual design because exposure to air pollution was defined based on averages of the cities, while individual information was collected on personal risk factors and the mortality outcomes.

Cohort studies have also been very important for evaluating the role of prenatal and early life environmental exposures on asthma [e.g., 46], respiratory illnesses [e.g., 47], lung development [44], and neurological outcomes in children and adolescents [e.g., 49]. A well-known example is the birth cohort study of more than 1000 children in the Faroe Islands in which the investigators identified infants at birth; used cord blood, cord tissue, and maternal hair to estimate prenatal exposure to methylmercury; and then followed the children through adolescence with periodic examinations to assess the effect of the methylmercury exposure on neurobehavioral function [50, 51]. The investigators showed that methylmercury exposure was significantly associated with deficits in motor, attention, and verbal neurobehavioral tests that persisted at least until 14 years of age. This study among others related to mercury exposure has been very influential in

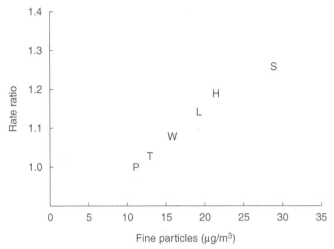

Fig. 6.5 Estimated adjusted rate ratios for total mortality and average PM$_{2.5}$ concentrations during 1974–1989 in six United States cities. Rate ratio for total mortality compared to Portage, WI (reference level). T=Topeka, KS; W=Watertown, MA; L=St. Louis, MO; H=Harriman, TN; S=Stubenville, OH; P=Portage, WI From [44]. Reproduced with permission from Dockery DW, Pope CA, 3rd, Xu X, Spengler JD, Ware JH, Fay ME, *et al.* An association between air pollution and mortality in six U.S. cities. *The New England Journal of Medicine.* 1993 329(24):1753–9.

shaping public health guidelines for consumption of fish that may contain methylmercury. Chapter 16 discusses the role of epidemiology in setting public policy.

6.2.5.1 Design of cohort studies

There are two basic types of cohort, defined according to the type of source population upon which study is based. A *fixed cohort* consists of a population of individuals who are identified at a point or interval of time and then followed over time. Fixed cohorts can also be defined on the basis of a specific event, such as exposure to a chemical spill. The cohort is considered fixed because cohort membership is defined at the time of entry. Examples include the community residents near Seveso, Italy, who were potentially exposed to dioxin or the persons enrolled in the Harvard Six Cities Study. A *dynamic cohort* allows the inclusion of members over time as they fit the selection criteria. An example of a dynamic cohort would be a community, exposed to an environmental hazard, into and out of which individuals could move during the follow-up period. The concept of a dynamic cohort is attractive because it reflects the constantly changing nature of populations. Dynamic cohort studies are most feasible in countries or regions in which population identification or registration records are routinely maintained.

The principal steps in conducting a cohort study are:

- identify and select the study population;
- classify the study population according to exposure status and other relevant risk factors;

+ follow the cohort members over time to determine the health outcome occurrence by exposure status subgroups.

Selection of study population

Cohort members must be *at risk* of developing the health outcome of interest. Therefore, when selecting the cohort the investigator must not include individuals who cannot develop the health outcome, and individuals who already have the outcome of interest, as well as persons who are not susceptible. For example, in a study of persons exposed to environmental tobacco smoke, potential cohort members may have to be screened at the beginning of the study to ascertain that they are free of respiratory disease.

The study population can be selected using one of two strategies. Subjects can be recruited into the cohort without regard to exposure status—the *census* strategy. Exposure status is determined after subjects have been enrolled into the cohort. This approach is useful if the exposure is likely to be common or if the aim of the study is to identify effects of more than one environmental factor. For example, Gold *et al.* [46] conducted a birth cohort study to determine the role of multiple risk factors for repeated wheeze in the first year of life. The investigators enrolled 499 families at the time of the child's birth and collected information on environmental exposures by administering questionnaires and conducting home visits to measure allergen concentrations in household dust. They evaluated the associations of multiple environmental and personal risk factors on wheeze during the first year of life. Exposure status was not known at the time of participants were enrolled in the study.

The alternative strategy is to select members for the cohort on the basis of their *exposure status*. This approach can be efficient because balanced numbers of exposed and unexposed subjects can be selected. The abovementioned Harvard Six Cities study used this approach by first selecting six US cities that were known to have different levels of air pollution, but were otherwise reasonably similar.

When planning a cohort study, identification of an appropriate *sampling frame* for selecting the study population is crucial. Sampling frames for cohort studies include population census lists, church parish registries, driver's licence lists, and telephone directories. The availability of useful sampling frames varies considerably among communities, which can affect the feasibility of doing a cohort study in particular communities.

Selection of a comparison group

The comparison group in a cohort study provides a measure of the health outcomes that occur in a population without exposure. As mentioned above, this group could emerge from the cohort by dividing members of the cohort by exposure status, in which case it is known as an *internal* comparison group. It is also possible to choose a comparison group from a broader sample of the source population which is known to be unexposed. In this case, the comparison group is an *external* comparison group.

The advantage of using an internal comparison group is that the various exposure groups within the same study population are more likely to be comparable than using an external comparison population. Yet identifying a large enough nonexposed group within a single cohort may not be possible. Moreover, by using an external comparison group, the investigator may be able to use existing data, rather than collecting new data, which can be cost-efficient. For example, a study could compare the number of deaths in an exposed community with the number of deaths—based on regional or national mortality rates derived from existing records—that would be expected under normal circumstances. The major challenge when selecting an external comparison group is to ensure that, apart from being nonexposed, it is comparable to the exposed population in every respect.

Population follow-up

Methods for following cohorts depend on the availability of adequate records. If mortality records are to be used, the investigators must identify appropriate sources of records to include in the study, e.g., national death registries or death certificates. Obtaining mortality records on a national basis may be costly. On the other hand, using regional records might not provide sufficient information on subjects who migrate during the follow-up period.

Follow-up studies of non-fatal health outcomes are no different in principle from mortality cohort studies, but since measurement of nonfatal health outcomes usually necessitates contact with the participants, more active methods are likely to be required to follow the study population. Direct contact would be necessary, for instance, to obtain information on outcomes such as respiratory symptoms or to measure lung function. Typically, in long-term cohort studies, investigators contact the participants periodically. So in designing a study, investigators must strike a balance between incurring higher costs as a result of more frequent follow-up intervals, and sustaining greater losses of information as a result of less frequent participant contact. That said, direct contact would be unnecessary if the health outcome could be determined from existing data sources, as in the case of hospitalization for a myocardial infarction. Particularly in some northern European countries with extensive procedures for linkage of population and health records, it is feasible to conduct follow-up of population cohorts using record linkage systems with no direct participant contact.

6.2.5.2 Historical cohort studies

A historical cohort study is conceptually identical to a prospective cohort study except that the study takes place after the causal events have unfolded. The investigator typically uses existing records to identify a cohort for some time in the past, to assign exposure status, and then to follow the cohort forward over time. Historical cohort studies are generally less expensive and take less time to complete than prospective cohort studies. However, existing records upon which historical cohort studies are based, may not provide accurate information. Even if information on the environmental factor of interest is available, information on confounding risk factors may not be. Moreover, exposure monitoring methods and diagnostic criteria may have changed, making it difficult to combine data that was collected some time ago with data that was collected more recently. Historical cohort studies tend to be used more commonly in occupational

studies than in environmental studies because employment records can be used to identify the cohorts and industrial monitoring data can often be used to estimate historical
exposures. Equivalent information is rarely available for the general population.

6.2.5.3 Strengths and limitations

The cohort study design is generally regarded as the most definitive of the observational
study designs, because the investigators identify the study population and then follow the
causal events as they unfold from exposure until the development of the health outcome.
Exposure status is determined before the health outcome events occur. Therefore, knowledge of health outcome risk cannot influence how exposure is classified. The temporal
relationship between exposure and health outcome is clearly determined. This study
design also allows for the analysis of multiple health outcomes in relation to an exposure.

However, cohort studies are not commonly undertaken in environmental epidemiology because they can be expensive, especially if the latency period between exposure and
the health outcome occurrence is lengthy. Furthermore, cohort studies can be inefficient
if the health outcome is rare. This is because the study population would have to be very
large in order for a sufficient number of outcome events to occur.

Although long-term cohort studies can be expensive and difficult to conduct, they
may be justified if evidence strongly suggests that a chronic health effect is associated
with an environmental exposure. For example, as previously mentioned, Dockery *et al.*
[44] evaluated the effects of air pollution on mortality for a 14- to 16-year follow-up
period, and in so doing demonstrated associations between fine particulate air pollution
and mortality. Their study was prompted by ecological and time-series studies that had
previously indicated such an association on a cross-sectional basis.

6.2.6 Experimental studies

Experimental studies differ fundamentally from observational studies in that the investigators or some other external agent (e.g., a governmental agency) determine who will be
exposed. Experimental studies are not common in environmental epidemiology because
most exposures that are of interest are potentially detrimental, rather than beneficial.
A *controlled human exposure* study can be undertaken to measure the effects of a potentially toxic substance on human subjects. However, such studies are generally considered
to be clinical rather than epidemiological studies as they typically take place in medical
research facilities, and include relatively few subjects.

Randomized controlled trials are experimental studies that are undertaken to evaluate a
new preventive or therapeutic regimen. Subjects who already have a disease or who are at
high risk of developing a disease are randomly allocated to groups which are then assigned
different treatments. Another group—the comparison group—receives no treatment or
an already standard treatment. After treatment, the groups are followed to determine
whether the experimental treatment affects the health outcome over time. Field trials are
similar to randomized controlled trials, but they involve disease-free persons who are
selected from a community and studied 'in the field' rather than in a hospital.

Randomized trials and field trials have been used to assess the value of new therapies in treating or preventing diseases of environmental origin. For example, Morgan *et al.* [52] enrolled more than 900 children 5 to 11 years of age with atopic asthma in seven large US cities in a randomized, control trial of environmental interventions. They recruited the children through medical clinics and emergency rooms. Following a baseline evaluation, the children were randomly assigned to either a control group or intervention group. The intervention included caretaker education and remediation for exposure to both aeroallergens and environmental tobacco smoke. During the subsequent year, the intervention group had fewer days with symptoms, and greater declines in the levels of allergens at home, compared to the control group. As another example, Rico, Rosado and colleagues [53, 54] enrolled 602 students in nine elementary school that were located near a medal foundry in Mexico. The students were randomly assigned to one of an iron, zinc, both, or placebo supplementation group, which was then followed for 6 months to evaluate effects on nutritional status and blood lead concentration. They found that iron supplementation improved iron status but did not reduce blood lead concentration. Blood lead decreased significantly in all groups, probably due a general decrease in lead pollution in the area, but was not significantly different across the groups – which demonstrates the value of having a placebo (nontreatment) control group in a randomized trial. Similarly, vaccination trials have been used to assess the efficacy of new vaccinations in preventing communicable diseases.

Environmental interventions are often applied to groups of subjects or communities. A *community trial*, in which communities rather than individuals are randomized for the intervention, may therefore be more appropriate. Community trials have included studies of communities to compare the effectiveness of different types of sewage treatment and water chlorination in preventing diarrheal disease, and of the addition of different fluorine concentrations to drinking-water supplies to prevent dental caries. A study of children living in New York in communities that were served by water supplies to which sodium fluoride had been added is a classical example of this approach [55]. The study observed a substantial decrease in the incidence of decayed, missing and filled (DMF) teeth among children in the treated community during the ten years following the onset of water treatment (see Table 6.4). For example, children 6–9 years of age living in Newburgh (fluoride-treated water supply) had 58 percent fewer DMF teeth than children living in Kingston, which did not have fluoride treated water.

Many community trials in environmental epidemiology do not include control communities, but they can still provide useful data on the potential benefits of interventions. The effectiveness of the intervention is evaluated by comparing community rates of health outcomes during the periods before and after the intervention. For example, Antó *et al.* [56] evaluated the effect of installing dust-control filters on silos in Barcelona, Spain, to reduce soybean dust released during the unloading of ships. They compared the number of visits to hospitals for asthma, intensive care admissions for asthma, and mean soybean serum IgE antibody concentrations in asthma patients for 60 months before and after installation of the filters, finding significant improvements in these health outcome

Table 6.4 Permanent teeth decayed, missing, or filled (DMF) per 100 children, ages 6–16, based on clinical and X-ray examination ten years after start of fluoridation — New York

| Age | Number of children | | DMF teeth per 100 children | | |
	Newburgh (treated)*	Kingston (comparison)	Newburgh (treated)*	Kingston (comparison)	% difference (N–K)/K*100
6–9	708	913	98	234	−58
10–12	521	640	328	699	−53
13–14	263	441	610	1170	−48
15–16	109	119	975	1649	−41

* Sodium fluoride was added to Newburgh's water supply.

Adapted from [53]. Reproduced with permission from Ast DB, Schlesinger ER. The conclusion of a ten-year study of water fluoridation. *American Journal of Public Health and the Nation's Health*. 1956 46(3):265–71.

measures following the intervention. Similarly, Clancy *et al.* [57] examined the standardized non-trauma, respiratory and cardiovascular mortality rates for 72 months before and after the ban of coal sales in Dublin, Ireland. They found that respiratory and cardiovascular mortality rates decreased more than the change in non-trauma (control outcome) mortality rates coincident with the ban on coal sales. Hedley *et al.* [58] examined the trend in deaths during a five-year period following restrictions on sulphur content of fill in Hong Kong. They demonstrated a significant decline in all deaths, especially respiratory and cardiovascular deaths, following the intervention. None of these studies had control groups, but they still provided evidence that the city-wide environmental interventions had beneficial effects.

6.2.6.1 Design of experimental studies

The essence of an experimental strategy consists in selecting two or more groups of participants randomly so that they are as comparable as possible. The exposure to the factor under study is then assigned to one of the groups, but not to the other (the comparison group), and the health outcomes for the groups then compared. As mentioned above, sometimes it is not feasible in a community intervention to have a formal control group, but it can still be helpful for the investigators to identify a comparison community that will not receive the intervention to help evaluate the effect of the intervention by comparing the patterns of health outcome occurrence in the two communities before and after the intervention. The steps of a formal experimental study are:

- identify a sampling frame, such as a roster of patients in a clinic;
- select potential participants based on explicit eligibility criteria;
- request the persons' participation in the study;
- randomly allocate the consenting, eligible participants into groups.

Random allocation or *randomization* of subjects is a key feature of a well-designed experimental study, although as previously mentioned some environmental studies are not able to randomize interventions across entire communities. The study groups must be as comparable as possible with respect to any factor that could influence the health outcomes. Random allocation is undertaken to minimize the potential for confounding or selection bias. Many techniques have been recommended for performing random allocation. Random number tables, for example, can be used to ensure that treatment assignment is random and not influenced by the subjects or investigators.

Once the study groups have been allocated, the experimental intervention is administered to one or more of them. If observation bias is to be minimized, neither subjects nor observers should know who receives the intervention. Subjects and observers should therefore be '*blinded*' with respect to the subjects' treatment status. In studies of clinical treatment or preventive regimens, subjects in the comparison group are commonly given a placebo which appears to be identical to the active treatment. Similarly, in experimental studies of environmental exposures, participants may not be informed as to when the experimental exposure will occur. Thus in experimental studies of indoor air pollution, investigators have manipulated the ventilation rate and amount of fresh air supplied to office buildings and requested the subjects to record their symptoms and health complaints in daily diaries [59, 60]. The participants did not know when the ventilation rates would be changed, which meant that this information could not influence their tendency to report symptoms.

An intervention is typically administered for a fixed period of time and the subjects or communities then followed to determine health outcome status. The methods for following up the study groups of experimental studies are similar to those used for following up the study groups of cohort studies.

A *cross-over design*, in which each subject serves both in the exposed group (at times of intervention) and the unexposed group (at other times), can also be applied in experimental studies. The health outcome status of each participant is compared during the exposed and unexposed periods. This was the approach taken in the aforementioned indoor air studies [59, 60]. Its advantage is that each participant serves as his or her own comparison, thereby minimizing the potential for confounding due to noncomparability. However, this approach can only be used effectively for studying rapidly reversible health effects with clear temporal relationships to the putative exposure. As with the indoor air studies, the crossover design can be useful for studying symptoms and subjective conditions, provided that participants record symptoms while they are blinded to their exposure status.

6.2.6.2 Strengths and limitations

Experimental studies are the most definitive study design since the investigators or some other external agent assigns the exposure. Experimental studies also make it possible to evaluate the effect of dose and study temporal relationships since exposure or treatment is assigned. However, individual experimental studies are limited in that they can be used only for the study of short-term, reversible effects of potentially harmful exposures, or of treatment, or of preventive interventions. Also, experimental studies require follow-up, so they share some of the limitations of cohort studies, namely, potentially high cost and loss to follow-up.

The community trial is an effective experimental study design if the problem to be studied could be affected by community-level intervention. Community trials raise some concerns, however. In common with ecological studies, it is not possible to determine whether group-level associations reflect individual-level effects accurately. Ethical issues of informed consent must also be considered before undertaking a community trial; requesting permission to administer the treatment from each community member is not always feasible. Finally, as individuals living in the same community tend to be relatively homogeneous, care should be taken to ensure that the statistical analysis of a community trial is adjusted for correlation within groups.

6.3 **Strategy in choosing a study design**

In order to choose an appropriate study design, the investigators must appreciate the relative strengths and limitations of the various study designs, which are discussed in Section 6.2, for each of the major types of study designs. After evaluating the strengths and limitations of the study design options, the investigators must consider several other factors before choosing a study design. These include the purpose of the study, the extent of exposure, the nature and frequency of the disease occurrence, and the availability of existing records of exposure and health outcome occurrence. Often the main determinants are the funding and feasibility of conducting a study, so investigators are rarely able to choose only the theoretically optimal study design, but rather they must consider study designs and methods that can address an issue within the constraints of funding and feasibility.

Descriptive studies are chosen when the purpose is to explore unknown but potential cause–effect relationships for the purpose of generating hypotheses. They are also used to quantify environmental health impacts when investigating known cause–effect relationships.

Analytic studies are often motivated by concern about specific environmental factors or disease occurrence. The investigator can use a cohort design if the motivation for the study is 'exposure-oriented' and a case-control design if it is 'disease-oriented', although the association between an exposure and disease occurrence can be evaluated using either study design. If the association between a specific environmental exposure and the occurrence of multiple diseases is being examined, a cohort design is appropriate, but if the association between a specific disease and multiple environmental exposures is being examined, a case-control design would be preferable.

If an analytical study design is favored, an exploratory analysis using existing records to develop more focused hypotheses can be undertaken. Indeed, a series of studies is often needed to refine and evaluate hypotheses about the role of environmental factors in disease occurrence. Investigators generally begin with ecological or cross-sectional studies before considering cohort or case-control studies. An example is the series of studies undertaken to determine the cause of asthma in Barcelona, Spain, which began with asthma outbreak investigations and eventually led to a community intervention study [55, 61, 62].

When evaluating the incidence of a health outcome, use of a case-control design to sample from the source population is usually more efficient than use of a cohort design to examine the entire source population. Sources of bias can prove harder to identify if a case-control strategy is used, but for many environmental studies, the overall effect of potential bias may not be greatly different between cohort and case-control designs. Environmental exposures commonly occur among dynamic populations. Therefore, a case-control study which samples from the experience of a dynamic population may be as feasible as a cohort design, for which identifying the exact source population would also be difficult because there is no readily available sampling frame.

The incidence rate of virtually all diseases in populations tends to be rare, so a case-control design is generally an efficient strategy. However, such a strategy may be ineffective if the exposure prevalence is also rare in the same population. There are three primary strategies for assessing the effects of *rare* exposures on *rare* health outcomes.

One option is to conduct a study with a very large source population. However, this approach is feasible only if existing databases can be used because the cost of obtaining new data on a very large study population would be prohibitive. Unfortunately, few datasets exist that include adequate information on both exposure and disease occurrence among appropriate populations. Studies based on very large populations can be conducted in countries that have excellent record linkage systems, although relatively few countries have such systems. Most commonly, use of existing data requires an ecological analysis.

An alternative strategy to study the effects of a low prevalent exposure on a rare health outcome would be to undertake a case-control study using a very large study population, but this would only be worthwhile if gathering of information on exposure status from the study participants was inexpensive. This approach is not used frequently because of the importance of obtaining valid measures of exposure, which generally require direct environmental or biological sampling, and tend to be expensive.

A third strategy would involve restricting the study population to a 'high-risk' population, that is, a population with a high proportion of exposed persons or high levels of exposure, or a population of individuals of greater susceptibility. However, this approach may limit the generalizability of the findings because the high risk population may not be representative of the general population.

A cohort study design can be an efficient means of evaluating the effect of a rare exposure, but this design is inefficient in ascertaining rare disease occurrence. Therefore, it is becoming increasingly common for investigators to combine the potential benefits of cohort and case-control studies by conducting nested case-control analyses within cohort studies. This approach is feasible because it is possible to collect and store many biological and environmental specimens for future analysis. Therefore, specimens can be collected on the whole cohort, but expensive laboratory analyses of these specimens can be conducted only on a subsample of cases and controls.

As with the nested case-control study, many variations of classical epidemiological study designs have developed over time as investigators have attempted to balance considerations of cost, feasibility, and validity to identify the appropriate study design and methods for an epidemiological study. It is important to understand the relevance, strengths and limitations of the various study design in order to select the most appropriate study design to address an environmental health issue.

6.4 **References**

[1] Künzli N, Tager IB. The semi-individual study in air pollution epidemiology: a valid design as compared to ecologic studies. *Environmental Health Perspectives.* 1997 **105**(10):1078–83.

[2] Beaglehole R, Bonita R, Kjellström T. *Basic epidemiology.* Geneva: World Health Organization 1993.

[3] Devesa SS. *Atlas of cancer mortality in the United States, 1950–9.* Bethesda, MD: National Institutes of Health, National Cancer Institute, 1999.

[4] Forman D, Burley VJ. Gastric cancer: global pattern of the disease and an overview of environmental risk factors. *Best Practice and Research.* 2006; **20**(4):633–49.

[5] Carlsen E, Giwercman A, Keiding N, Skakkebaek NE. Evidence for decreasing quality of semen during past 50 years. *BMJ (Clinical Research edn).* 1992 **305**(6854):609–13.

[6] Parkin DM, Khlat M. Studies of cancer in migrants: rationale and methodology. *Eur J Cancer.* 1996 **32A**(5):761–71.

[7] Parkin DM, Iscovich J. Risk of cancer in migrants and their descendants in Israel: II. Carcinomas and germ-cell tumours. *International Journal of Cancer.* 1997 **70**(6):654–60.

[8] Evrard AS, Hemon D, Billon S, Laurier D, Jougla E, Tirmarche M, *et al.* Ecological association between indoor radon concentration and childhood leukaemia incidence in France, 1990–1998. *Eur J Cancer Prev.* 2005 **14**(2):147–57.

[9] John EM, Phipps AI, Davis A, Koo J. Migration history, acculturation, and breast cancer risk in Hispanic women. *Cancer Epidemiol Biomarkers Prev.* 2005 **14**(12):2905–13.

[10] Pang JW, Cook LS, Schwartz SM, Weis NS. Incidence of leukemia in Asian migrants to the United States and their descendants. *Cancer Causes Control.* 2002 **13**(9):791–5.

[11] Gushulak B. Healthier on arrival? Further insight into the "healthy immigrant effect". *Cmaj.* 2007 **176**(10):1439–40.

[12] Montana E, Etzel RA, Allan T, Horgan TE, Dearborn DG. Environmental risk factors associated with pediatric idiopathic pulmonary hemorrhage and hemosiderosis in a Cleveland community. *Pediatrics.* 1997 **99**(1):E5.

[13] Habiba A. Acute idiopathic pulmonary hemorrhage in infancy: case report and review of the literature. *Journal of Paediatrics and Child Health.* 2005 **41**(9–10):532–3.

[14] Chen CJ, Wang CJ. Ecological correlation between arsenic level in well water and age-adjusted mortality from malignant neoplasms. **Cancer Res.** 1990 **50**(17):5470–4.

[15] Lin RT, Takahashi K, Karjalainen A, Hoshuyama T, Wilson D, Kameda T, *et al.* Ecological association between asbestos-related diseases and historical asbestos consumption: an international analysis. *Lancet.* 2007 **369**(9564):844–9.

[16] Khanjani N, English DR, Sim MR. An ecological study of organochlorine pesticides and breast cancer in rural Victoria, Australia. *Archives of Environmental Contamination and Toxicology.* 2006 **50**(3):452–61.

[17] Coyle YM, Hynan LS, Euhus DM, Minhajuddin AT. An ecological study of the association of environmental chemicals on breast cancer incidence in Texas. *Breast Cancer Research and Treatment.* 2005 **92**(2):107–14.

[18] Kouznetsova M, Huang X, Ma J, Lessner L, Carpenter DO. Increased rate of hospitalization for diabetes and residential proximity of hazardous waste sites. *Environmental Health Perspectives.* 2007 **115**(1):75–9.

[19] Bernard A, Carbonnelle S, de Burbure C, Michel O, Nickmilder M. Chlorinated pool attendance, atopy, and the risk of asthma during childhood. *Environmental Health Perspectives.* 2006 **114**(10):1567–73.

[20] Nickmilder M, Bernard A. Ecological association between childhood asthma and availability of indoor chlorinated swimming pools in Europe. *Occupational and Environmental Medicine.* 2007 **64**(1):37–46.

[21] Morgenstern H. Ecologic studies. In: Gail MH, Benichou J, eds. *Encyclopedia of epidemiologic methods.* Chichester and New York: Wiley 2000: xxi, 978.

[22] Greenland S, Morgenstern H. Ecological bias, confounding, and effect modification. *Int J Epidemiol.* 1989 **18**(1):269–74.

[23] Arif AA, Shah SM. Association between personal exposure to volatile organic compounds and asthma among US adult population. *International Archives of Occupational and Environmental Health.* 2007 **80**(8):711–19.

[24] Wright JM, Schwartz J, Dockery DW. Effect of trihalomethane exposure on fetal development. *Occupational and Environmental Medicine.* 2003 **60**(3):173–80.

[25] Fujino Y, Guo X, Shirane K, Liu J, Wu K, Miyatake M, *et al.* Arsenic in drinking water and peripheral nerve conduction velocity among residents of a chronically arsenic-affected area in Inner Mongolia. *Journal of Epidemiology / Japan Epidemiological Association.* 2006 **16**(5):207–13.

[26] Behrens T, Maziak W, Weiland SK, Rzehak P, Siebert E, Keil U. Symptoms of asthma and the home environment. The ISAAC I and III cross-sectional surveys in Munster, Germany. *International Archives of Allergy and Immunology.* 2005 **137**(1):53–61.

[27] von Ehrenstein OS, Poddar S, Yuan Y, Mazumder DG, Eskenazi B, Basu A, *et al.* Children's intellectual function in relation to arsenic exposure. *Epidemiology (Cambridge, Mass).* 2007 **18**(1):44–51.

[28] Carta P, Flore C, Alinovi R, Ibba A, Tocco MG, Aru G, *et al.* Sub-clinical neurobehavioral abnormalities associated with low level of mercury exposure through fish consumption. *Neurotoxicology.* 2003 **24**(4–5):617–23.

[29] Yokoo EM, Valente JG, Grattan L, Schmidt SL, Platt I, Silbergeld EK. Low level methylmercury exposure affects neuropsychological function in adults. *Environ Health.* 2003 **2**(1):8.

[30] Krewski D, Lubin JH, Zielinski JM, Alavanja M, Catalan VS, Field RW, *et al.* A combined analysis of North American case-control studies of residential radon and lung cancer. *J Toxicol Environ Health A.* 2006 **69**(7):533–97.

[31] Provost D, Chantagrel A, Lebailly P, Jaffre A, Loyant V, Loiseau H, *et al.* Brain tumors and exposure to pesticides: a case-control study in southwestern France. *Occupational and Environmental Medicine.* 2007 **64**(8): 509–14.

[32] Weihkopf T, Becker N, Nieters A, Mester B, Deeg E, Elsner G, *et al.* Sun exposure and malignant lymphoma: a population-based case-control study in Germany. *International Journal of Cancer.* 2007 **120**(11):2445–51.

[33] Pesch B, Ranft U, Jakubis P, Nieuwenhuijsen MJ, Hergemoller A, Unfried K, *et al.* Environmental arsenic exposure from a coal-burning power plant as a potential risk factor for nonmelanoma skin carcinoma: results from a case-control study in the district of Prievidza, Slovakia. *Am J Epidemiol.* 2002 **155**(9):798–809.

[34] Pan XL, Day HW, Wang W, Beckett LA, Schenker MB. Residential proximity to naturally occurring asbestos and mesothelioma risk in California. *American Journal of Respiratory and Critical Care Medicine.* 2005 **172**(8):1019–25.

[35] Goldberg SJ, Lebowitz MD, Graver EJ, Hicks S. An association of human congenital cardiac malformations and drinking water contaminants. *J Am Coll Cardiol.* 1990 **16**(1):155–64.

[36] Tonne C, Melly S, Mittleman M, Coull B, Goldberg R, Schwartz J. A case-control analysis of exposure to traffic and acute myocardial infarction. *Environmental Health Perspectives*. 2007 **115**(1):53–7.

[37] Lu Y, Zeger SL. On the equivalence of case-crossover and time series methods in environmental epidemiology. *Biostatistics (Oxford, England)*. 2007 **8**(2):337–44.

[38] Künzli N, Schindler C. Case-crossover studies. *Epidemiology (Cambridge, MA)*. 2005 **16**(4):592–3.

[39] Zanobetti A, Schwartz J. The effect of particulate air pollution on emergency admissions for myocardial infarction: a multicity case-crossover analysis. *Environmental Health Perspectives*. 2005 **113**(8):978–82.

[40] Yamazaki S, Nitta H, Ono M, Green J, Fukuhara S. Intracerebral hemorrhage associated with hourly concentration of ambient particulate matter: case-crossover analysis. *Occupational and Environmental Medicine*. 2007 **64**(1):17–24.

[41] Peters A, von Klot S, Heier M, Trentinaglia I, Hormann A, Wichmann HE, *et al.* Exposure to traffic and the onset of myocardial infarction. *The New England Journal of Medicine*. 2004 **351**(17):1721–30.

[42] **Bertazzi PA, Zocchetti C, Pesatori AC, Guercilena S, Sanarico M, Radice L.** Ten-year mortality study of the population involved in the Seveso incident in 1976. *Am J Epidemiol* 1989 **129**(6): 1187–200.

[43] **Bertazzi PA, Pesatori AC, Zocchetti C.** The Seveso accident. In: Elliott P, Cuzick J, English O, Stern R, (eds.) *Geographical and environmental epidemiology: methods for small-area studies*. Oxford: Oxford University Press, 1992:342–58.

[44] Dockery DW, Pope CA, 3rd, Xu X, Spengler JD, Ware JH, Fay ME, *et al.* An association between air pollution and mortality in six U.S. cities. *The New England Journal of Medicine*. 1993 **329**(24):1753–9.

[45] Laden F, Neas LM, Dockery DW, Schwartz J. Association of fine particulate matter from different sources with daily mortality in six U.S. cities. *Environmental Health Perspectives*. 2000 **108**(10):941–7.

[46] Gold DR, Burge HA, Carey V, Milton DK, Platts-Mills T, Weiss ST. Predictors of repeated wheeze in the first year of life: the relative roles of cockroach, birth weight, acute lower respiratory illness, and maternal smoking. *American Journal of Respiratory and Critical Care Medicine*. 1999 **160**(1):227–36.

[47] Ly NP, Rifas-Shiman SL, Litonjua AA, Tzianabos AO, Schaub B, Ruiz-Perez B, *et al.* Cord blood cytokines and acute lower respiratory illnesses in the first year of life. *Pediatrics*. 2007 **119**(1):e171–8.

[48] Gauderman WJ, Avol E, Gilliland F, Vora H, Thomas D, Berhane K, *et al.* The effect of air pollution on lung development from 10 to 18 years of age. *The New England Journal of Medicine*. 2004 **351**(11):1057–67.

[49] Bellinger DC, Stiles KM, Needleman HL. Low-level lead exposure, intelligence and academic achievement: a long-term follow-up study. *Pediatrics*. 1992 **90**(6):855–61.

[50] Debes F, Budtz-Jorgensen E, Weihe P, White RF, Grandjean P. Impact of prenatal methylmercury exposure on neurobehavioral function at age 14 years. *Neurotoxicology and Teratology*. 2006 **28**(5):536–47.

[51] Grandjean P, Weihe P, Jorgensen PJ, Clarkson T, Cernichiari E, Videro T. Impact of maternal seafood diet on fetal exposure to mercury, selenium, and lead. *Archives of Environmental Health*. 1992 **47**(3):185–95.

[52] Morgan WJ, Crain EF, Gruchalla RS, O'Connor GT, Kattan M, Evans R, 3rd, *et al.* Results of a home-based environmental intervention among urban children with asthma. *The New England Journal of Medicine*. 2004 **351**(11):1068–80.

[53] Rico JA, Kordas K, Lopez P, Rosado JL, Vargas GG, Ronquillo D, *et al.* Efficacy of iron and/or zinc supplementation on cognitive performance of lead-exposed Mexican schoolchildren: a random-ized, placebo-controlled trial. *Pediatrics.* 2006 **117**(3):e518–27.

[54] Rosado JL, Lopez P, Kordas K, Garcia-Vargas G, Ronquillo D, Alatorre J, *et al.* Iron and/or zinc supplementation did not reduce blood lead concentrations in children in a randomized, placebo-controlled trial. *The Journal of Nutrition.* 2006 **136**(9):2378–83.

[55] Ast DB, Schlesinger ER. The conclusion of a ten-year study of water fluoridation. *American Journal of Public Health and the Nation's Health.* 1956 **46**(3):265–71.

[56] Antó; J, Sunyer J, Reed C, Sabria J, Martinez F, Morell F, *et al.* Preventing asthma epidemics due to soybeans by dust-control measures. *The New England Journal of Medicine.* 1993 **329**:1760–3.

[57] Clancy L, Goodman P, Sinclair H, Dockery DW. Effect of air-pollution control on death rates in Dublin, Ireland: an intervention study. *Lancet.* 2002 **360**(9341):1210–14.

[58] Hedley AJ, Wong CM, Thach TQ, Ma S, Lam TH, Anderson HR. Cardiorespiratory and all-cause mortality after restrictions on sulphur content of fuel in Hong Kong: an intervention study. *Lancet.* 2002 **360**(9346):1646–52.

[59] Jaakkola JJ, Tuomaala P, Seppanen O. Air recirculation and sick building syndrome: a blinded crossover trial. *Am J Public Health.* 1994 **84**(3):422–8.

[60] Menzies R, Tamblyn R, Farant JP, Hanley J, Nunes F, Tamblyn R. The effect of varying levels of outdoor-air supply on the symptoms of sick building syndrome. *The New England Journal of Medicine.* 1993 **328**(12):821–7.

[61] Antó JM, Sunyer J. Epidemiologic studies of asthma epidemics in Barcelona. *Chest.* 1990 **98**(5 Suppl):185S-90S.

[62] Antó JM, Sunyer J, Rodriguez-Roisin R, Suarez-Cervera M, Vazquez L. Community outbreaks of asthma associated with inhalation of soybean dust. Toxicoepidemiological Committee. *The New England Journal of Medicine.* 1989 **320**(17):1097–102.

Chapter 7

Data analysis

Lianne Sheppard

7.1 Concepts of data analysis and hypothesis testing

Data analysis is the process of summarizing data and using it to gain insight or draw conclusions from a study. The goal of data analysis is to reveal the patterns of interest in the data, ideally without these patterns being clouded by bias or random error. There are multiple steps to data analyses, including data cleaning, descriptive analyses, inferential analyses, and sensitivity analyses. While every data analysis process should include some description, inferential analyses are typically the primary goal. Inferential analyses relate the sample (study population) to a source population. For many environmental epidemiological studies, this involves quantifying the size of the effect in the presence of random error. Not all errors are random, and statistical inference does not protect against systematic error, i.e., bias, in the data or the analysis. Systematic error must be addressed scientifically throughout the design and conduct of a study using appropriate study design and choice of study population, proper alignment of the statistical model with the study design, selection of suitable control variables to be incorporated into the analysis, quality control procedures, and data cleaning. Strategies to reduce systematic error, including confounding, at the study design stage were discussed in Chapter 6.

Data analysis can be descriptive or inferential, and most data analyses include both approaches. *Descriptive analysis* is an exploration of the data and the relationships found in it. It is useful as a preliminary step in all analyses, and can be the end goal of hypothesis-generating and descriptive studies. Sometimes the term '*exploratory data analysis*' is used instead. Descriptive analysis is used to understand the basic properties of each variable and patterns that appear in the data. It is always valuable to visualize the data. Not only does this process help to identify outliers, coding errors, and distributional forms for variables, but in some cases the primary study results are so obvious from the descriptive analyses alone that further analysis is not needed. A rule of thumb is that 90 percent of the results can be detected from the descriptive analyses 90 percent of the time. However, environmental exposures are typically low-level and may induce subtle effects, so environmental epidemiology is one discipline where this rarely holds.

Inferential analysis is intended to draw scientific inference about a particular contrast from a sample to a population. It provides a framework for the scientist to generalize beyond the data at hand. Tools for inferential analysis include hypothesis testing and estimation.

Analysis in practice is often confused between the descriptive and inferential goals. Often exploratory analysis is substituted for inferential analysis and then the results are reported as though an inferential analysis was done. This can overstate the research findings and result in a literature that becomes biased towards false positive results. This is particularly problematic in environmental epidemiology, where the effect sizes of interest may be small and of the same order as the bias due to model selection. There are two main approaches to addressing the multitude of potential models in analyses. One is to write down an analysis plan in advance with a limited number of *a priori* hypotheses. Analysis proceeds without restriction and includes testing of those hypotheses along with exploring of alternative models, checking the sensitivity of primary analyses to different assumptions, and screening of additional hypotheses. The written report from the analysis makes inferences based upon the *a priori* written hypotheses and incorporates a discussion of the more extensive analyses as sensitivity and supporting analyses. The second approach is to explicitly account for all possible models. With Bayesian model averaging the analyst puts a 'prior' probability on all models and then bases inference on the 'posterior' probability of the result.

The data analysis must be true to the study design and its goals at inception. As studies become more complex, it becomes more difficult to understand whether the analysis is properly aligned with the study design. Different statistical modeling choices will lead to different uses of the data and parameter interpretations. Particularly in environmental epidemiology where the exposure effect is typically small, subtle differences in the framing of models or changes in the choice of confounding variables can have a large impact on the parameter estimate and the ability to detect the effect of interest. Understanding key sources of variation in the data is one step in the process of determining the appropriateness of the statistical analysis. It is particularly important to understand the primary sources of variation for the exposure. For instance, how do the data vary over time, over space, within individuals, or between individuals? What sources of variation are important in this study design? Do the data as collected fix or collapse over one or more dimensions? How does one's ability to collect detailed information over these dimensions affect one's ability to capture the key sources of variation in the data? Exposure variation can be confounded differently at different levels of analysis. At some levels the ability to control for confounding may be so challenging that it is better to remove that source of variation from the results. This can be done by design or through modeling. For instance, seasonal variation is a major confounder in studies of the acute effect of air pollution on health outcomes. Time-series studies remove seasonal variation through inclusion of a smooth function of time in the model (see Chapter 8, Section 8.1). Case–crossover studies control for this source of confounding by design by restricting the time period in the referent set.

7.1.1 **Hypothesis testing and reporting**

Hypothesis testing is a form of inferential analysis. Hypothesis tests are framed in terms of a statistical model based upon an underlying probability model. The probability model is assumed to apply to the data and has parameters that are estimated using the data. Hypotheses are stated in terms of null and alternative values of the parameter of interest. The null value of the hypothesis is the value the investigator wants to disprove. Inference is based on a conditional probability, the probability that a statement about the parameter of interest is true, given the null hypothesis value of that parameter is correct. For example, suppose the null hypothesis is H_0: $\mu=0$. When testing the null hypothesis that an estimate of the mean μ is zero, the p-value is the conditional probability of observing a result as extreme or more extreme than the estimate. The conditional probability restricts attention to the probability distribution for the estimate that is centerd at the null hypothesis value for μ. When the p-value is smaller than the significance level of the test (α, often taken to be 0.05), then the hypothesis is rejected. When indeed the null hypothesis is true, the hypothesis has been falsely rejected and a Type I error has been committed. Significance levels are chosen to be low to limit the occurrences of Type I errors. Many introductory textbooks (e.g.,[1]) give details on statistical hypothesis testing.

Hypothesis testing is at the core of the scientific method because it sets out to disprove unsatisfactory hypotheses in favor of alternative, more satisfactory hypotheses. However, inference should not be based solely on significance testing. Hypothesis tests quantify results in the presence of random error, but do not address systematic error. Assessment of systematic error is a separate activity based on judgment. Statistically significant hypothesis tests are often interpreted as 'clinically significant'. The clinical significance or scientific meaning of results should be interpreted from understanding of the scientific context and not based on the statistical findings alone. Because the size of a difference that will be found to be statistically significant depends upon the sample size, it is possible to have statistically significant differences that are not scientifically meaningful, and vice versa.

Often the reporting of hypothesis test results is reduced to a binary quantity of significance vs nonsignificance based on whether the p-value is larger or smaller than the preselected significance level α. P-values depend upon three quantities: the sample size, the mean difference of the statistic from the null hypothesis value, and the variance of the statistic. All components of the p-value contain valuable information. When reporting results, the least informative result is the presence or absence of statistical significance. Reporting the p-value alone also hides information. The most informative result to report is the point estimate and a measure of its uncertainty, such as its confidence interval. Primary focus should be on the result thought to be least confounded. Interpretation of the study results should be put into the context of the magnitude and precision of the primary point estimate [2]. When studies find no difference, the magnitude and precision of the estimates will help distinguish null findings (failing to reject the null hypothesis with a confidence interval that is sufficiently wide that it includes many scientifically meaningful differences) from negative results (where in addition to failing to reject the null hypothesis, it is also possible to rule out meaningful effects).

7.2 Analysis planning

Initial planning of analyses has two major advantages: preservation of the inferential strength of the analysis and minimization of the effort that is required to conduct the analysis. An analysis plan is a description of the scientific objectives of the study, the data to be analyzed, and the data analysis approach. The process of creating the analysis plan ensures the investigative team thinks through the scientific and statistical issues of the analysis in advance. The inferential strength of the study is preserved when the primary and secondary *a priori* hypotheses are tested and reported as such. A pre-specified plan provides structure for presentation of the results and helps the investigator protect against the tendency to report the most statistically significant findings as the primary focus of the study interpretation. Finally, an analysis plan can save significant data analysis effort by limiting the objectives and clearly outlining the steps of the analysis, thus preventing extra effort that can result from analyses lacking a clear focus and direction.

Figure 7.1 shows a template for an analysis plan. It is often most practical to develop a separate analysis plan for each paper planned for a study. The plan includes a summary of the scientific justification and objectives of the study, a detailed list of testable statistical hypotheses, a description of the variables available, a detailed list of analyses to be conducted, dummy tables and figures, and administrative details. A good analysis plan has a thoughtful characterization of the study and the scientific question(s). General scientific ideas are stated and then translated into specific question(s) that can be tested with statistical analyses. An important step in the analysis plan is to frame statistical questions from scientific questions. The statistical questions are the hypothesis statements. Important features of the analysis are determined by testable hypotheses. The inferential analyses flow from the hypotheses, the study design, and the variables collected in the study. The types and roles of variables indicate which statistical tests should be chosen and the underlying assumptions needed for the selected test(s).

7.2.1 Further analysis planning details

One of the challenges investigators often face during analysis planning is the difficulty of limiting the research focus to a single primary hypothesis. Since the inferential strength of the study is weakened by an undisciplined approach to hypothesis testing and results reporting, prioritization of hypotheses during analysis planning is an important step. Each separate inferential analysis should be classified as hypothesis testing, hypothesis screening, or exploratory or hypothesis-generating. One or at most two analyses should be designated as the primary analyses and can be classified as hypothesis-testing analyses. When there are three or more related hypothesis tests to be conducted and none can be selected as primary, these analyses are hypothesis screening analyses. Often hypotheses for hypothesis screening analyses are more diffusely stated than for hypothesis

Title:

Brief background:

Objectives:

    Broad objective

    Specific objectives (specific aims)

Testable hypotheses:

Variables: Create a table with columns for

    Variable name

    Scientific meaning

    Use in the analysis (e.g., response, exposure, treatment, confounder, effect modifier)

    Measurement units or coding

    Type of data (e.g., binary, nominal, ordinal, count, continuous)

Other important features (may need multiple columns; e.g., missing data count or pattern,

    restricted range, limit of detection, recoding scheme)

Other Data and Study Details:

Statistical Analysis:

    Descriptive analyses

    Inferential analyses

    Sensitivity analyses

Other Considerations:

Skeleton Tables and Figures:

Plan of Action:

Roles, Responsibilities and Deadlines:

Revision History:

Fig. 7.1 Analysis plan template.

testing analyses. For instance, an investigator might ask which variables in a set of predictor variables are important to include in a regression model. Or, they might screen a range of exposure metrics to determine which one to report in an epidemiological study. Hypothesis screening analyses will have greater inferential strength when correction for multiple testing is used. A completely *exploratory* or *hypothesis-generating* analysis is one where there are no specific prior hypotheses and the investigator wants to just look at the data to see what they find. The term 'fishing' is often used for this type of analysis. Note that when there is a primary hypothesis with additional related analyses that the researchers wish to explore, these additional hypothesis tests can be conducted as sensitivity analyses when their primary purpose is to deepen the understanding of the primary hypothesis testing analysis. Primary interpretation of the results is based on the primary hypothesis testing analysis. The results of the sensitivity analysis are interpreted in the context of the primary hypothesis test and do not stand alone.

The definitions of hypothesis testing, hypothesis screening, and hypothesis generating or exploratory tests lie along a continuum indexed by the inferential strength of the analysis. Since the classical framework for hypothesis testing is designed for a single hypothesis to be tested from a single dataset, it is not well-suited to testing multiple hypotheses. Multiple testing increases the probability of rejecting the null hypothesis when it is true. The theory of hypothesis testing controls the Type I error (by choosing a small significance level) but does not eliminate it. Thus, because the overall Type I error increases as the number of tests increases, if one does enough analyses, one would expect to reject the null hypothesis even when it is true. The purpose of labeling each hypothesis in an analysis is to explicitly recognize the underlying continuum of inferential strength and encourage the analyst to address it in advance of the analysis. During the analysis planning stage, scientists are asked to 'place their bets' on one or two clearly stated prior hypotheses. When investigators are unwilling to do this (most often because they believe they don't know enough), the subsequent analyses should not be classified as hypothesis testing. This results in weaker inferential strength of the conclusions that can be drawn from the analyses.

Since investigators want to make the most out of all the time and effort that goes into collecting data, a single analysis plan can describe analyses for each degree of inferential strength. The primary scientific question(s) relating to the primary study objective would be categorized as hypothesis testing analyses. It is not unusual to have several alternate exposure or outcome variables that are also of scientific interest and could be listed as secondary objectives for a hypothesis screening or sensitivity analysis. Finally, there could be additional data collected that might show some interesting relationships, but where the investigators have no prior experience with which to base their hypotheses. Such analyses would fall into the exploratory category.

Often, the approach to actually carrying out each of the above types of analyses is identical. Namely, the analyst describes the data, makes a comparison, and follows this by computing a point estimate and confidence interval or test statistic that is compared to a reference distribution under a null hypothesis (often the default null hypothesis of no difference, or a mean of zero). The distinction between the types of analyses lies in the number of hypotheses tested and the case that can be made during study interpretation and discussion of the results. *Be careful not to overinterpret study results when there were no or too many prior hypotheses.* One of the main purposes of the analysis plan is to help researchers use their awareness of the pitfalls of multiple testing to prevent later overinterpretation of their study results.

7.2.2 Analysis plan example—Port Alberni, Canada

The following example will be used to demonstrate concepts discussed in this chapter, beginning with an analysis plan.

Background and introduction: In the late twentieth century research was showing associations between air pollution exposures and health effects. Policies were being put in place to regulate air pollutants because of adverse health effects. However, in 1991, Canada had no Federal or Provincial air quality objectives for inhalable particulate matter. Vedal and colleagues [3] collected cross-sectional data from school children from Port Alberni, Vancouver Island, to help inform Canadian policy.

Objectives: The goal of this study was to determine whether there is scientific information to suggest that Canadian regulatory policy for air pollution should be changed. The specific objective was to assess whether there was an association between particulate matter air pollution and respiratory health. Respiratory outcomes include symptoms, illness, and lung function. For this analysis, the investigators will concentrate on the symptom data.

Testable hypotheses: The primary hypothesis is to estimate the association between particulate matter (PM_{10}) and prevalence of wheeze on most days, and to test whether this estimate is different from zero. Estimates of interest will be adjusted for important confounding and precision variables, specifically race, gender, and parental smoking. Secondary analyses will also assess the prevalence of any symptoms, cough, congestion or phlegm lasting three months per year, occasional wheeze, wheeze with shortness of breath, and wheeze with play. Secondary analyses will further estimate effects for alternate exposure metrics, specifically total suspended particulate (TSP) and submicron particles.

Variables: The data indicated in Table 7.1 will be used in the analysis.

Other data and study specifics:

1. All school children in the Port Alberni area in grades 1 through 6 were invited to participate.
2. Exposure data were interpolated from annual averages of measurements made every 6 days from 13 sites using a distance-weighted average of the three sites closest to the subject's home and school. Subject-specific estimates were time-weighted averages of the school and home values.
3. Health outcomes were obtained from questionnaires administered to the child's parent or guardian between January and April 1989.

Statistical analysis

Exploratory analyses

1. Each variable will be checked for missing data and univariate statistics evaluated for reasonable ranges or frequencies. Categories for pollutant data summarization will be developed after examining pollutant distributions.
2. The association of potential confounders and pollution exposure will be evaluated. The analyst will use graphical displays (e.g., side-by-side box plots) and tables for categorical variables.
3. The analyst will produce descriptive tables characterizing the population by demographic features.
4. The analyst will assess the crude association symptoms and pollution by tabulating the prevalence in pollution categories.

Inferential analyses

1. – Primary analysis: Logistic regression for the 'wheeze on most days' outcome and PM_{10} entered linearly as the primary predictor. Adjustment variables include race, gender, parental smoking.

2. – Secondary analyses: Repeat the primary analysis using alternate outcome and exposure variables as listed in the testable hypotheses section.

3. – Residual analysis will be done for the primary analysis model. The analyst will plot squared standardized Pearson or deviance residuals versus fitted values (estimated probability) and plots of the effect of deleting separate covariate patterns on the values of the estimated coefficients [see 3]. Any large values from these plots will be investigated. If necessary, modifications will be made to the primary analysis and results compared. For instance, predictor variables may be transformed or identified points will be dropped. If the conclusions change significantly the details of this analysis will be reported. For instance, if dropped data lead to different conclusions and the investigators cannot find a good scientific reason to exclude data, both analyses will be reported; otherwise only one analysis will be reported (the original analysis if conclusions don't change, the new analysis *only if* the investigators have a scientifically defensible reason to drop data and note that in the methods section).

Sensitivity analyses

The two primary purposes of the sensitivity analyses will be to assess the adequacy of the confounding control by considering a different or richer confounding model and to determine whether there is any evidence that the pollution exposure effect should have a different functional form.

Confounding

1. All primary analyses will be evaluated to determine whether additional confounding terms are appropriate. In particular, the investigators will assess the additional contribution of age.

2. All primary analyses will be evaluated to determine whether other functional forms of the included confounders are appropriate. In this case most confounders are categorical, so this investigation will be very limited.

Assessment of the functional form of the exposure term

1. The analyst will assess the dose–response relationship of the pollutant variable by considering alternate functions, specifically a group linear model, and a general smooth function.

Other considerations: Use this section to discuss any other important issues that haven't been presented yet. Examples include a power analysis, or concerns related to missing data, measurement error, and changes in instrumentation over time.

Skeleton table and figures: Skeleton tables are like Tables 7.3 to 7.6—shown in section 7.3.5—with all titles, headings, captions, legends, reference lines, and labels, but no data. There are no skeleton figures for this example.

Plan of action: First conduct exploratory analysis, followed by any data cleaning and clarification. Then conduct inferential and sensitivity analyses.

Roles, responsibilities, and deadlines: Not applicable.

Revision history: None yet.

7.3 Data analysis process

The major steps to data analysis are to conduct descriptive, then inferential, then sensitivity analysis. Often integrated into the beginning of a data analysis is data cleaning – the process of verifying, validating, and correcting data in the dataset – since the initial descriptive analyses often identify additional data cleaning needs that were not identified prior to data analysis.

7.3.1 Descriptive analysis

Data analysis always begins with an exploratory or descriptive analysis. Each descriptive analysis has at least one purpose and at least one purpose should be listed in the analysis plan. The general purpose of the exploratory analysis is to gain appreciation for broad patterns in the data, and look for errors, outliers, or other data anomalies. There are a number of purposes for an exploratory data analysis. The first is to identify errors in the data that may inspire additional data cleaning. Errors can be due to particularly unusual measurements (such as out of range data) or unusual combinations of measurements. Problematic data (e.g., outliers) should be reviewed for accuracy and corrected as needed. Outliers should only be omitted from the data analysis if there is a well-founded scientific justification. Otherwise, their effect should be assessed during sensitivity analysis. A second purpose is to allow the data analyst to verify their understanding of the measurements. Third, identification of patterns of missing data is important preparation for later steps of the analysis. Fourth, description of the study population is often the main focus of the first table in a published paper and is yet another important goal of descriptive data analysis. A fifth reason is to verify assumptions that will be needed for planned inferential analyses. A sixth purpose of descriptive analysis is to identify important confounding variables. Identification of predictors or surrogates of the response are two additional purposes of the analysis. Finally descriptive analyses can be used to characterize the form of functional relationships.

Descriptive analyses include tabular and graphical summaries. Graphical univariate summaries include box plots and histograms. Bivariate displays include scatterplots and side-by-side box plots. Tables of statistics that include means and standard deviations or percent for categorical variables are routine. In any given setting, it may be informative to expand such tables to include other descriptive statistics (e.g., median, quartiles, deciles, range). In studies where there are multiple sources of variation (e.g., individuals, areas, time periods) summaries should be chosen to highlight the most pertinent source of variation relative to the study design and goals, as well as to give an overall appreciation of the relative sources of variation within and between the individuals, areas, and time periods. For instance, panel studies recruit a cohort of individuals and study them repeatedly over time (see Chapter 8, Section 8.2). Traditionally in this design panel

Table 7.1 Variables used in the analyses—Port Alberni study example

Variable name	Scientific meaning	Use in the analysis	Measurement units	Type of data	Other important features
id	Identification number	Label	NA	Nominal	
Male	Subject's sex	Confounder	0 = Female 1 = Male	Binary (nominal)	
Race	Subject's race	Confounder	1 = White 2 = Native American 3 = East Indian 4 = Asian 5 = Other	Categorical (nominal)	
Asthma	Current diagnosis of asthma	Possible precision or effect modifier	0 = No 1 = Yes	Binary (nominal)	
Msmoke	Mother smokes?	Possible confounder	0 = No 1 = Yes	Binary (nominal)	
Fsmoke	Father smokes?	Possible confounder	0 = No 1 = Yes	Binary (nominal)	
Age	Age of subject	Confounder	Year	Continuous	
Anysx	Presence of any symptoms	Outcome	0 = No 1 = Yes	Binary (nominal)	Includes any indication of cough, congestion, phlegm, and wheeze
Wmost	Wheeze on most days	Outcome	0 = No 1 = Yes	Binary (nominal)	
Wsob	Wheeze with shortness of breath	Outcome	0 = No 1 = Yes	Binary (nominal)	
Wplay	Wheeze with play	Outcome	0 = No 1 = Yes	Binary (nominal)	
Cof3	Cough 3 months per year	Outcome	0 = No 1 = Yes	Binary (nominal)	
Cong	Congestion 3 months per year	Outcome	0 = No 1 = Yes	Binary (nominal)	
TSP	Total suspended particulate	Exposure	$\mu g/m^3$	Continuous	Interpolated value
PM$_{10}$	Particles less than 10 microns in diameter	Exposure	$\mu g/m^3$	Continuous	Interpolated value
SUB	Submicron particles	Exposure	$\mu g/m^3$	Continuous	Interpolated value

members are all studied at the same time, but resource limitations often dictate that individuals are staggered over a long time period. Therefore it is possible to have exposure variation within and between panel members. Often the interpretation of interest will focus on the within-individual variation but the design and nature of the exposure may mean exposure is not identical for all subject-times.

Data description can reveal features of the data that may present technical statistical issues. Ideally the data are structured to allow the easiest analysis and most precise statistical inference with a reasonable sample size. Desirable features include equal information about all groups being investigated, the measure of response within each group has a nice symmetric distribution with no long tails or outliers, and there are no missing data. Descriptive analysis can identify potential problems that may inhibit sound scientific interpretation or limit the generalizability of the results. For instance certain missing data patterns can result in certain subgroups not being represented, thus restricting inference about those groups. Data description may suggest the possibility of less precise inference because of limited variation in exposure variables, or too much association between predictor variables. The analyses may also suggest that more sophisticated statistical methods are required because of data features such as repeated measurements on the same sampling unit (implying correlated responses), unequal variances across comparison groups, nonlinear effects and interactions.

Data description can also show complexities of the data that may affect interpretation of study results. For instance, nonlinear dose–response relationships can be discovered through descriptive or sensitivity analyses. Historically, epidemiologists would divide continuous predictor variables into categories and plot these as a function of outcome as a way of understanding dose–response relationships and allowing for nonlinear relationships. An alternative approach is smoothing. Smoothing and categorization are just different ways of putting covariates into a regression model. Categorization assumes the same effect for all members of the category and different effects for different categories. Modern computing and smoothing algorithms allow data analysts to do the same kinds of exploration of dose–response relationships but more flexibly by fitting smooth functions of continuous predictors and assessing their association with outcome. Some approaches to smoothing allow arbitrary relationships, while others are constrained (e.g., to be monotonic).

7.3.2 Inferential analysis

The next step in the data analysis process is to conduct an inferential analysis. Inferential analyses allow generalizations from the sample (study population) to the broader population by identifying and explaining associations, or discriminating between individuals and predicting new observations based on these features. In contrast to descriptive analyses, all inferential analyses are based on an underlying model. Models, such as regression models, are useful tools for simplifying reality. They allow the analyst to use data to make predictions and draw conclusions. With the exception of mechanistic models, many models are chosen because of their ease of use and interpretation, and not based on assumptions about the form of the underlying natural relationship.

Typically, environmental epidemiological studies address questions about the effects of environmental exposures. The goal of these studies is explanation. Interest centers on estimating the health effect of the environmental exposure in the absence of important sources of bias. Explanatory analyses are typically regression models and interest is in interpreting regression coefficients. For instance, the goal may be to draw inference about a particular environmental exposure that can explain some of the differences observed in the outcome. In this regression analysis, the health outcome is the dependent or outcome variable and the environmental exposure is the independent variable or predictor. An explanatory analysis can estimate the crude effect of exposure on the outcome using just those two variables, or it can estimate the adjusted effect by incorporating additional predictors to reduce bias and increase precision.

Regression underlies most epidemiological study analyses. Even simple one- or two-sample t-tests can be framed as regression models. Relative to early epidemiological tools for adjustment, such as the Mantel–Haenzel test, regression can be viewed as a more sophisticated approach to stratification that allows for more flexibility and the ability to use information more efficiently. The regression model provides a structure for combining information across strata. The model structure can provide useful simplification of the relationship between a predictor and the outcome, but if poorly understood or chosen, can impose structure not well suited to the data. The form of the regression (i.e., the transformation of the expected outcome), typically known as the model for the link function, varies by study design, but the basic framework still holds that an outcome is associated with one or more predictors. Typically a linear function (or more generally an additive function) is assumed on the exposure scale, and then the outcome is transformed with a link function to allow plausible patterns for the outcome scale.

A standard linear regression model is

$$Y_{ki} = \beta_0 + X_{ki}\beta_1 + \varepsilon_{ki}$$

Where Y_{ki} is the disease outcome, β_0 the intercept, X_{ki} the regression coefficient to be estimated, β_1 the exposure variable, and ε_{ki} the random error term.

Generalized linear models use more complex link functions than the identity link used for linear regression. For instance, a binary outcome can only take the values of 0 and 1, and its expected value (p) will range between 0 and 1. A linear model for this outcome will allow for values larger than 1 and smaller than 0. The logistic transformation of the expected value ($\log(p/(1-p))$) is typically used for binary regression by equating this to the linear predictor (a linear combination of covariates times parameters to be estimated). This form of the model constrains predicted values for p to be between 0 and 1.

Multiple regression refers to multiple predictors. *Multivariate models* typically refer to multiple correlated outcomes. Repeated outcome assessment on the same person over time, e.g., FEV_1, is an example of a multivariate outcome. Often these are addressed by expressing the outcome as a single measure at each time and incorporating a dependence model to allow for the correlation between repeat measures within the same person.

These concepts are used when fitting generalized estimating equation (GEE) or longitudinal data analysis models. The GEE model specifies the mean model (i.e., the regression model) and the dependence model separately. Many other multivariate models, such as random effects models, do not explicitly separate specification of the mean model from the dependence model.

Regression models most commonly used in epidemiology are linear, logistic, Poisson, and proportional hazards. Studies with continuous outcomes, such as cross-sectional or panel studies, rely on linear regression. Studies with binary outcomes, including case-control and case-crossover studies, use logistic regression. Poisson regression is used for studies with count outcomes, including air pollution time-series studies (see Chapter 8.1). Studies with time to event outcomes (also called survival outcomes) use survival analysis methods in large part so censoring of observations can be accommodated appropriately. Most often this is proportional hazards regression because this model makes no assumptions about the form of the baseline hazard function. With some loss of information, these data can also be recoded to binary data (e.g., five–year survival) and then analyzed using logistic regression.

In regression, it matters which variables are in the model since the other variables in the model influence the interpretation of the regression coefficient of interest. This means confounding variables must be chosen appropriately, measures of the outcome should not be included, and statistical significance of the candidate variables is not the most important criterion for model selection. It doesn't matter how predictive an association model is; there can be important predictions in an association model even though there is significant unexplained variation (i.e., small R^2 in a linear regression model).

Choice of confounders in an explanatory analysis should be based on scientific grounds rather than predictive ability. Statistical significance is not a reason to include or exclude confounding variables. Ideally models should adjust for confounding variables as richly as possible in order to remove residual confounding. A good practice is to fit and report three models for estimating the effect of an exposure. The first is the model with the exposure as the only predictor. (Due to small effect sizes and relatively larger confounding effects, this model may not be useful in environmental epidemiological investigations and is not always reported.) The second model also includes the full set of prespecified confounders according to current research experience. The final model includes an expanded set of confounding variables. Exposure effect estimates are reported for all three models so readers can see the effect of confounding control on the exposure estimate.

Models can be either confirmatory or exploratory. Confirmatory analyses attempt to answer the scientific question that the study was designed to address. Confirmatory analyses follow a detailed *a priori* protocol. The variables chosen to be in the model are specified in advance. This protects the interpretation of the *p*-values and the inferential strength of the study. In contrast, exploratory analyses make use of hard-won data to further understanding, explore relationships, and suggest additional hypotheses for study. The variables chosen to be in the model depend upon the relationships found in the data. Interpretation of exploratory analyses must be cautious because the results are likely to be overstated (e.g., the p-values are likely to be inflated). It is important to distinguish between the different goals of data analysis, particularly when writing up the results of the analysis. Interpretation of a confirmatory analysis can be strong, i.e., results can be stated to confirm or refute a prior hypothesis. A written analysis plan is a particularly important tool when confirmatory analysis is the goal.

7.3.3 Ecological and multi-level data

7.3.3.1 Ecological data

Studies with group-level information can be analyzed at the individual or group level. Sheppard [4] categorizes types of analyses based on the nature of the exposure data and how the outcome is incorporated into the analysis (see Table 7.2).

When the goal is to make inference about individuals, ecological studies have many possible sources of bias due to using group-level predictors and analysis. Ecological biases can be due to specification bias, between- and within-group confounding, contextual effects, lack of mutual standardization, measurement error, and effect modification [5]. The term ecological fallacy is a broad one that refers to the possibility of fallacious inference for effects on individuals. Semi-individual studies are nearly individual-level studies because most of the predictors and the outcome are available at the individual level. In such studies the predictor of interest (typically the exposure) is only available at the group level. For inference about exposure effects, semi-individual studies with nonlinear link functions can still suffer from specification bias. Individual-level studies do not suffer from biases specific to designs with limited individual-level information, but these analyses must incorporate predictors that can vary within and between groups, and also they must take into account the clustering that can occur due to shared outcomes, often as a result of effects on outcome that are not incorporated into the analysis. Two-stage and multilevel analysis approaches are most common. Two-stage analyses explicitly conduct the first stage analysis at the individual level, summarizing results for further analysis at the second stage. Multilevel analyses conduct the entire analysis in one step.

7.3.3.2 Multilevel modeling

Multilevel models incorporate predictors from multiple levels of observation into a single analysis. For studying the effects of environmental exposure, this often means

Table 7.2 Categorization of studies by exposure and outcome

		Exposure	
		Individual	Group
Disease summary/Analysis approach	Individual	Individual	Semi-individual
	Group	Aggregate	Ecological

inclusion of city or area-specific information in the analysis. The challenge in conducting such analyses is deciding how to incorporate information from multiple levels. Distinction is made between individual- and group-level predictors; sometimes both versions of a single predictor are included in the analysis. Blakely and Woodward [6] classify group-level variables as aggregate, contagion, environmental, structural, and global. An aggregate variable is the most common type. It is a group-level summary variable derived from information about individuals in the group and is well suited to being incorporated into a multilevel analysis. Mean income is an example of an aggregate variable. Environmental variables are properties of the environment that can be measured on the individual or group level. Annual average ambient air pollution concentration obtained from a single monitor is an example. It can be very helpful to view environmental variables as potentially measured at the individual level. Even when they aren't measured at the individual level, they can still be viewed as having an individual-level analog. For example, ambient air pollution measured only at a single location is an environmental variable that can be assumed to be representative of the group exposure. Also it can be viewed as an aggregate variable with measurement error and this is a helpful perspective in the analysis.

The basic multilevel model can be written in common regression notation. Suppose we have $I = 1,\ldots,I$ individuals in $k = 1,\ldots,K$ areas. Let X_{ki} represent exposures that vary with individuals and Y_{ki} represent the outcome. The notation allows both X and Y to vary both within and between groups. The standard regression model $Y_{ki} = \beta_0 + X_{ki}\beta_1 + \varepsilon_{ki}$ becomes a multilevel model when we allow β_0 and β_1 to vary by area (β_{0k} and β_{1k}). Using conventions followed by Diez-Roux [7], the multi-level (first stage) model is $Y_{ki} = \beta_{0k} + X_{ki}\beta_{1k} + \varepsilon_{ki}$. For the second stage we assume a model for β_{0k} and β_{1k}, specifically $\beta_{0k} = \gamma_{00} + \gamma_{01}G_k + u_{0k}$ for the intercept and $\beta_{1k} = \gamma_{10} + \gamma_{11}G_k + u_{1k}$ for the slope. We assume u_{0k}:$N(0,\tau_{00})$, u_{1k}:$N(0,\tau_{11})$, $cov(u_{0k}, u_{1k}) = \tau_{01}$, and G_k are group-level predictors that vary by area. The overall model has both systematic and random components and can be written all-together as

$$Y_{ki} = \beta_{0k} + X_{ki}\beta_{1k} + \varepsilon_{ki}$$

$$= \gamma_{00} + G_k\gamma_{01} + u_{0k} + X_{ki}(\gamma_{10} + G_k\gamma_{11} + u_{1k}) + \varepsilon_{ki} \qquad (0.1)$$

$$= \gamma_{00} + G_k\gamma_{01} + X_{ki}\gamma_{10} + G_kX_{ki}\gamma_{11} + u_{0k} + X_{ki}u_{1k} + \varepsilon_{ki}$$

Here all the terms involving γ summarize the systematic component, and all the remaining terms summarize the random component. The basic model can be extended to include confounders Z_{ki} in addition to exposures X_{ki}. Confounders can act at the between or within group level and control at the appropriate level is necessary to remove residual confounding.

Fitting multilevel models can be challenging both technically and with respect to interpretation. Using the multilevel model notation and fitting a full random effects model will produce a multilevel analysis. A stratified analysis eliminates all the separate random effects and fits a separate intercept (fixed effect) for each area. Fitting of intermediate versions of the full multilevel model is possible by eliminating components of the general model, such as removing variations across groups in the slope (either in the fixed or random effects, or both). Different approaches to the analysis give different interpretations of the exposure effect parameter γ_{10}. For instance, the stratified analysis gives an average of within-area slopes, while the random effects analysis also includes information from the relationship between areas in the slope estimate.

One strategy for fitting multilevel models with exposures that vary both between and within areas is to use mean-balanced predictors. Mean-balanced predictors are individual-level variables with mean 0 within an area. Using the above notation, a mean-balanced version of the exposure of interest would be $(X_{ki} - \bar{X}_k)$ where $\bar{X}_k$ is the arithmetic average of the exposure for area k. In general, multilevel models with mean-balanced predictors are preferable because they have more stable parameter estimates, are easier to interpret (because more predictors are orthogonal), and have better behavior of the random effects [8]. Furthermore, with incorporation of both the individual-level and group-level exposure in the analysis (preferably using a mean-balanced version for the reasons suggested above), the multilevel model can estimate the contextual effects of exposure, if present. Contextual effects are the effect of a group-level variable on an individual outcome. In formula 0.1 above, when G_k is replaced by $\bar{X}_k$, γ_{01} is a contextual effect. Contextual effects are not always of scientific interest, and in environmental epidemiology it is reasonable to assume there are no contextual effects. However, even when there are no hypothesized contextual effects, they may 'show up' because of uncontrolled individual-level confounding, uncontrolled area-level confounding, or exposure measurement error at the individual or group level. Thus it can be useful to incorporate them in the analysis, even if there are no hypothesized contextual effects.

Multilevel models are complex and many factors need to be considered in fitting them. The complexity includes all issues in ordinary observational studies, but now at multiple levels. In addition, multilevel analyses must also assess cross-level issues, including cross-level effects (e.g., contextual effects), cross-level confounding, and cross-level effect-modification. Exposure variation is crucial to being able to estimate exposure effects in multi-level studies. This feature should be considered at the design stage. In addition, variation of exposure both between and within areas should be reported as part of the descriptive analysis. The complexity of multilevel studies challenges researchers to think carefully about what their model is saying and what they want it to say.

7.3.4 Sensitivity analyses

Sensitivity analyses are 'what if' analyses of the study results where different assumptions are made or different analyses procedures are used. Their purpose is to determine whether the results are particularly sensitive to the 'what if' scenario. They allow the investigators to convince themselves that they trust the results of the inferential analyses. Sensitivity analyses include analyses that check underlying assumptions beyond those already conducted as part of the descriptive analyses. For instance, an analysis that is adjusted for age could evaluate the sensitivity of the primary results to a different approach to adjusting for age in the analysis. Sensitivity to single observations can be evaluated by removing them and re-running the analyses to see how much the results change. Sensitivity to adjustment for additional confounders can be determined by comparing the primary effect estimate from a new analysis with added confounders to the primary result. New conditions can also be evaluated, such as exploring whether there is any effect modification.

7.3.5 Cross-sectional data analysis example—Port Alberni data

Descriptive analyses: Most of the data in this study are categorical, so frequencies and percentages by category are the summaries of interest. The particulate matter exposures are continuous and their univariate distributions can be summarized using histograms. Because exposure was assigned using only a few monitor measurements over space, many subjects share similar exposure values. Thus the histograms are jagged and show higher frequencies concentrated at some values. There is also evidence of positively skewed exposures with much larger range in the top quartile of the data as compared to the lowest quartile (standard deviation of 7.1 vs 1.6 in the fourth versus first quartiles of PM_{10}). Table 7.3 gives the characteristics of study subjects for demographic features, exposure, and outcome variables. There are small differences between groups in PM exposure categories with relatively more minority children living in the highest pollution areas and slightly fewer males. Larger proportions of parents smoke in the higher pollution areas as compared to lower pollution areas. There is no evidence of differences in age distributions across exposure categories. As for outcome variables, the highest exposure category has the highest proportion of each outcome, with the exception of 'wheeze with play'.

Inferential analyses: Table 7.4 shows estimates of odds ratios and 95 percent confidence intervals for a 10 µg/m^3 increase in PM_{10} in both crude and adjusted analyses. These two analyses give nearly identical estimates. There is evidence of an increase in prevalence of wheeze with increased PM_{10} exposure. Residual analysis suggested the one Asian subject who wheezed was highly influential on the entire set of parameter estimates. Since the estimates for the Asian and the 'other' race categories were very similar, the investigators refit the models using the combined categories. This gave a result for the PM_{10} effect nearly identical to the original analysis, but with better residual behavior. Secondary analyses for TSP and submicron particles are shown in Tables 7.5 and 7.6.

Sensitivity analyses: Age was the only additional potential confounder and inclusion of it in the model did not change the exposure effect estimates. Assessment of the shape of the concentration–response model for the primary analysis of wheeze most days on PM_{10} suggested the linear concentration–response model was adequate.

Table 7.3 Characteristics of study subjects, exposures and outcomes according to quartile of PM_{10} exposure — Port Alberni study example

Characteristic	Quartile of PM_{10} concentration ($\mu g/m^3$)				Overall
Male gender (%)	53.7	51.9	47.3	46.8	49.9
Race (%)					
White	84.5	85.2	90.3	73.9	83.5
Native American	0.9	4.2	2.9	7.7	3.9
East Indian	9.3	5.7	3.1	11.5	7.4
Asian	0.9	1.3	0.6	1.8	1.1
Other	4.4	3.7	3.1	5.1	4.1
Age (year)	9.3 ± 1.8	9.4 ± 1.8	9.2 ± 1.8	9.4 ± 1.8	9.3 ± 1.8
Mother smokes? (%)	31.2	30.0	35.4	36.2	33.2
Father smokes? (%)	25.7	22.7	20.5	28.9	24.5
Any asthma? (%)	4.7	6.0	6.2	6.0	5.8
PM_{10} ($\mu g/m^3$)	16.3 ± 1.6	20.0 ± 0.8	23.2 ± 1.4	34.2 ± 4.2	23.4 ± 7.1
Wheeze most days? (%)	6.9	8.2	6.2	8.8	7.5
Any symptoms? (%)	37.2	43.1	40.5	43.7	41.1
Cough (%)	16.4	17.2	17.6	21.2	18.1
Congestion (%)	12.4	15.7	14.7	18.1	15.2
Wheeze w/SOB (%)	13.7	17.4	16.1	18.7	16.5
Wheeze w/play (%)	7.9	12.6	10.8	12.3	10.9

Table 7.4 Estimated odds ratios for prevalence outcomes associated with an exposure increase of 10 $\mu g/m^3$ of PM_{10} — Port Alberni study example

Outcome (%)	Number of cases (n = 2188)	Unadjusted	Adjusted*
Wheeze most days?	165	1.25 (1.01, 1.54)	1.25 (1.01, 1.55)
Any symptoms?	900	1.13 (1.00, 1.27)	1.13 (1.00, 1.28)
Cough	396	1.24 (1.07, 1.43)	1.24 (1.07, 1.44)
Congestion	333	1.24 (1.06, 1.45)	1.24 (1.06, 1.46)
Wheeze w/SOB	360	1.16 (0.99, 1.35)	1.16 (0.99, 1.35)
Wheeze w/play	238	1.22 (1.01, 1.46)	1.22 (1.01, 1.46)

*Adjusted for gender, race, parental smoking (both mother and father)

Table 7.5 Estimated odds ratios for prevalence outcomes associated with an exposure increase of 10 µg/m³ of TSP — Port Alberni study example

Outcome (%)	Number of cases (n = 2188)	Unadjusted	Adjusted*
Wheeze most days?	165	1.22 (1.03, 1.44)	1.22 (1.03, 1.45)
Any symptoms?	900	1.12 (1.01, 1.22)	1.12 (1.02, 1.23)
Cough	396	1.18 (1.05,1.33)	1.19 (1.05, 1.34)
Congestion	333	1.21 (1.06, 1.45)	1.21 (1.07, 1.38)
Wheeze w/SOB	360	1.13 (1.07, 1.28)	1.16 (1.02, 1.32)
Wheeze w/play	238	1.23 (1.07, 1.43)	1.24 (1.07, 1.44)

*Adjusted for gender, race, parental smoking (both mother and father)

Table 7.6 Estimated odds ratios for prevalence outcomes associated with an exposure increase of 10 µg/m³ of submicron particles — Port Alberni study example

Outcome (%)	Number of cases (n = 2188)	Unadjusted	Adjusted*
Wheeze most days?	165	1.32 (0.89, 1.97)	1.32 (0.88, 1.97)
Any symptoms?	900	1.15 (0.92, 1.43)	1.14 (0.92, 1.42)
Cough	396	1.43 (1.09, 1.89)	1.42 (1.07, 1.87)
Congestion	333	1.37 (1.02, 1.83)	1.35 (1.00, 1.82)
Wheeze w/SOB	360	1.23 (0.92, 1.63)	1.27 (0.95, 1.70)
Wheeze w/play	238	1.38 (0.99, 1.94)	1.39 (0.98, 1.96)

*Adjusted for gender, race, parental smoking (both mother and father)

7.4 Combining study results: meta-analysis of observational studies

Meta-analysis is combination of information from different sources: traditionally meta-analyses are of published studies. Most often these meta-analyses rely only on published data, but sometimes the authors are able to assemble and reanalyze the data from all the studies in a uniform fashion. Meta-analysis can also be done using new unpublished data to combine results from multiple cities or areas within a study. This use of meta-analysis techniques is becoming more common in environmental epidemiology [e.g., 9, 10]; these techniques avoid many of the challenges inherent in combining information from published studies.

Meta-analysis is the process of combining separate effect estimates from published data to produce an overall effect estimate and standard error. When using published data, a first step in such an analysis is a systematic review. From there the analyst determines whether there is consistency of the evidence. If this assessment suggests it is warranted, estimates from multiple studies are combined. While there is disagreement about the value of meta-analysis, many scientists believe it is a mechanism for objective appraisal of evidence and quantification of uncertainty. The combination of information from multiple studies increases power and allows subgroup analyses to be done that would be impossible within a single study. Heterogeneity between studies can be evaluated and it may be possible to find predictors of the heterogeneity (using a technique called meta-regression).

The systematic review is the process of assembling the evidence from the literature. Since a systematic review is data collection in its own right, it should follow a prespecified data collection protocol. The aims of the meta-analysis need to be clearly defined, the search process and criteria outlined, and the study inclusion criteria delineated. The information to be collected from each study must be specified and can be summarized using a data extraction table that lists each item to be extracted, including authors, study design, study population, sample size, major exposure and control variables, primary results (including effect estimates and their uncertainty), discussion of study quality, and comments on any other important features of the study. One difficulty with systematic reviews is assessing study quality, and determining the appropriate criteria for inclusion based on quality. It is also very difficult to incorporate information about quality into the analysis. For that reason, many authors emphasize that meta-analysis should focus more on description of results and investigation of uncertainty rather than on reporting overall estimates. For guidance on conducting systematic reviews, see the Cochrane collaboration (http://www.cochrane.org), the NHS Center for Reviews and Dissemination at the University of York (http://www.york. ac.uk/inst/crd/report4.htm) and various articles and textbooks [e.g., 11, 12, 13]. Meta-analysis is distinct from subgroup analysis [14]. Subgroup analysis compares results of stratified (i.e., separate) analyses for each subgroup. Such analyses should be interpreted as hypothesis-generating except when a very limited number of subgroup analyses are specified in advance.

Combining results of studies requires that the meta-analyst select an effect estimate. Common estimates are the relative risk, odds ratio, or risk difference. The analyst selects a fixed or random effects model for the meta-analysis. The fixed effect model assumes every study has the same constant underlying effect whereas the random effect model assumes the effect from each study comes from a distribution of underlying effects with a constant mean. The fixed effect model is the so-called pooled analysis that uses data as though they come from a single study [15]. Pooled analyses are only appropriate when there is no heterogeneity between studies. Assessment of heterogeneity of studies is done by assessing the assumption of a single constant effect for all studies using a chi-square test. It is generally advised to use a random effects model even if the chi-square test of homogeneity is not rejected. This advice is based on the low power of the chi-square test, along with the fact that often fixed and random effect estimates are different even when the chi-square test does not reject. Furthermore, the random effects model reduces to the fixed effect model when there is no between-study variation in effects.

For the random effects model there are several different approaches to estimation. No single approach is correct; each has its own features. The moment-based DerSimonian and Laird [16] approach is simplest to implement and doesn't require iteration. It also does not give an estimate of the uncertainty of the heterogeneity parameter. Maximum likelihood is used for estimation in the fixed effects model. In the random effects model, maximum likelihood makes the strong assumption that the heterogeneity parameter is known, so therefore the restricted maximum likelihood approach to estimation is preferred. This procedure is iterative, requiring reliance on statistical software. A fully Bayesian analysis also requires specialized software. It allows for additional parameter uncertainty through incorporation of prior distributions for all the parameters.

Many investigators argue that investigation of between-study heterogeneity is the most interesting feature of meta-analysis. In most meta-analyses, examination of sources of heterogeneity should be an exploratory objective [see, e.g., 17]. A *forest plot* is a simple graphical tool to display between study differences (see Figure 8.3). This plot gives the effect size and 95 percent confidence intervals drawn horizontally for each study listed vertically. The null hypothesis value is shown with a vertical line. The size of the boxes for the effect sizes are often scaled proportional to the inverse variance of the study estimate. The pooled estimate and 95 percent confidence interval is given at the bottom of the plot. An *influence plot* shows the square root of the study's weight (its inverse variance) versus the square root of its heterogeneity measure, i.e., its contribution to the chi-square test of homogeneity. Meta-regression is the process of investigating the heterogeneity between studies using study-level predictors in a regression model. Often this is called the second stage model. A simple linear regression model is assumed for the effect estimates with the overall effect estimate represented by the intercept and an explanatory variable represented as a predictor. A weighted regression model should be fit to preserve the weights of each study.

Study quality can affect the results of a meta-analysis. This could affect a subset of the studies or the collection of studies available for analysis. For instance, should unpublished studies or studies that have not been peer reviewed be included in the meta-analysis? Are researchers less likely to publish the results of their study when they are not statistically significant? What role do confounding and selection bias play in the published results? *Sensitivity analysis* and *funnel plots* are two tools that can be used to assess the impact of the studies included in the meta-analysis on the meta-analysis results. One or a few studies in a meta-analysis can be dropped in a sensitivity analysis to assess the robustness of the pooled effect estimate to differing assumptions about which studies belong in the population of studies. Publication bias due to failure to publish nonsignificant results can be assessed via a funnel plot. These plots depict the study-specific inverse standard error on the x axis vs the effect estimate on the y axis, both similarly transformed so the effect estimate is approximately normally distributed. A horizontal line is drawn at the pooled effect estimate. In the absence of publication bias, the population of studies should display a funnel shape with the top of the funnel aligned with larger variability in effect estimates between studies for smaller inverse standard errors. Systematic exclusion of studies with negative effect estimates will result in skewed funnel plots with a disproportionately large number of small studies with large positive effect sizes included. However, random variation, particularly when the number of studies is relatively small, can also result in a skewed appearance of these plots, so publication bias is not the only possible source of asymmetry. Methods are available to correct for publication bias, but these all rely on assumptions that are difficult to justify; a better approach is to report the evidence for bias without correction and to review the systematic review procedures critically.

7.5 **Finally**

This chapter described the various methods for data analyses in environmental epidemiology and laid out a systematic approach. Of course, there are other approaches and methods. The chapter did not go into great technical details of statistical analyses. The aim was to keep it accessible for non-statisticians. Future details can be found in the many statistical textbooks that exist. Furthermore, more and more environmental epidemiologists work in teams with statisticians because of the complexity of the statistical analyses, and rely on their expertise for the actual analyses. These types of collaborations are therefore essential for high-quality environmental epidemiological studies, and are very much encouraged, specifically by funding agencies.

7.6 **References**

[1] van Belle G, Fisher L, Heagerty P, Lumley T. *Biostatistics: a methodology for the health sciences, 2nd edn.* Hoboken, NJ: Wiley-Interscience 2004.

[2] Cummings P, Rivara FP, Koepsell TD. Writing informative abstracts for journal articles. *Arch Pediatr Adolesc Med.* 2004 **158**(11):1086–8.

[3] Vedal S, Blair J, Barid M. Adverse respiratory health effects of ambient inhalable particle exposure. *Air and Waste Management Association Annual Meeting preprint*, 1991, 91–180: 1–16.

[4] Hosmer DW, Lemeshow S. *Applied logistic regression, 2nd edn.* New York: Wiley 2000.

[5] Sheppard L. Insights on bias and information in group-level studies. *Biostatistics (Oxford, England).* 2003 **4**(2):265–78.

[6] Greenland S. Divergent biases in ecologic and individual-level studies. *Stat Med.* 1992 **11**(9):1209–23.

[7] Blakely TA, Woodward AJ. Ecological effects in multi-level studies. *J Epidemiol Community Health.* 2000 **54**(5):367–74.

[8] Diez-Roux AV. Multilevel analysis in public health research. *Annu Rev Public Health.* 2000 **21**:171–92.

[9] Schildcrout JS, Heagerty PJ. Regression analysis of longitudinal binary data with time-dependent environmental covariates: bias and efficiency. *Biostatistics (Oxford, England).* 2005 **6**(4):633–52.

[10] Schildcrout JS, Sheppard L, Lumley T, Slaughter JC, Koenig JQ, Shapiro GG. Ambient air pollution and asthma exacerbations in children: an eight-city analysis. *Am J Epidemiol.* 2006 **164**(6):505–17.

[11] Dominici F, McDermott A, Daniels M, Zeger SL, Samet JM. Revised analyses of the National Morbidity, Mortality, and Air Pollution Study: mortality among residents of 90 cities. *J Toxicol Environ Health A.* 2005 **68**(13–14):1071–92.

[12] Dickersin K, Berlin JA. Meta-analysis: state-of-the-science. *Epidemiol Rev.* 1992 **14**:154–76.

[13] Stroup DF, Berlin JA, Morton SC, Olkin I, Williamson GD, Rennie D, *et al.* Meta-analysis of observational studies in epidemiology: a proposal for reporting. Meta-analysis Of Observational Studies in Epidemiology (MOOSE) group. *Jama.* 2000 **283**(15):2008–12.

[14] Woodward M. *Epidemiology: study design and data analysis, 2nd edn.* New York: Chapman & Hall/CRC 2005.

[15] Bigger JT. Issues in subgroup analyses and meta-analyses of clinical trials. *J Cardiovasc Electrophysiol.* 2003 **14**(9 Suppl):S6–8.

[16] Lievre M, Cucherat M, Leizorovicz A. Pooling, meta-analysis, and the evaluation of drug safety. *Curr Control Trials Cardiovasc Med.* 2002 **3**(1):6.

[17] DerSimonian R, Laird N. Meta-analysis in clinical trials. *Control Clin Trials.* 1986 **7**(3):177–88.

[18] Mosteller F, Colditz GA. Understanding research synthesis (meta-analysis). *Annual Review of Public Health.* 1996 **17**:1–23.

Chapter 8

Special study designs and analyses in environmental epidemiology

8.0 Introduction

Mark Nieuwenhuijsen

This chapter deals with more special designs in environmental epidemiology. A number of these designs are data intensive (time-series, spatial epidemiology and cluster analyses) and use specific statistical methods. These studies generally rely on routinely collected environmental or health data and have a history of statistical method development. The time-series studies specifically make use of temporal variability in both environmental and health data to examine any relationship, while spatial epidemiological studies specifically make use of spatial variability in environmental and health data. However, this does not mean that time-series studies ignore spatial variability and spatial epidemiological studies ignore temporal variability, but they use it in a different way. Time-series studies and spatial epidemiological studies generally tend to make use of long(er) time periods and areas large(r), respectively. Cluster analyses studies focus specifically on the identification of increased risk of disease within short time periods or small areas.

In studies of short-term effects of an environmental exposure, time-series data have been extensively used to assess the short-term association between a series of exposure measurements (e.g., daily measurements of ambient particles) and a series of health outcome measurements (e.g., the daily number of respiratory admissions). Time-series data are often aggregated over a time period, e.g., one day. In this sense the studies may be thought of as ecological. Another related design is having a number of individual time-series, each with repeated measurements on a specific individual. The individual measurements may concern the health outcome only or both outcome and exposure. The analysis of these individual time-series can either preserve the separate measurements by individual with appropriate methodology or aggregate the data. To clarify the terminology, the name of 'time-series study' will be preserved for the time series, which are aggregated by their definition and the term 'panel study' used for situations where there are individual time-series of repeated measurements, irrespective of the analysis method used. Since the basic concepts are similar, they will be discussed in adjacent sections.

The meaning of 'short' may of course vary, so 'short-term' is defined as the effects of exposure over a few days, typically up to about 40. For effects observed after longer time periods, it is very difficult to separate seasonal effects, often characteristic of many environmental exposures and relevant outcomes, from the effects under study.

The time-series and panel studies have advantages concerning confounding and other biases: in both designs the same population is used as exposed and control population (e.g., on days of high and low exposures respectively) and thus confounding by personal characteristics is eliminated. They also have limitations which mainly concern the data quality and availability (for time-series studies) and the length of follow-up and size of the panel (for panel studies).

Short-term versus chronic effects is an issue for spatial epidemiological studies and cluster investigations. Diseases with a long latency time are more difficult to study because of movement of subjects. Furthermore, confounding and case ascertainment may make the interpretation of studies more difficult.

All the above designs have their strengths and limitations and these will be discussed in the specific sections. Furthermore, a fairly detailed description of the statistical techniques that are used will be given. The application of these designs has led to fruitful collaboration between statisticians and epidemiologists.

The last section of the chapter deals with gene–environment studies. After the epidemiological transition, i.e., the shift of mortality from infectious to chronic diseases (such as cardiovascular diseases and cancer), health professionals and researchers attempted to apply to chronic diseases the same approach used to understand and treat infections. The attempt to identify a single etiological agents (such as a bacterium), and to develop an appropriate therapy (like antibiotics) or preventive measures (like vaccines) has proven to be a simplistic approach for chronic diseases. The majority of chronic diseases seem to be determined by many different risk factors, only few of them necessary for developing the disease, and each contributing for a relatively small proportion (with notable exceptions such as cigarette smoking for lung cancer and human papilloma virus—HPV—for cervical cancer). This evidence led to the great majority of chronic diseases being defined as multifactorial. Cancer for example can arise through the role of different external exposures, different somatic mutations or other genetic acquired alterations and genetic predisposition. The gene–environment studies have led to fruitful collaboration between genetics and epidemiologists. The recognition of the role of both genes and environment has led to a whole new area of research, and again the development of new statistical techniques. The section on gene–environmental interaction provides an introduction to the topic and an overview of recent developments.

8.1 Time-series studies

Klea Katsouyanni and Biota Touloumi

8.1.1 Introduction

The time-series design investigates the relationship between an exposure and an outcome variable—each measured and aggregated over the same time units (e.g., days, weeks) during a specified time period. The measurements of each variable constitute a time series. For example, in Figure 8.1, the daily number of natural deaths and the PM_{10} and O_3 concentrations for one city are plotted against time for the study period [1].

The time-series design has been applied extensively in air pollution epidemiology. The evidence that severe episodes of air pollution, such as the December 1952 London episode, had important short-term effects originated from such studies [2]. Widespread use of the design and substantial development of the methodology started in the 1980s [3–5] and has increased since then. During the early 1990s, several time-series studies in the US set the stage for a renewed discussion of air pollution effects on health. In Europe, the multicenter Air Pollution and Health: a European Approach (APHEA) Network started in 1993. The APHEA study was one of the first large-scale studies that involve the combination of data from several locations across Europe, making it feasible to investigate heterogeneity of effect estimates across the study locations [6–9]. In 1996, the National Morbidity Mortality and Air Pollution Study (NMMAPS) study was initiated in the US, which studied the short-term effects of air pollution in the 100 largest US cities. The results of these large multicity studies have been instrumental in decisions for air quality management and standard setting.

8.1.2 Rationale, concepts and methods of the design

8.1.2.1 Time considerations

The objective of a time-series design is to assess the short-term changes in the health outcome series which follow changes in exposure. The health outcome variable may respond (change) immediately after the change in exposure, or it may change one or more days following the changes in exposure. The time periods between the change in exposure and the consequent change in outcome are called lags. Thus, 'lag 0 effects', usually means same day effects; 'lag 2', the effects two days later; etc. It is natural to hypothesize that the effect of a specific exposure may be distributed over more than one lag. Thus the study of 'lagged' effects is interesting and, statistically, several approaches have been developed. The exposure and outcome time series often display an annual seasonal pattern or other periodic patterns which are consistent (see, for example, Figure 8.1). They may also display unique peaks due to known or unexplained factors. Although the control or adjustment of seasonal patterns is an issue which has been addressed, it is generally accepted that with this design only effects that are short term can be studied, because the effects after a period of time (usually thought to be slightly over a month) of an environmental exposure, may hardly be separated from seasonal effects [10, 11]. In Table 8.1, the percent increase in the daily cardiovascular number of deaths associated with an increase of $10\mu g/m^3$ in PM_{10} concentrations at different lags is shown [12].

8.1.2.2 Exposure data

The time-series design may be applied to exposures with short-term variability. It has been applied to the study of air pollution, meteorological variables and other time-varying exposures. Time-series studies of air pollution have mainly used routinely measured air pollutants. For example, measurements from ambient air pollution monitoring stations have been used for gaseous pollutants such as NO_2 [13–15], ozone [16, 17],

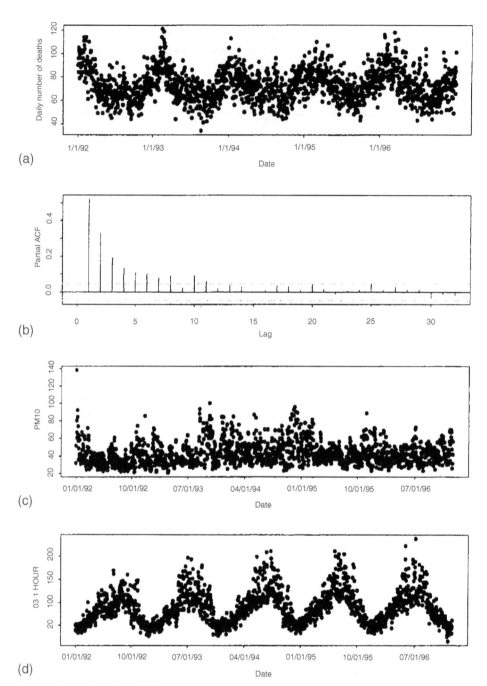

Fig. 8.1 Time series plot of daily total number of deaths in the Athens area from 1 January 1992 to 31 December 1996 (a) and the corresponding partial autocorrelation function (PACF) plot (b). Time series plot of PM_{10} (c) and O_3 (d) in the Athens area are also known. From [1]. Reproduced with permission from Rossi G, Schindler C, Schwartz J, Katsouyanni K, Touloumi G, Atkinson R, *et al.* Analysis of health outcome time series data in epidemiological studies. *Environmetrics.* 2004 **15**(2):101–17.

Table 8.1 Results for the combined (based on 10 European cities) estimated PM_{10} effect on cardiovascular (CVD) mortality on the same and previous day (lags 01) and with 20, 30 and 40 days of delay using an unrestricted distributed lags model.

	Daily increase in CVD mortality *	
Lag	Percent	(95% CI)
0–1	0.69	(0.31, 1.08)
20 days	1.34	(0.89, 1.79)
30 days	1.72	(1.20, 2.25)
40 days	1.97	(1.38, 2.55)

* increase per $10\mu g/m^3$ increase in PM_{10} concentrations.

Adapted from [12]. Reproduced with permission from Zanobetti A, Schwartz J, Samoli E, Gryparis A, Touloumi G, Peacock J, *et al*. The temporal pattern of respiratory and heart disease mortality in response to air pollution. *Environmental health perspectives*. 2003 111(9):1188–93.

SO_2 [18], and CO [19], and for particulate matter indicators such as PM_{10} [8, 20], black smoke [6], and $PM_{2.5}$ [21]. A few research studies have set up their own monitoring sites to measure specific exposures [22]. The effects of meteorological variables have been studied with this design and specifically daily average, minimum or maximum temperature, relative humidity [23] and daily synoptic classification patterns [24] are commonly used as explanatory variables. A few investigations of other environmental exposures have been reported, e.g., the effects of daily variations in water turbidity, a measure of water quality, on various health outcomes [25, 26].

In order to obtain good quality daily measurements over a long period of time, the use of routinely measured variables has been preferred over variables measured within a specific study. Routinely available measurements, usually implemented for the surveillance of air or water quality or for recording the weather patterns, are often quality controlled and they cover a wide area and long time periods. However, there are disadvantages to their use in epidemiological studies: the substances monitored have been chosen by criteria (e.g., political or environmental) often independent of health considerations; they may not include indices which are most interesting for health research; and they do not allow an estimation of interindividual variability in exposure within the population concerned.

8.1.2.3 Outcome data

The health outcome indices used in time-series studies are also based on routinely collected data and typically concern outcomes based on death registration (e.g., total or cause-specific daily number of deaths); or on hospital admissions (e.g., total or cause-specific daily number of emergency admissions) or visits (e.g., for asthma attack). These routinely collected data have the advantage of covering large populations and long time periods but are subject to errors in data recording (e.g., errors in the diagnosis of cause of death or admission or the International Coding of Disease (ICD) coding) and often do not represent the aspects of health that the investigators would like to study.

8.1.2.4 Confounding

Behavioral variables or personal characteristics that often are potential confounders in other epidemiological study designs do not present as much of a problem in time-series studies. Such behavioral or personal characteristics in a population may be associated with the outcomes studied, e.g., the proportion of smokers or the age structure in a population is associated both with mortality and with morbidity indices. However, these associations tend to reflect long-term effects. Furthermore, there is usually no reason to expect that these behavioral variables or personal characteristics would be associated with the temporal change in environmental exposures under study: e.g., the smoking 'load' in a population on a particular day is not associated with outdoor air pollution levels or to temperature (at least under the usual range of exposures) or to the quality of water, and certainly the age structure of a population will not change with short-term fluctuations of environmental exposure. Therefore, the only potential confounding variables for the exposure–outcome associations investigated with the time-series design are those with short-term temporal variability associated with the exposure and the outcome under study.

The most important of such confounders, which may well have a strong confounding effect, are the seasonal or other periodic patterns or long-term trends of both exposure and outcome. In Figure 8.1(a), for example, a strong seasonal pattern with higher daily counts of death during the winter is evident. On the other hand, the two pollutants shown in Figure 8.1(b) and 8.1(c) (namely, PM_{10} and O_3) have different seasonal patterns, with O_3 concentrations having a strong seasonal pattern with higher levels during the summer and PM_{10} having less pronounced seasonal pattern with relatively higher levels during the winter. The adjustment for these seasonal patterns has occupied a large proportion of the discussion on how to address the statistical analysis in time-series designs [1, 10, 11].

Other confounders may be relevant for specific studies following the same principle: for example in air pollution studies, meteorological variables are important confounders [27] and vice versa, in studies investigating the effects of meteorological variables, the levels of air pollutants may be important [28]. As an example, Table 8.2 shows the reduction of temperature effects in Monterrey, Mexico, when adjustment for air pollutants was included in the model [29].

Also other chronological variables, such as the day of the week, may be important confounders as they are often associated with health outcomes (morbidity and mortality) and with some of the exposures which may be studied.

8.1.2.5 Population selection (sensitive subgroups)

The whole population is a mixture of subgroups (e.g., people of different age groups or with different underlying chronic health problems), some of which may be less or more sensitive to the effect of a specific environmental exposure. It is interesting to investigate

Table 8.2 Percent change in daily mortality and 95% confidence intervals (CI) at 35–36°C apparent temperature relative to 25–26°C (3-day lagged moving average) under different model specifications in Monterrey 1996–99.

Model covariates	All age mortality	
	Percent change	95% CI
Base model: day of week, public holidays, season[a]	27.2	(20.0, 34.7)
Base model plus ozone and PM_{10} (lags 0–2)	20.4	(13.3, 28.1)

[a] 18 df for seasonal natural cubic spline.

Adapted from [29]. Reproduced with permission from O'Neill MS, Hajat S, Zanobetti A, Ramirez-Aguilar M, Schwartz J. Impact of control for air pollution and respiratory epidemics on the estimated associations of temperature and daily mortality. *Int J Biometeorol*. 2005 50(2):121–9.

the data concerning the more sensitive subgroups. Often such data are not available, i.e., routine statistics typically concern only the whole population, but in some situations it is possible to study sensitive subgroups. For example in hospital admission data comorbidities may be noted, or mortality data may be provided by age groups or by SES [30, 31]. In Figure 8.2, the increase in the relative risk for death with age, in São Paolo, Brazil, is shown [31].

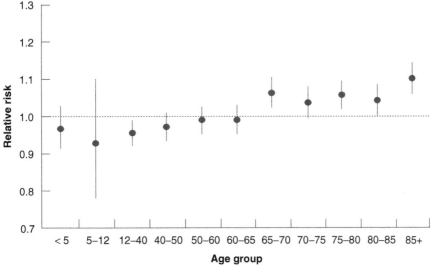

Fig. 8.2 Relative Risks (95% CI) for all cause mortality for an increase from the 10th to the 90th percentile in levels of PM_{10} according to age group, in São Paolo, Brazil 1991–1993. From [31]. Reproduced with permission from Gouveia N, Fletcher T. Time series analysis of air pollution and mortality: effects by cause, age and socioeconomic status. *J Epidemiol Community Health*. 2000 54(10):750–5. With permission by Oxford University Press.

8.1.2.6 Combination of results from various locations and investigation of effect modification

It is important to investigate the consistency or the heterogeneity of the effects of the same exposure across different populations. Consistency is generally thought of as a criterion for causality and an estimate of the consistency of effects across studies may provide valuable information. On the other hand, the magnitude of an effect may reflect characteristics of the environment or of the population in a specific area which act as effect modifiers. Therefore, studying determinants of heterogeneity is also very useful. Standard methods of meta-analysis as well as second stage models or meta-regression or Bayesian hierarchical modeling may be used [31–33].

Here it should be noted that the effect estimates calculated from time-series studies may be small in size (weak effects) but are often statistically significant, since the large number of observation units (e.g., the days) and the large populations studied result in small standard errors. Similarly the usual χ^2 tests for heterogeneity in time-series designs

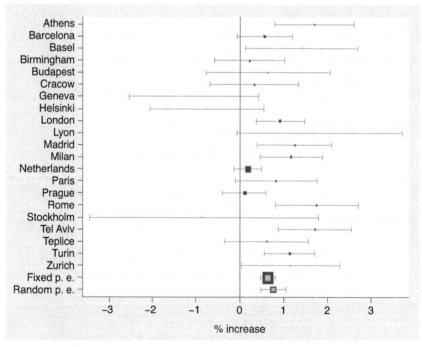

Fig. 8.3 Percentage increase in the daily number of cardiovascular deaths and its 95% confidence interval (CI) associated with an increase of 10μg/m³ in the levels of PM₁₀ (average of lags 0 and 1) in each city, estimated using penalized splines. The size of the point representing each increase is inversely proportional to its variance. From [37]. Reproduced with permission from Analitis A, Katsouyanni K, Dimakopoulou K, Samoli E, Nikoloulopoulos AK, Petasakis Y, *et al.* Short-term effects of ambient particles on cardiovascular and respiratory mortality. *Epidemiology (Cambridge, MA).* 2006 17(2):230–3.

yield statistically significant differences between the individual estimates even in situations of relative consistency, due to the high statistical power of this analysis. Therefore, one should explore heterogeneity based not on statistical significance, but on more descriptive measures [34]. The aforementioned APHEA study in Europe [8, 9, 35] and NMMAPS study in the US [20, 36] are examples of time-series studies that used data from multiple cities to yield combined effects and to explore heterogeneity. In Figure 8.3 a forest plot of the effects of PM_{10} on the daily number of cardiovascular deaths in 21 European cities from the APHEA project is shown. Table 8.3 shows effect modification patterns from the same data set. It may be seen that in warmer and drier cities the PM_{10} effects are higher; they are also higher in cities with a lower mortality rate and where annual NO_2 concentrations are higher [37].

8.1.3 **Analytical strategy and statistical methods**

The time-series type of analysis was first introduced in the seventeenth century and was used until the early twentieth century by mathematicians and physicists with the objective of describing phenomena. In the late twentieth century, time-series models were largely developed in the context of econometrics with the aim of description and prediction or forecasting. Models developed for the purpose of prediction apply transformations to the dependent variable which yield estimates that are hard to interpret. Therefore, this methodology was not appropriate for the main objective of epidemiological research, i.e., understanding the magnitude of the effect of an exposure on an outcome and the estimation of the dose–response pattern. The time-series modeling approach needed modifications for use in epidemiological time-series studies, and much development has taken place in the last 20 years.

Table 8.3 Results of second stage regression models, investigating the role of potential modifiers* of the estimated effects of PM_{10} on cardiovascular deaths

Effect modifier in model[β]	25th percentile[a]		75th percentile[a]	
	% increase	(95% CI)	% increase	(95% CI)
Annual temperature	0.24	(0.03, 0.46)	0.97	(0.77, 1.17)
Annual humidity	1.12	(0.88, 1.36)	0.50	(0.34, 0.67)
Age standardized mortality rate	1.02	(0.68, 1.35)	0.83	(0.21, 0.84)
Mean NO_2 over 24 hours	0.20	(−0.03, 0.44)	0.94	(0.74, 1.14)

* These are variables characterizing each city. Only effect modifiers reducing the heterogeneity by >10 percent are presented.

[a] Increase in CVD number of deaths associated with an increase of 10µg/m³ in the daily PM_{10} concentration, estimated using fixed effects model, for a city with levels of the corresponding effect modifier equal to the 25th and 75th percentiles of its distribution.

[β] The effect modifiers were included alternatively in the model. Adapted from [37]. Reproduced with permission from Analitis A, Katsouyanni K, Dimakopoulou K, Samoli E, Nikoloulopoulos AK, Petasakis Y, et al. Short-term effects of ambient particles on cardiovascular and respiratory mortality. Epidemiology (Cambridge, MA). 2006 17(2):230–3.

Typically, in epidemiological time-series studies, the outcome variable consists of daily counts over several years of a health indicator, such as deaths or admissions in various diagnostic and age groups. Modeling such data is challenging since usually the aim is to identify and quantify a relatively small effect in the presence of strong confounding. The outcome series often exhibit seasonal and long-term trends (see for example Figure 8.1a). Therefore the major statistical challenge is to adequately control for time-varying risk factors [38, 39].

In earlier studies, Generalized Linear Models (GLM) and in particular Poisson regression techniques with parametric functions of time-varying factors (linear, quadratic or sinusoidal curves of differing periodicities) were used to analyze epidemiological time-series data [10, 40, 41]. However, in the last decade, these standard regression techniques have been almost fully replaced by the more local and flexible Generalized Additive Models (GAM) with nonparametric smoothing functions for modeling nonlinear relationships of time-varying factors [1, 8, 20, 42].

To analyze the data a model of the following general form is applied:

$$\eta_t = \ln(\mu_t) = \ln\left[E\left(Y_t\right)\right] = \alpha_0 + \sum_{j=1}^{q} f_j(X_{tj}) + \beta\, E_t + \sum_{d=1}^{p} \beta_d Z_d \tag{1}$$

with health counts variances $v_t = \varphi \mu_t$, where Y_t denotes the observed count of the relevant health outcome on day t, β the effect estimate for the exposure of interest, X_{tj} the time-varying predictor variables and potential confounders, f_j smooth functions of these variables to allow for non-linear relationships and Z_d other nontime varying cofactors. μ_t is the expected count of the relevant health outcome and φ the overdispersion parameter estimated from the Pearson's χ^2 statistic as described in McCullagh and Nelder [43]. Depending on the specification of the smoothing functions (parametric or nonparametric) model (1) leads to GLMs or GAMs.

One of the confounding variables is usually time, which is considered as a proxy for any omitted variables with separate temporal trends. The smooth function of time will filter out the effect of these unknown variables. However, other known covariates, including the exposure of interest, may also display temporal trends. Therefore, the choice of the degree of smoothness should be based on eliminating confounding effects from seasonal and longer-term trends but retaining as much as possible short-term fluctuations, part of which may be causally associated with short-term fluctuations in the exposure variable. Other known time-varying covariates include meteorological factors such as the mean daily temperature and relative humidity or dew point.

Among the nonparametric smoothers, the most commonly used ones were *loess* [1, 8] and *smoothing splines* [20, 42]. While initially nonparametric smoothers were preferred to parametric ones as they could provide a more flexible and 'localized' fit to the data, recent reports have questioned their suitability for a fixed number of degrees of freedom [44, 45]. The main issues raised were related to the way GAMs are implemented in statistical software which could lead to bias with underestimated variances and overestimated exposure effect estimates. Although methods to overcome these problems exist [44, 46, 47], a return to GLM using natural splines as smoothers has been proposed. Penalized splines (PS) with natural or B-splines bases [48–50] have become the most popular choices recently [11]. Several approaches to choose the optimal number of degrees of freedom have been proposed: use of fixed number of degrees of freedom based on biological knowledge or previous work [20, 42], and use of data-driven methods. A general rule could be to use the PS method with a large number of effective dfs (e.g., 8–12 per year) as the basic, relatively conservative, analysis whereas the PS and natural splines in combination with partial autocorrelation function (PACF) could be applied to provide a reasonable range of the effect estimate. Final models should be checked (e.g., through residuals' PACF plot) for presence of serial correlation. If present, adjustment using autoregression models [51] should be applied.

8.1.3.1 Distributed lags models

One issue in epidemiological time-series data is how to choose the appropriate lag structure for the exposure variable. Many authors use data to select the most relevant lag. However, it has been shown that to select the most significant lag among a set of possible lags, overstates the chance of finding a significant association [52]. One alternative is to pre-specify the lag of the exposure based on previous knowledge. In air pollution epidemiology for example, it has been shown that same and previous day concentrations of, e.g., particulate matter are the most relevant lags for predicting mortality [53] and, therefore, the average of these two lags is used in most studies [1]. Another alternative is to use distributed lags models [54]. These models are used to estimate associations between the health outcome on a given day, and exposure several days prior. In such models the term bE_t in equation (1) is replaced with

$$\theta \sum_{l=1}^{L} w_l E_{t-l} , \quad \sum_{l=1}^{L} w_l = 1$$

where θ measures the cumulative effect and w_l the contribution of the lagged exposure E_{t-l} to the estimation of θ.

8.1.3.2 Dose–response curves

At a given lag, the shape of the dose–response curve between the exposure of interest and the health outcome can be investigated by modeling the health outcome as a smooth function of the exposure. Nonparametric (e.g., loess [55]) or parametric (e.g., cubic splines [36, 56]) smoothers can be used. When cubic splines are used, the number and the location of the knots are usually fixed in advance based on prior knowledge [36] or on exploratory analysis [56]. To estimate the exposure–response curves for PM_{10} and total cardiovascular and respiratory mortality, Samoli *et al.* [56] used a cubic spline function with 2 knots set at 30 and 50 mg/m^3 based on explanatory analysis. Alternatively the number and location of the knots number and location can be estimated from the data using Reversible Jump Monte Carlo Markov Chain (RJMCM) [57, 58].

Threshold models are a specific case in which it is assumed that the exposure effect is negligible below a certain level k. In such cases, the exposure variable E_t in equation (1) is replaced with $(E_t–k)^+$ where $(x^t = x$ if $x \geq 0$ and 0 otherwise) and k the change in slope level. Level k can be fixed or estimated from the data using Bayesian methods [36].

8.1.4 Advantages and limitations

The time-series design is relatively cheap and easy to apply since it uses data already recorded for other purposes. This advantage is weakened when exposure measurements are actually done within a study in order to improve exposure assessment. The aggregate nature of the required data makes it easier to get permission from ethical committees. The fact that data are already recorded offers the possibility of obtaining long time series at small additional costs, thus allowing increased statistical power. The design is free from confounding by all variables which do not vary according to the time period of aggregation (e.g., one day). Those variables which may act as potential confounders (e.g., meteorological or chronological variables) are also routinely recorded and readily available.

The time-series design also has limitations. Often the data available are not optimal for an epidemiological study. Thus for exposure, the monitoring may be based on one site and may misclassify the population exposure. With regard to the outcome, for example, emergency admissions may not be available, so the investigators may have to rely on total admissions, which include planned admissions (which are not relevant for the study of short-term effects). Because of the aggregate nature of the data, individual variability in sensitivity or other characteristics cannot be studied. Finally the results may prove to be sensitive in modeling choices, especially those concerning the adjustment of seasonal and long-term patterns in the data.

Several model uncertainties exist. Ignoring uncertainties due to model choice can lead to over-confident inferences and predictions [59, 60]. Dominici *et al.* [61] give a detailed statistical review for studies investigating the health effects of air pollution. Despite the recent developments in statistical methods, biases due to residual confounding can never be completely ruled out in observational studies.

8.2 Panel studies

Klea Katsouyanni and Giota Touloumi

8.2.1 Introduction

Panel studies are prospective studies that follow a usually small group of individuals intensively over a short time period (typically a few months) with the objective to study short-term effects of a time-varying environmental exposure on health outcomes. Over the time period of a study, repeated observations (e.g., every day) are made on both exposures and outcome variables, as well as potential confounders. This study design yields time-series data for each individual subject. It shares the common objective as time-series studies of studying short-term effects and it uses similar analytical methodology, but there are also important differences between panel studies and time-series studies.

The most important difference is the availability of individual measurements. The time considerations are the same as those mentioned for time-series studies.

Panel studies have been widely used to study the short-term health effects of air pollutants on sensitive subjects. Children, and especially symptomatic or asthmatic children, have been investigated in single location studies in many parts of the world. The main outcomes studied were respiratory function indices and respiratory symptoms [62–68]. Similarly, panel studies for the acute effects of air pollution have been conducted with adult or elderly subjects, and the main outcomes studied were respiratory symptoms, lung function, cardiovascular and inflammatory endpoints [69–76]. The panel study design allows a more thorough characterization of indoor exposures, and indoor studies have been reported as well [77–79].

Panel study designs have also followed the general trend in environmental epidemiology for investigators to organize multi-location projects, especially in Europe. There are reports of meta-analyses for effects on children [67, 80] and a large multipanel study on children, the PEACE study [81]. Also, multicenter panel studies on adults have reported results, like the ULTRA study [82, 83], and others are still ongoing, e.g., the AIRGENE study [84].

8.2.2 Rationale, concepts and methods

8.2.2.1 Exposure data

The nature of the exposures studied, i.e., the short-term variability, is shared with the time-series studies. However, the panel study approach allows individual assessment of exposure where relevant. This exposure assessment can be quite intensive, including the use of personal monitoring of multiple environmental agents. Typically these studies also incorporate the use of a diary or GPS device to track the subjects' location and activities during the monitoring period. This combination of environmental monitoring and time-activity tracking allows the investigators to determine sources of exposures, confounders and effect modifiers. For example, the time spent outdoors or the area of residence may be important modifiers of the individual's exposure to air pollution, and drinking tap or bottled water is an important determinant of exposure to poor-quality community water.

8.2.2.2 Outcome data

Health outcomes are assessed continuously during the study period, so the assessment is similar to repeated cross-sectional measurements of health status. Like cross-sectional studies, the primary outcomes of interest in panel studies tend to be symptoms, physiological indicators of health status, or measures of minor morbidity. As discussed in Chapter 4, routinely collected health data are quite limited in most countries of the world. Some countries have better health information systems, but these data sources are still limited to identifying clinical events, such as hospitalizations. However, environmental exposures can have short-term effects on symptoms, minor morbidity, respiratory function, inactivity, medication use, and absenteeism from work or school to a larger proportion of the population compared with effects on hospital visits and admissions or death. These subclinical health outcomes are of interest in environmental epidemiology and they may be studied using a panel study design. For example, panel studies have been used to study respiratory function indices [75, 81] and subclinical cardiovascular end points, such as heart rate variability [85].

8.2.2.3 Confounding

Confounding by time-varying factors applies in panel studies, in a similar way as in time-series studies. Additionally in panel studies, personal behavior characteristics may act as confounding variables as they are associated both with exposure and outcome (e.g., staying indoors when it is extremely cold or hot or very polluted; using drugs on demand in heavy pollution). Since the panel study investigates each individual separately, it is possible to collect the relevant information on all potential confounders via a carefully designed protocol [75].

8.2.2.4 Population selection

Because of the intensive follow-up of panels, it is difficult to enrol large populations. Therefore, investigators typically try to maximize the statistical power by studying sensitive individuals. For example, panel studies have focused on children, the elderly, asthmatics, myocardial infarction survivors, etc. It is important when investigators do choose to study sensitive populations for them to be careful when generalizing from the sensitive study population to the larger general population.

Another consideration in population selection is that these studies can be quite demanding on the participants, since they may have to wear personal monitoring devices and be asked to complete diaries or time-activity logs. Thus, people who agreed to participate in such studies may not be typical of the general population. The analysis of these studies is based on comparison of the same subjects across time (see next section), so selective participation should not bias the study findings, although it may limit generalizability. Investigators typically have to spend considerable effort to identify and enrol study subjects who are likely to complete the full study protocol.

8.2.2.5 Analysis

For the analysis of panel studies, the data may either be aggregated or analysed individually. In the former case, the data are ecological and the same analytical methods as for time-series studies are used (see section 8.1); in the latter case, more complex modeling must be used.

Multilocation studies and investigation of effect modification

The combination of results from the study of various panels from different locations and the influence of effect modifiers with contrasting distribution between locations can be applied in a similar way as in time-series studies, although statistical power is smaller. The individual nature of data in panel studies also allows the study of effect modification within panels. For example, Figure 8.4 shows the odds ratios for incident shortness of breath associated with $10\mu g/m^3$ increase in $PM_{2.5}$ and 10,000 particles/cm^3,

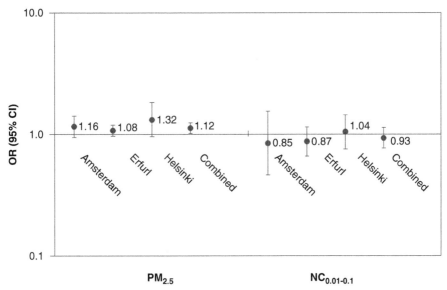

Fig. 8.4 Odds ratios for the relation of incident shortness of breath to increases in PM$_{2.5}$ and number concentrations of particles in the size range of 0.01–0.1 μm (NC$_{0.01-0.1}$) among elderly subjects with a history of coronary heart disease, ULTRA Study, winter 1998–1999. The odds ratios (OR) shown are for an increase of 10 μg/m^3 in PM$_{2.5}$ and an increase of 10 000 particles/cm^3 in NC$_{0.01-0.1}$ (5-day average). Bars, 95% confidence interval (CI). From [86]. Reproduced with permission from de Hartog JJ, Hoek G, Peters A, Timonen KL, Ibald-Mulli A, Brunekreef B, *et al*. Effects of fine and ultrafine particles on cardiorespiratory symptoms in elderly subjects with coronary heart disease: the ULTRA study. *American Journal of Epidemiology*. 2003 157(7):613–23.

in three European cities, within the ULTRA project [86]. In this study, the odds ratios for the relation of symptoms to air pollution, adjusted for time trend, respiratory infections, and meteorological variables, were mostly homogeneous across the centers. A 10 μg/m^3 increase in PM$_{2.5}$ was positively associated with the incidence of shortness of breath (OR = 1.12, 95% CI: 1.02, 1.24), but there was no apparent association between small particle concentration and shortness of breath.

8.2.3 Analytical strategy and statistical methods

In panel studies individual data are collected and, almost always, the health outcome of interest is measured repeatedly over time. Therefore, the study design of panel studies is similar to that of cohort studies. The difference between the two designs is that the cohort study generally evaluates the effects of exposures on single incident event (e.g., death or onset of disease), while a panel study generally evaluates the short-term effects of time-varying exposures. Also the study periods are generally quite different, although it is not a requirement of the study designs. Panel studies usually last for a few months or a year, while cohort studies can last for several years. Because of the similar data structure, similar statistical methods for data analysis can be used in cohort and panel studies, although cohort studies tend to be analysed using survival methods in which each subject is treated as one independent observation (see Chapter 7). The analytical methods would be similar to that of a cohort study that collects repeated data on subjects during the follow-up period.

In panel studies the response variable is either binary (e.g., onset of a symptom) or continuous (e.g., pulmonary function) measured several times in each individual. At a given time, exposure measurements can be either ecological (i.e., come from one fixed site and be the same over all individuals) or subject-specific when personal monitors or other individual estimates are used. For example, in a panel study in Alpine, California, designed to investigate associations between air pollutants and asthma in asthmatic children, Delfino *et al.* [87] followed 28 asthmatic children daily from March through April 1996. Figure 8.5 shows the time plots of selected pollutant measurement across the days of this study.

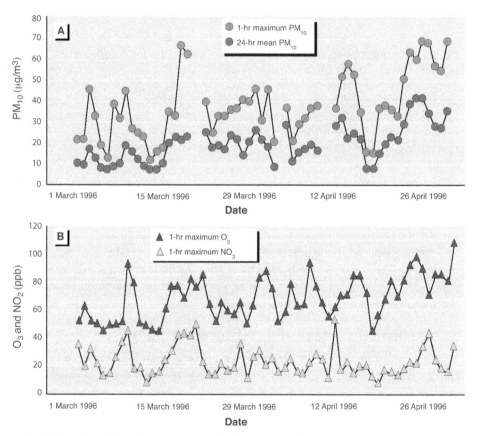

Fig. 8.5 Time plot of air pollutant exposures, (A) PM$_{10}$ and (B) O$_3$ and NO$_2$, Alpine California, panel study, March through April 1996. From [87]. Reproduced with permission from Delfino RJ, Zeiger RS, Seltzer JM, Street DH, McLaren CE. Association of asthma symptoms with peak particulate air pollution and effect modification by anti-inflammatory medication use. *Environ Health Perspect.* 2002 110(10):A607–17.

Traditionally, repeated measurements within a subject are assumed to be correlated, whereas measurements in different individuals are assumed to be independent. Two classes of models are commonly used for data analysis:

Marginal models (MM) are one class of models, in which the regression of the response on the exposure variables is modeled separately from the within-subject correlation. In other words, a MM has a generalized linear model for its expectation while it incorporates the dependence between observations as a nuisance parameter in the residual error of the model. Zeger *et al.* [88] have investigated MM for longitudinal data and have developed the Generalized Estimation Equation (GEE) to estimate the regression parameters. MM utilizing GEE have been applied in air pollution epidemiology to investigate the relationship between symptoms in paediatric asthmatics and air pollution [87]. In Table 8.4 the results of this study regarding the effect of air pollution on children's asthmatic symptoms are presented. The table shows that the odds ratio for experiencing

Table 8.4 ORs for risk of asthma symptoms from a 90th percentile increase in pollutants or aeroallergens in those who report a respiratory infection compared with those who do not have respiratory infections

Pollutant and aeroallergen variables	Air pollutant level[b]	OR(95% CI)[c]
1-hr max PM_{10} lag 0	51 $\mu g/m^3$	4.88 (1.31–18.2)
8-hr max PM_{10} lag 0	38$\mu g/m^3$	6.78 (1.38–33.3)
24-hr max PM_{10} lag 0	25$\mu g/m^3$	4.68 (0.71–30.7)
3-day moving average 1-hr max PM_{10}	51$\mu g/m^3$	11.1 (1.10–112)
3-day moving average 8-hr max PM_{10}	38$\mu g/m^3$	10.1 (1.42–72.0)
3-day moving average 24-hr mean PM_{10}	25$\mu g/m^3$	2.67 (0.60–11.8)
1-hr max O_3 lag 0	43 ppb	3.27 (1.00–10.7)
8-hr max O_3 lag 0	36 ppb	2.72 (0.67–11.0)
1-hr max NO_2 lag 0	34 ppb	3.46 (0.45–26.6)
8-hr max NO_2 lag 0	20 ppb	6.72 (1.73–26.1)
12-hr fungi lag 0	4,644 particles/m^3	6.38 (1.03–39.6)
24-hr pollen lag 0	732 particles/m^3	0.95 (0.16–5.74)

Max, maximum. Effect modification of respiratory infection in children not on anti-inflammatory medications, Alpine, California, panel study, 1 March through 30 April 1996.

[a] The asthma symptom severity score was dichotomized to a) no symptoms or symptoms not bothersome or not interfering with daily activities, versus b) symptoms interfering with daily activities.

[b] 90th percentile minus the minimum.

[c] Per increase to 90th percentile concentration of pollutant or aeroallergen given the presence vs. absence of a respiratory infection from GEE models including the pollutant or aeroallergen, an indicator variable for respiratory infection and a product term between them. Models involve 12 subjects with 678 person-days of O_3 and NO_2 observations, 622 person-days of PM_{10} observations, and 666 person-days of aeroallergen observations.

From [87]. Reproduced with permission from Environmental Health Perspectives. Delfino RJ, Zeiger RS, Seltzer JM, Street DH, McLaren CE. Association of asthma symptoms with peak particulate air pollution and effect modification by anti-inflammatory medication use. *Environ Health Perspect.* 2002 110(10): A607–17.

asthma symptoms during a day time period was positively associated with several measures of PM_{10} and ozone exposure. The associations were generally stronger for PM_{10} with the strongest odds ratio equal to 10.1 for the 3-day moving average 8-hour maximum PM_{10} measure.

Random effects models (RE) are a second class of models, which assume that the dependence between measurements comes as a result of some subject-specific random effect, conditional on which, the measurements within subjects are assumed independent. Thus, RE models allow for random deviations of an individual's response curve from the expected curve for the population to which the individual belongs. RE models not only describe the covariance between repeated measurements but also explain the source of this covariance [89, 90]. RE models have a long history in air pollution epidemiology [91–93].

MM and RE models can be easily fitted using most of the widely available statistical software such as SAS, Stata and S-plus. However, it should be emphasized that the two classes of models are different. The effect estimates derived from MM and RE models could differ substantially. The interpretation of the effect estimates also differs substantially. MM effect estimates are interpreted as population averages, while in RE they express changes in a typical individual. For more discussion on the issue, see Diggle *et al.* [89], Breslow and Clayton [90], Zeger *et al.* [88] and Fitzmaurice *et al.* [94].

A historically popular method to analyze panel data is to aggregate over all measurements on time (day) *t* to estimate a panel average. Examples include the percentage of persons with symptoms on a given day. A disadvantage of this approach is that such models ignore the longitudinal nature of the data and assume that outcomes on successive days are independent. Although these models have been discouraged since the early seventies [95], they continue to be used. However, in recent decades special adjustments are undertaken. For example, aggregated outcomes are weighted by the number of reporting subjects each day, whereas additional correction for autocorrelation is made when necessary [81, 93, 96]. As an alternative to RE models, an indicator variable for each subject has been used to control for individual differences in the frequency of symptoms [86].

In panel studies, adjustment for time-varying confounders is important. Methods similar to those described in the time-series section could be applied in principle, although their application, especially when RE models are used, is not trivial. Additional variables that do not vary within individuals (e.g., demographic characteristics, baseline health status) can be incorporated into the model to improve its efficiency. The most challenging and difficult statistical issue to deal with in panel (as in longitudinal) studies is missing outcome data due to dropout. The effect of ignoring missing data on statistical inferences depends on the underlying missingness process (*i.e.*, whether the probability of dropout depends and how on the health outcome or not). Laird [97] gave a detailed discussion of how the missingness process can affect inferences about the response variable. Care is needed since ignoring missing data due to dropout could lead to seriously biased effect estimates [97, 98]. Several methods to deal with missing data in specific cases have been proposed [99–103] but their implications are not trivial and they have rarely been applied in environmental panel studies.

8.2.4 **Advantages and limitations**

The main advantage of panel studies is the fact that individuals are studied and individual measurements are available. This allows the study of refined hypotheses and effect modification and the identification of sensitive subgroups. However, the requirements of participation increase the burden of the subjects and may affect compliance and alter their behavior. Additionally the intensive follow-up increases the cost per subject and limits the number of participants. As a result, the statistical power decreases. Furthermore, their statistical analysis is much more complicated than time-series studies.

8.3 **Spatial epidemiology**

Lars Jarup and Nicky Best

8.3.1 **Introduction**

Spatial epidemiology is the description and analysis of geographical variations in disease with respect to environmental, behavioral and sociodemographic risk factors, encompassing disease mapping, geographic correlation studies, disease clusters and clustering [104]. There have been substantial developments in computing, Geographical Information Systems (GIS), and spatial statistics during the last decade, improving study designs in geographical epidemiological studies. In many countries, high resolution, geographically referenced health data and, albeit to a lesser extent, environmental data are available, which facilitates spatial analyses at a small-area scale. These data increase the possibilities of investigating geographical relations between environmental and other factors and disease. However, there are several pitfalls in the spatial epidemiological approach, including the large random component that may dominate disease rates across small areas. This can be dealt with using Bayesian statistics to provide 'smooth' estimates of disease risks, but sensitivity to detect areas at high risk is limited when expected numbers of cases are small. Furthermore, data quality is of crucial importance; data errors can result in apparent disease excess in one or more locations in the study area. Arbitrary boundaries (commonly administrative areas), which are often used in spatial epidemiology, may yield incorrect and misleading results. This problem is known as the modifiable area unit problem (MAUP) [105] and is fundamental in spatial epidemiological study design.

8.3.2 **Study design**

There are four major study types in spatial epidemiology: disease mapping, geographical correlation studies, cluster detection (discussed in Section 8.4) and 'point source' studies. Disease mapping is primarily used for descriptive studies based on geographical features, while geographical correlation studies are ecological studies that are based on comparisons of geographical units. Examples have been given in previous chapters. These study designs are well suited to explore unusual clusters or patterns of disease in an area (with or without any prior hypothesis) and create new hypotheses, which can be further analysed using other (epidemiological) tools. Point-source studies may also add to the evidence of causality, if, for example, a clear exposure–response pattern can be demonstrated in relation to a point, line or area source (e.g., a chemical plant).

8.3.2.1 Disease-mapping studies

Descriptive studies based on disease mapping may provide baseline data on health patterns and may elucidate changes in disease patterns over time. Disease mapping may also be useful in an initial exploration of relationships between exposure and disease. As mentioned in Chapter 6, maps of cancer incidence and mortality, computed on a global scale by the International Agency for Research of Cancer (IARC), are readily interpretable. For example, maps of lung cancer show a clear gradient between high rates in affluent countries and low rates in developing countries, which mainly reflects differences in exposure to tobacco smoke, which is (still) more prevalent in affluent parts of the world. Other large-scale maps, such as the atlases of cancer mortality produced by the US National Cancer Institute (NCI) are also relatively easy to interpret (http://www3.cancer.gov/atlasplus/type.html). The NCI county-specific maps have been very useful in identifying cancer disease patterns with the location of major industries by means of ecological studies [106]. Examples include nasal cancer in areas with furniture manufacturing, lung cancer in counties with petrochemical manufacturing, bladder cancer where chemical industries were located, and oral cancer in regions where snuff use was common.

However, accurate *small area* disease maps are usually much more difficult to produce and interpret in a meaningful way. For example, increase in prostate cancer incidence during recent years has been reported for many countries, possibly linked to environmental exposures. Exposure to environmental carcinogens is likely to be unevenly spatially distributed, potentially giving rise to variations in disease occurrence, which may be detectable in a spatial analysis. A Small Area Health Statistics Unit (SAHSU) study did not show any marked geographical variability at a small area (electoral ward) scale in Great Britain, arguing against a geographically varying environmental factor operating strongly in the etiology of prostate cancer [107] (Figure 8.6). However, caution needs to be exercised in the interpretation because of factors mentioned above, such as latency time and migration. Although little is known about the latency time from exposure to an (environmental) agent and the occurrence of prostate cancer, it can be assumed that the latency (induction) time is long, probably in the order of decades. Given the high probability of substantial migration in and out of the study area over a long time period any risk patterns are likely to be obscured due to misclassification of exposure.

The choice of statistical methods for small area disease mapping is very important. Standardised Incidence or Mortality Ratios (SIR, SMR) are commonly used as estimates of disease risk in epidemiological studies. The statistical assumption underlying these estimates is that the observed disease counts, y_i, in each area arise from a Poisson distribution with mean $r_i E_i$, where E_i is the age and sex standardized expected number of cases in area i and r_i is the relative risk of disease in that area. It can then be shown that the SIR (SMR) is the maximum likelihood estimate of r_i. The standard error of this estimate is inversely proportional to the square root of E_i. The latter tend to be low for rare diseases in small areas, but can vary by an order of magnitude or more over the study region due to differences in population density and age structure, leading to risk estimates in different areas that have very different degreees of precision.

A criticism that is sometimes raised against mapping indirectly standardized relative risks (SIRs, SMRs) is that any two SIRs (SMRs) are not directly comparable since they are not based on the same standard population. This is theoretically correct, but in practice, using SIRs (SMRs) to compare risks between two or more areas will only be misleading if the age and gender structure of the area populations are extremely disparate, a situation which is unlikely to occur in practice [108]. The imprecision of directly standardized rates when calculated on small area scale is a far more serious problem [109].

Statistical smoothing of risk estimates based on Bayesian inference methods has been recommended by statisticians for some time, and this technique is increasingly being used in spatial epidemiology. Bayesian smoothing works by taking a form of weighted average of the SIR (SMR) in a particular small area and the overall risk for either the whole study region (leading to global smoothing) or for a local region surrounding the small area (local smoothing). The resulting smoothed risk estimates for each area are more precise and more robust against false positive estimates than are unsmoothed SIRs (SMRs), and hence lead to more meaningful and interpretable disease maps, as illustrated by the comparison of unsmoothed and smoothed relative risks of prostate cancer in Great Britain [107] (see Figure 8.6). Formally, the statistical model for Bayesian smoothing has the following general form:

$$y_i \sim Poisson\,(r_i E_i)$$
$$\log r_i \sim Normal(m, v)$$

where m and v represent the overall mean log relative risk for the whole study region and the between area variance in log relative risks, respectively. Non-informative prior probability distributions are usually assumed for these parameters. A widely used alternative to the above model is to replace the independent normal distribution for the log r_i with a spatially correlated distribution, such as the intrinsic conditional autoregressive (CAR) distribution [110, 111]. The CAR model has the form:

$$\log r_i \,|\, r_j \sim Normal(m_i, v_i); \quad j \neq i$$
$$m_i = \sum_{j \neq i} w_{ij} \log r_j \,\Big/ \sum_{j \neq i} w_{ij}$$
$$v_i = s \,\Big/ \sum_{j \neq i} w_{ij}$$

where w_{ij} are weights usually defined to be 1 if areas i and j are adjacent and zero otherwise, leading to m_i being the average log relative risk in the areas neighboring area i. s is an overall scale parameter controlling the variance of the log relative risks.

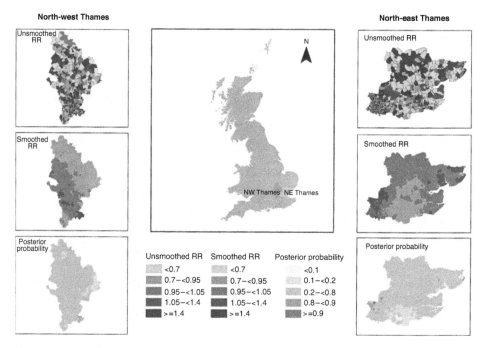

Fig. 8.6 Unsmoothed and smoothed risk estimates of prostate cancer in the north-west and north-east Thames area, UK. From [107]. Reproduced with permission from Jarup L, Best N, Toledano MB, Wakefield J, Elliott P. Geographical epidemiology of prostate cancer in Great Britain. *Int J Cancer.* 2002 97(5):695–9.

Concerns have been voiced that Bayesian risk estimates may tend to oversmooth variations in disease risk, particularly if the data are very sparse, and it is important to make sure that true excess risks have not been smoothed away by using these methods. Richardson *et al.* [112] considered this problem using a large simulation study. They found that Bayesian risk estimates have high specificity (>90 percent for most scenarios considered) but relatively low sensitivity (often below 60 percent) unless the true excess risks are large (relative risks above 3) or the expected counts high (>50). Further empirical work is needed to address whether these findings hold in a wide range of geographical settings, but it is clear that care must be taken not to overinterpret any *lack* of spatial variation in a disease map in much the same way as epidemiologists and statisticians already caution against overinterpretation of apparent clusters.

Relative risks in disease maps are almost exclusively shown as point estimates, not taking into account the uncertainty in the risk estimates. Maps display information about geographical variations in risk in a powerful way. Therefore, techniques need to be developed to map uncertainty in risk estimates logically and understandably, making it easy for readers to understand, without the need for an in-depth statistical knowledge. One possibility when using Bayesian smoothing methods is to map the posterior probability of the relative risk exceeding a pre-specified threshold in any area. Assuming the threshold is set as unity, the posterior probabilities may be interpreted as the strength of (statistical) evidence of excess risk in each area [107, 112].

As noted above, maps of the same raw data can result in very different visual patterns depending on the resolution and aggregation choice [113]. Thus, it is important to select the appropriate size of units and the relevant aggregation method to highlight the features of interest. Detailed general guidelines are difficult to suggest, since selection of geographical units will depend on the circumstances in the study region, such as the availability of data at different geographical levels.

Although variation in rates across a map may reflect real differences in disease occurrence, such variation may commonly reflect data quality, for example in the diagnosis, case ascertainment, or the estimation of population denominators. Best and Wakefield [114] showed an example of breast cancer incidence in south east England in the 1980s and 1990s, where an apparent decreasing south-to-north trend in risk was largely attributable to under-ascertainment of cases by the cancer registries covering the southern part of the study region.

Visualization (e.g., choice of color schemes) is very important for the perception of cancer maps, which is often ignored. For example, red symbolizes 'danger' for many people, whereas green may stand for 'no hazard', which will influence the intuitive interpretation of the mapped risks. Since a good map of bad data looks better than a bad map of good data, it is essential that the investigators make sure that not only the data and the analysis are valid and accurate, but also are presented in a sensible way.

Recently, it has been proposed that Bayesian smoothing methods be extended to map geographical patterns of joint variation in two or more diseases that are hypothesized to share similar environmental risk factors (see [111] for a short review). The statistical models used are similar to a spatial factor analysis model, where the relative risk of disease k in region i, r_{ik}, is modeled as the sum of a shared latent factor, f_i, that is common to all diseases, and a disease-specific residual e_{ik} that captures spatial variation in risk of disease k that is not shared with other diseases. This joint mapping approach has several advantages. Identification of common geographical variations in risk of multiple diseases provides stronger evidence of the presence of an underlying environmental risk factor than does mapping of a single disease. Precision of small area risk estimates can also be improved, due to the extra information about the common spatial patterns contained in data from more than one disease. Examples of the application of these methods include Knorr-Held and Best [115] who identified patterns of high shared risk of oral and esophageal cancers in Germany that coincided with regions having high smoking and alcohol consumption rates.

Feltbower et al. [116] used a different joint mapping method, based on a multivariate version of the Bayesian CAR model, to investigate whether the observed international correlations in incidence of acute lymphoblastic leukemia and type 1 diabetes were also seen at the small area level. They found much weaker evidence of geographical correlation between the two diseases at this scale, part of which could be explained by the effects of deprivation and population density. Hansell *et al.* [117] used joint disease mapping methods for a different purpose. Their goal was to investigate small area variations in chronic obstructive pulmonary disease (COPD) mortality that may have been related to historically high levels of air pollution. To account for confounding by smoking, they used a joint spatial analysis of COPD and lung cancer mortality, and interpreted the shared pattern of risk as reflecting mainly smoking-related risks, and the residual pattern of risk specific to COPD as reflecting COPD-specific environmental risk factors, such as air pollution.

8.3.2.2 Geographical correlation studies

In an ecological or geographical correlation study, the unit of analysis is an aggregate population and information is collected on group level rather than on individuals. The association between summary measures of disease and exposure is then analysed. The statistical model typically takes the form of a log-linear Poisson regression:

$$y_i \sim Poisson(r_i E_i)$$
$$\log r_i = b_o + \sum_k b_k X_{ik}$$

where y_i, r_i and E_i are defined as before, and X_{ik} is the summary (e.g., average) value of exposure k in area i. For example, y_i may represent annual number of breast cancer cases in country i and X_i may be mean fat consumption for adult females in that country. Ecological studies have often found a positive correlation between these two variables, which might lead one to conclude that fat consumption is a risk factor for breast cancer. However, a well-known error in this reasoning is the so called ecological fallacy [118], which occurs when conclusions are drawn about individuals from group-level data, since group-level relationships may not necessarily hold for individuals. In the above example, it is not possible to infer that the individual women with breast cancer actually had a high fat consumption.

As discussed in Chapter 6, ecological studies based on geographical correlation are often thought of as *hypothesis generating* because of the problems of inferring causality at an individual level as mentioned above, but ecological studies have also been important in developing and exploring hypotheses of great public health importance. For example, the association between living near a landfill site and giving birth to a child with a congenital anomaly was studied in Great Britain [119]. A database on all known landfill sites was compiled and potential exposure assigned on the basis of distance from landfill sites. Analyses were performed on different types of landfill sites (licensed to carry hazardous waste or household waste) using area level data on socioeconomic confounding (Carstairs' index). A major finding was that 80 percent of the British population lives within 2 km of a landfill site, which posed the unusual problem of having a much larger 'exposed' population in relation to the 'reference'. The findings indicated small excess risks of congenital anomalies near landfill sites, interestingly also before opening of the sites. The authors noted that the large heterogeneity between landfill sites and the likelihood that the effect of any emissions would be greatest close to the sites, causal effects related to particular landfill sites might have been greatly diluted. However, there are no known causal mechanisms that might explain the findings, and there is considerable uncertainty as to the extent of any possible exposure to chemicals found in landfills. Further understanding of the potential toxicity of landfill emissions and possible exposure pathways is needed in order to help interpret the epidemiological findings. A further study using the same exposure database investigated the incidence of selected cancers near landfill sites [120]. No excess risks were found for any of the cancers. It should be emphasized that latency time and migration issues as mentioned above may well have obscured any real excess risks.

Recently, interest has focused on ecological designs that combine aggregate level data on the general population with individual-level survey data. One of the main sources of bias in ecological studies is failure to account for *within-area* variation in the exposures of interest. In order to avoid the ecological fallacy, it is necessary to integrate or average the individual-level disease-exposure relationship for each area. For the multiplicative relationships typically assumed in epidemiology, this leads to a more complex regression model at the aggregate level that depends not only on the mean exposure in the area, but also on the within-area variability of the exposure. It is often possible to obtain information on the joint *within-area* distribution of potential risk factors from sample surveys or from high density environmental monitoring schemes and/or models. In such situations, methods proposed by, for example, Richardson *et al.* [121] and Prentice and Sheppard [122], can be used to combine such data with area-level health outcomes in order to estimate the appropriate integrated aggregate-level regression model. For example, if a single exposure variable is assumed to be normally distributed within areas, and the disease outcome is relatively rare, the following ecological regression model can be assumed:

$$y_i \sim Poisson\,(r_i E_i)$$
$$\log r_i = b_o + b_1 X_i + 0.5 b_1^2 V_i$$

where X_i and V_i are the area mean and within-area variance of the exposure variable, respectively.

Whitaker *et al.* [123] proposed a related approach for use in situations where samples are available for each area that contain information on both exposures and health outcomes for the same individuals. In a simulation study, Jackson *et al.* [124] showed that combining such individual-level samples with aggregate data on health outcomes and exposures via a pair of linked regression models (one at the individual level and one at the aggregate level) led to a reduction in bias over a standard ecological regression analysis, and also improved power compared to analysis of the individual-level data alone. They applied this method to a study of socioeconomic risk factors for self-reported limiting long-term illness, using aggregate (electoral ward) data on risk factors and health outcome from the 1991 UK census, plus samples of individual-level data collected in some wards from respondents to the Health Survey for England 1994–98.

8.3.2.3 Point source studies

Programs such as the Small Area Health Statistics Unit (SAHSU) of Imperial College, London, conduct studies to investigate health risks associated with point sources of pollution, such as industrial plants. Circular areas around the point source have traditionally been used as surrogates for exposure, using different distances from the source to define potential exposure zones. Better exposure estimates can be obtained, for example, by using dispersion modeling. One limitation is that data are usually available only for the current exposure situation, making assessment of chronic health outcomes (which often have long latency times between exposure start and diagnosis) difficult. Nevertheless, dispersion modeling was recently used in a study of mercury exposure (see Chapter 3, Figure 3.6) and kidney disease mortality, showing a clear exposure response pattern between modeled mercury levels in ambient air and kidney disease mortality [125].

8.4 Investigation of disease clusters

Daniel Wartenberg

8.4.1 Introduction

Disease clusters are aggregations of similar or related diseases in specific groups of people. They are local outbreaks of disease, usually chronic disease, that raise concerns because there appear to be more observed cases of disease than is typical in populations of similar size and demographics. Clusters often are identified initially based on the number of cases occurring in a given time period, in a certain geographic area, or in a specified population subgroup, such as a workforce, a social or recreational club, or even within a group taking the same pharmaceutical. They are a common occurrence, with more than 1000 cluster reports filed each year with state health departments in the United States [126–128]. Cluster investigations can be large, costly and time-consuming tasks, and yet concern about the occurrence and cause of clusters is understandable.

Identification of perceived clusters often is controversial because investigations are costly and successes in finding the underlying risk factors have been rare, but the impact of those successes has been dramatic, such as banning pharmaceuticals or changing industrial practices. While no one doubts the occurrence of clusters nor the impact of identifying their causes, debate continues about the effectiveness of cluster investigation strategies for differentiating among those situations that are attributable to the normal random variation of disease incidence, those attributable to a specific cause, and those that remain unresolved. The most controversial clusters are those with suspected environmental etiology, which are difficult to resolve often due to lack of adequate information, particularly about exposures to possible risk factors. The divergence of opinions range from communities demanding investigations through political and media contacts to some public health authorities who have argued against such investigation, regardless of the context, except in the most extreme circumstances [129]. They argue that since most investigations have not resulted in the detection of new hazardous agents or etiologies, such studies are not a good use of money and other government resources.

8.4.2 **Motivation for conducting cluster investigations**

There are two main reasons to study reported or suspected disease clusters. First, cluster investigations are warranted because of the concern raised when someone contracts a serious illness, and when this concern is compounded by the observation of several cases of the same illness in a small group, small geographical area or some other type of associ- ation of individuals. People want to know why this happened and what can be done. They want to know whether it is just a unfortunate twist of fate, of which they are unlucky recipients, and that over time the disease rates will return to normal, or whether there is an identifiable cause suggesting an intervention that may be able to prevent addi- tional people from being exposed to a specific disease-causing agent, thereby decreasing the future risk and the number of new cases of disease. For example, a cluster may be due to genetic predisposition, such as increased risk of female breast cancer among those with the *BrCa I* and *II* genes [130]. Among members of this group, not much can be done to reduce risk except to surgically remove the target organ. Or, a cluster may be due to an undetected exposure to a known etiologic agent, such as the unusually high rates of nonoccupational mesothelioma due to community exposure to asbestos, as in Manville, New Jersey [131]. In this case, environmental clean-up and indoor air quality controls may have reduced risk had they been implemented at the time of first exposures. In each such instance, the situations are tragic on a personal level, although scientifically clusters attributable to known etiologies are neither surprising nor remarkable. People seek explanations from health authorities, wanting to know why their family, their friends, their neighbors, or their coworkers appear to have a disproportionate amount of this specific disease compared to the number of cases typically observed in a population of this size.

Second, but far less frequently, clusters may be worth investigating because they provide new clues to a previously unknown etiology, or even a new disease. Although rare, these discoveries have led to actions that limit or prevent exposures to these disease- causing agents, thereby decreasing or eliminating additional cases of these disease. For example, in the late 1950s and early 1960s, thalidomide, a pharmaceutical that was given to pregnant women to treat morning sickness, resulted in an unusual excess of serious birth defects, including phocomelia. The first report was based on the observation of three cases [132]. As a result of this observation, use of this drug was suspended, although recently it has been re-approved for treatment of multiple myeloma, under strict controls to prevent any possibility of birth defects. In 1971, Herbst and cowo- rkers [133] reported the observation of eight cases of adenocarcinoma of the vagina in women aged 15–22 in Massachusetts, US, and implicated as the cause maternal use of diethylstilbestrol (DES), a pharmaceutical that is a synthetic, nonsteroidal oestrogen. This pharmaceutical is no longer in use, although it continues to cause health effects in the children and grandchildren of users. In 1972, the observation of three cases of angiosar- coma of the liver among polyvinyl chloride production workers was used to implicate vinyl chloride monomer as the risk factor in a worker population [134]. The industry implemented a workplace clean-up to eliminate worker exposures to vinyl chloride.

In 1977, an unusually high rate of male infertility in a pesticide manufacturing facility was used to identify dibromochloropropane (DBCP) as the cause of another workplace cluster [135]. In each of these cases, the agent implicated was not known to cause these serious adverse health effects prior to the detection of the cluster. After confirming the etiology suggested by the cluster, and where possible, interventions were introduced reduce the future disease burden.

Cluster investigations also have uncovered new diseases, such as Lyme disease, first reported in 1977 [136]; Legionnaire's disease, first reported in 1977 [137]; and HIV/AIDS, first reported in 1981 [138]. The identification of Lyme disease arose from the observation of a geographical cluster of childhood arthritis. Lyme disease has been linked to a bacterial infection acquired from the bite of an infected tick that was prevalent in that geographical area, and has now become far more widespread in the US. The identification of Legionnaire's disease arose from the detection of several cases of severe pneumonia, several of which were fatal, at a Legionnaire's convention held outside of Philadelphia in the US, and eventually determined to be due to bacterial contamination of water in a hotel's air conditioning system. Additional clusters, or outbreaks, of Legionnaire's disease have been recurring sporadically. HIV/AIDS was first detected due to five cases of *Pneumocystis carinii pneumonia*, two of which were fatal, in previously healthy patients, even though the disease is almost exclusively limited to severely immunocompromised patients. This devastating disease has taken on global, epidemic proportions. Even though studies subsequent to the clusters confirmed the etiology of these three diseases, prevention programs have had limited to moderate success.

On the other hand, it is important to recognize that the vast majority of cluster investigations conducted by public health authorities in response to concerns about disease clusters have ultimately proved to be fruitless [139, 140]. So the nature and extent of cluster response remains a major controversy.

8.4.3 **Investigative and analytical strategies**

To help explain the nature of cluster studies, Quartaert and colleagues have suggested a three-stage typology: cluster response, cluster monitoring and cluster research [141]. Cluster response is the short-term response to concerned citizens, typically based on the analysis of data directly related to cluster reports and its comparison to larger regional data. Cluster monitoring is the ongoing collection of analysis of data to identify changes in risk factors and/or disease (i.e., surveillance) for early detection of possible regional or local clusters. Cluster research is the conduct of traditional epidemiologic studies to evaluate etiologic hypotheses based on observed clusters.

8.4.3.1 **Cluster monitoring: using typical cluster report data**

Given the public health importance of following up reports of disease clusters, it is important to have a clear, efficient and effective process for doing so. Because the nature of the problem is different to that addressed in most epidemiological studies, most strategies for the investigation of reported local excess disease are different from traditional epidemiology. First, typical cluster reports may include only a few to a few dozen cases. From a statistical perspective, the small number of cases makes it difficult to exclude random variation as a plausible explanation for the observation, no matter what the disease or the rate of occurrence in the comparison population. All that may be known is the names and maybe the residential addresses of the cases. Second, the population within which the cases were observed may not be well defined, making rate calculations unreliable. For example, for a geographical cluster, it may not be known whether the cases come from a specific block in a neighborhood, are residents in the same town, work together, or have spent time in the same environment. The person reporting the observed excess may define the population by circumscribing the cases, even though had others outside this boundary been diagnosed with the same disease, word would have spread and they would have been included in the suspect group of cases. This underestimates the population at risk and inflates the apparent magnitude of the excess. Without a clearly and systematically defined population at risk (or under consideration), it is hard to determine whether the reported cluster has an unusual rate of disease. Third, at the time of the report, there is often no reliable exposure and risk factor information. Without that information, one cannot easily identify an appropriate comparison population, determine the possible risk factors that the cases experience or estimate the degree of exposure across the cases. Further, collecting this important information can be difficult, costly and time-consuming. In short, the limited data available from preliminary cluster reports often precludes rigorous analysis. Therefore, the analysis of cluster reports is often seen as a preliminary, hypothesis-generating exercise designed to help determine whether more rigorous follow-up investigations are warranted and to educate people so that they understand the situation and plans for follow up (i.e., cluster response in Quataert et al.'s typology). These analyses also have been called *pre-epidemiology*, to differentiate them from more traditional epidemiological research and so that reports are not overinterpreted [142].

8.4.3.2 Designing a cluster investigation

There are many ways to design a cluster investigation, depending on the characteristics of the cluster report, nature of the data available, and the time and resources available for the investigation. Most often, preliminary analyses are conducted based on the data reported, using methods specifically designed for such situations. These will be described below. In the best circumstance, if these results are positive, one would use these results to generate a relatively specific hypothesis for investigation with a traditional epidemiological study design. Several government public health programs, as well as many independent investigators [143–145], have developed and implemented investigation protocols, often based in part on the one developed by the US Centers for Disease Control and Prevention [146, 147], that include both the preliminary pre-epidemiology assessments (i.e., cluster response, in Quataert et al.'s typology) and planning for the possibility of more rigorous epidemiological investigation (i.e., cluster research, in Quataert et al.'s typology). In general, the steps are:

1. collect information from the original source of the cluster report regarding the cases and possible risk factors and/or etiology;

2. evaluate the data reported by:

(i) validating the cases and their diagnoses,

(ii) defining and characterizing the population at risk and the space–time extent of the cluster, determining an appropriate reference population, and

(iii) determining the biological and statistical plausibility of an excess, typically using methods specifically designed to assess disease clusters;

3. assess the feasibility of conducting an epidemiologic study based on the cluster-generated hypothesis;

4. conduct the etiological study.

There are no clear, generally accepted criteria by which scientists decide whether or not to conduct the etiologic study, and the decision is complicated. Factors that are considered typically include: the number of cases observed in the cluster, the magnitude and statistical significance of the disease excess, the background rate of the disease, the latency of the disease, the magnitude (above background) and prevalence of the suspected exposure(s), the plausibility that the exposure(s) caused the observed disease, availability of relevant data (e.g., exposure data, data on potential confounding factors), the public health impact of the problem, and the estimated time and resources it would take to conduct the study. Political pressure and community concern also may play a role. In a survey conducted in the US, about one percent of the initial cluster reports resulted in such epidemiological cluster research studies [127].

8.4.3.3 Statistical methods

There are many statistical methods available to conduct the pre-epidemiology phase of cluster investigations. This review covers only a limited number of these. Note that sometimes tests are conducted to look for temporal patterns, sometimes for spatial patterns, and sometimes for simultaneous space–time patterns. Several, but not all, methods can be adapted for these different situations. The reader is referred to Kulldorff [148] for a more extensive discussion of the methodology. The methods can be grouped into four main classes: goodness-of-fit tests, cell-occupancy methods, distance-based methods, and moving window methods. This section considers each in turn and, for brevity, provides a limited number of examples of specific methods.

1. Goodness-of-fit tests (of probability models)

The most basic test for an apparent local disease excess is to assess whether the observed number of cases fits a specified statistical distribution. Often, this is the first assessment made before other resources are allocated, because it is so easy and quick to do. The test assesses whether the observed number of cases is greater than would be found in a population of similar size and demographics, given the background rate of disease, assuming a specific statistical distribution of cases. Most often, the assumed distribution is a Poisson distribution. For that model, one can calculate, for a given population with a specified background or comparison disease rate λ, the probability of seeing exactly n cases by using the following formula:

$$Pr(n) = \frac{\lambda^n}{n!} e^{-\lambda}$$

Then, by summing probabilities for 0 cases to one less than the number observed, and subtracting this total from 1, one derives the probability of seeing at least as many cases as were observed. Note that the limitation of this approach is that it does not address where or when the cases occurred, other than within the overall space–time limits chosen. If the calculated probability is large, say greater than 0.05, some interpret the observation to be likely due to normal variability and not worthy of further follow up.

2. Cell occupancy (cell count) methods

Cell occupancy tests address whether there is a disproportionate number of cases in any geographic or temporal subregion of the observation space [149, 150]. To do this, one must define the full extent of the study area both geographically and in terms of time, and then subdivide it into smaller, disjoint, equal size blocks with carefully defined geographic and temporal boundaries. Then, the cases are assigned to the blocks, and the data are summarized in a variety of ways, determining whether the number that are 'close' is greater than expected [149]. For example, one could calculate whether the sum across all spatial blocks of largest number of cases in any single time block within each spatial block, is greater than expected [150]. If so, that would suggest some type of spatial or space–time cluster. Two limitations of the method are that it is highly dependent on the definition of the space–time blocks and the homogeneity of expected risk across blocks. One way for investigators to address this is to modify the space–time boundaries of individual blocks, based population size, demographic characteristics and other factors, so that they all have equal risk, and then conduct a similar statistical analysis. That way each block would be expected to have a similar number of cases. This approach, and the successive enhancements, is used less frequently today.

3. Distance-based methods

Distance-based methods compare the distances between cases, assessing whether or not the distribution of cases appears random. In one of the early methods proposed by Knox, the spatial and temporal distances between all possible pairs of cases were calculated and dichotomized into two groups, close or near [151]. Then, these distance categories were cross-classified in a 2×2 table, and the observed number of pairs that were close in both space and time were tested under the hypothesis of a Poisson distribution. The underlying statistical assumption is that the distribution of cases in space is independent of that in time. One limitation of this method is the need to define the critically 'close' space and time distances and, typically, it is a somewhat arbitrary decision.

Mantel [152] proposed a generalization of Knox's method in which functions of the actual interpoint distances were used rather than Knox's close or far dichotomization. He recommended using an inverse transformation, possibly with an offset, so that small distances between cases were given more weight than large distances between cases. The test statistic for this approach is the sum over all possible pairs of the product of the function of the temporal distance and the function of the geographic distance. Mantel points out that this is essentially a regression of the function of one type of distance on the other.

$$X = \sum_i \sum_j f(t_{ij}) g(s_{ij})$$

Where f(-) and g(-) are functions of time and space distances;
For example $f(t_{ij}) = 1/t_{ij}$ and $g(s_{ij}) = 1/s_{ij}$

Cuzick and Edwards [153] propose a related method using cases and controls, in which nearest neighbours are assigned to each case and each control, and then the number of case–case pairs, case-control pairs, and control–control pairs are compared. An excess of case–case pairs would suggest clustering. This method can be implemented with any number, say k, nearest neighbors. This method is different from several other distance methods in that it needs both cases and controls, rather than only cases, but is less arbitrary than many others by using nearest neighbors in place of artificial cutoffs or transformed distances. Jacquez [154] describes a modification of the Mantel method, similar to Cuzick and Edwards. The method uses the number of pairs of cases that are k-nearest neighbors in both space and time to assess clustering. It also removes the arbitrariness of Mantel's inverse transformation with offset. He shows that in addition to being less arbitrary, this test also is more sensitive that either the Knox or Mantel tests. A related, but not strictly distance-based method, sometimes used to assess disease patterns and clusters, is spatial autocorrelation [155]. Spatial autocorrelation methods, such as Moran's I and Geary's c, assess whether geographic units that are adjacent or near one another also have similar values for a specified unit-specific index, such as a disease rate.

Some additional distance-based methods examine the distance of cases and controls from putative risk factors [156, 157]. These tests are called focused tests, and Waller and Lawson have shown that the score test is uniformly the most powerful test for these situations.

4. Moving window methods

Moving window methods are a set of approaches that define the dimension of a cluster that they are seeking to detect, the window, and then move the window across the entire time, space or space–time data field, scanning for areas that exceed a specified threshold, often set based on data outside the window. This approach was first used by Naus [158] in looking at time-series data. He sought to find the line segment of specified length with the greatest number of events over a long time period. Openshaw [159, 160] generalized this approach to two dimensions with his so-called Geographical Analysis Machine (GAM). He used a circle with a pre-specified radius to scan a spatial grid in search of the grid point at which the circle contains more cases than the specified threshold. The radius of the circle was specified to be slightly greater than the distance between grid points. Rather than being proposed as a rigorous, statistical approach, Openshaw suggests that this method should be used as a screening tool for an automated surveillance program, to identify areas for possible follow-up investigation.

Rushton and Lolonis [161] developed a similar approach for case-control data, using a circle with a radius slightly smaller than the grid spacing, the method of overlapping local case proportions. Statistical testing is based on Monte Carlo simulations, to adjust for multiple comparisons, although there is some inherent bias due to the overlap of circles in the assessment. Kulldorff [162–166] developed a similar method, called the spatial scan statistic, but based it on a different inferential framework using likelihood ratio statistics and Monte Carlo simulations for statistical significance testing. In this case, the specifics of his simulation approach do not have the same limitation as that of Rushton and Lolonis, and provide valid tests of clustering and the most likely cluster. Kulldorff also has extended the method to the assessment of space–time clustering. His software is available as freeware, and it is being used widely.

8.4.3.4 Further characterization of methods

The tests described above, which are simply an arbitrary sample of the more than 100 methods available for assessing disease clusters, also can be divided into groups that describe their substantive purpose and compared in terms of their sensitivity or statistical power [167]. A full description of the methods and the specific characteristics is beyond the scope of this chapter. For context, the following is a brief summary of these groupings. Tests can be dichotomized into tests of global clustering vs cluster detection. Global clustering methods assess whether there is any clustering overall in data, or possible accumulating small increments of clustering across the entire data field, which might be relevant for infectious disease assessment. Cluster detection methods, on the other hand, seek to detect the presence of a specific local disease excess, identify its location, and test its statistical significance. These methods are more appropriate for environmentally related clusters. Cluster detection tests can be further dichotomized as focused or general, in terms of how clustering is defined. General cluster detection tests identify disease excesses based on the proximity of cases to each other (and possible controls) in a localized area, as described above, while with focused cluster detection tests, the clustering is defined as excess disease within close proximity to an exposure source [156, 168]. Some methods can be adapted for either purpose.

8.4.4 Interpreting results of cluster investigations

8.4.4.1 Statistical interpretations

There are a variety of generic considerations one should address when interpreting the results of an analysis of disease cluster data. First, there is the method by which the data are collected: passive (e.g., self-reported) or active (e.g., routine assessment of incidence data). To date, most, if not all, entities rely on local residents, astute physicians and the media to identify local disease excesses. This is a passive reporting system from the perspective of a government public health authority. Unfortunately, this is a biased approach, statistically, in that these observations are based on informal evaluations conducted in each community as neighbors talk to one another about their lives. Therefore, those that garner attention have been screened out of thousands and thousands of potential study areas that do not appear unusual. Just due to random fluctuations, one would expect a statistically significant excess from out of every 20 assessments, or thousands each year [169]. For these assessments, one also does not know if those reporting the cluster have drawn the boundaries specifically around the known cases, rather than identifying a region of concern and the calculating a disease rate, sometimes called the 'Texas Sharpshooter' approach. Even with this *ad hoc* screening, there likely are many areas where no such assessment is made, leading to an undercount. Further, there is no guarantee that a true cluster will be detected and reported to a health department. The only obvious solution to these concerns of false positives and false negatives is to routinely and rigorously review disease incidence data, such as cancer registry records, i.e., cluster monitoring in Quataert *et al.*'s typology, yet no health department in the US actively does so [170].

8.4.5 Managing public concern about clusters

Members of the public are concerned about clusters because they perceive them as a very serious problem, the extent of which is unknown. Often, they believe that the situation could have been averted by greater vigilance, its expansion still can be limited, and a similar occurrence still can be prevented elsewhere. It is a personal tragedy to have a family member or friend fall seriously ill. In situations where environmental contamination is the suspected cause of the disease, the public is worried that these observations may be a harbinger of impending environmental disease catastrophes, a sentinel to be heeded. It may seem callous at best—unacceptable at worst—to family members and friends when scientists dismiss a cluster of disease as normal, 'expected' or uninterruptible, or if the scientists suggest to these aggrieved relatives that they wait until there are enough data available for further analysis.

Media reports of clusters often heighten concern, and distress government officials due to the uncertainty surrounding possible causation. Nonetheless, these reports are stories of great human interest and tragedy, stories that connect with their readership, and often involve blame. Not as involved with the larger scientific issues, reporters are more concerned about journalistic issues such as accurate reporting and human interest, even if in the end, the cluster can explained by routine factors such as demographics and individual behaviors. Their publishers look for stories with human drama and political intrigue to sell papers, and clusters often are true reports of disease that involve personal tragedy for a family or workplace. They may involve blame, with the pattern of those falling ill suggesting a source of the disease, which may be related to the workplace exposures or the environment contamination. Further, in situations where the community is particularly distressed by the disease, residents often resort to political pressure to elicit a response. That also is newsworthy. These factors all lead to a good story for a reporter and newspaper sales for the publisher, whether or not the situation is, in fact, not due to environmental contamination or other troubling causes.

Government officials are concerned about disease clusters in terms of balancing the competing goals of cluster response and other health department programs, and the availability of resources to be responsive to community concerns. They want to respond to valid public health problems but do not want to squander precious resources on wild goose chases. Many see prevention of unnecessary disease, where possible, as an important goal and responsibility. However, government officials must balance the many disease prevention and health management issues facing them, in terms of the staff time and resources required to address them, with the utility of the likely ambiguous outcome of even a limited cluster investigation. They have to decide which cluster reports warrant follow-up and which do not in the context of their entire disease prevention and health management programs and mandates. As currently practiced, disease cluster reports usually receive limited evaluation and response unless the data presented are strongly compelling or there is substantial external pressure (e.g., from political or media sources).

Scientists often view the disease cluster issue as one of ascertaining reasonable certainty. Afraid to cry wolf too often and lose their credibility, scientists often are reluctant to render an opinion about the validity and implications of a reported cluster until they reach an acceptable level of certainty that the occurrence of these cases is unusual statistically and that there is at least one plausible explanation for their occurrence at this place at this time, such as a known, toxic exposure. This level of scientific certainty is an extremely difficult standard to achieve, and suggests a strong bias toward false negative reports over false positive reports. Even the routinely accepted statistical criterion, determining that the chance that an observation could be attributed to random variation is less than 1 in 20 (analogous to flipping five heads in a row with an evenly weighted coin), is a very high standard to achieve, particularly in light of the small number of cases typically reported as a cluster.

In summary, most cluster investigations are considered exploratory and hypothesis-generating, rather than more traditional hypothesis testing activities. Yet, historically, they have played a crucial role in identifying previously unknown local disease excesses, previously undetected exposure situations putting people at risk to known hazards, and previously unknown hazards and carcinogens. Conversely, such investigations have been able to assist in the vindication of situations believed to be hazardous but where the interpretation had not allowed for the impact of well-known risk factors. On the other hand it is important to remember that many cluster investigations that have been conducted have not led to any conclusive results, but have raised considerable anxiety and consumed enormous resources. It is therefore very important to consider the consequences in detail before starting any investigation, and draw on the lessons learned from many previous investigations. Finally, routine monitoring, or surveillance and assessment, provides an opportunity for a rigorous and systematic approach for diffusing much of the controversy surrounding clusters.

8.5 Gene–environment interactions

Valentina Gallo and Paolo Vineis

8.5.1 Introduction—genetics and diseases

A sequence of DNA bases encoding for an amino acids sequence is generally defined as a 'gene'. An allele is one of a series of two or more different genes that occupy the same position (locus) on a chromosome. In the gene, the DNA bases sequence can be divided in group of three ('triplets'); each triplet corresponds to one amino acid or to a 'stop sequence' that ends the chain. The mechanism that turns the information contained in the DNA into a protein is a two-step process: the first step is the transcription (from DNA to RNA) which occurs in the nucleus of the cell; the second step is the translation (from RNA to an amino acid chain) which occurs in the cell cytoplasm. This apparently simple process is modulated by numerous factors inside and outside the cell, giving rise to a complex pattern of gene expression. In addition to factors affecting gene expression, the DNA sequence itself can change in response to a number of factors affecting the length, the structure, and the function of the corresponding protein. Changes in the DNA sequence affecting the nucleotide sequence are called 'mutations' and can be divided into four main categories: deletions (when one or more pair bases is taken off from the DNA chain); insertions (when one or more pair bases are added to the DNA chain); translocations (when a piece of DNA is moved from one part to an other of the chain) and inversions (when a piece of DNA is reversed). Mutations can arise from the process of DNA copying (which is carried out when DNA duplicates at the moment of cell division) which is rarely error-free; and from environmental factors such as radiation and other agents called mutagens. Every cell in the body has a complex system which might identify and repair genetic mutations when they arise in its DNA, but some mutations may escape this control system. Not all the mutations, however, imply a protein modification: many sequences of DNA are 'silent' (do not actively encode for proteins), and some mutations in a coding sequence can also be silent (do not cause changes in protein composition or function) because different triplets encode for the same amino acid.

The relationship between genetic make-up and disease is quite complex. Every individual can carry, in their own genetic make up, a gene variant (genotype) inherited from one or both parents, which determines a disease (phenotype). This is clearly the case of monogenic diseases and their transmission follows Mendel's laws. In addition to monogenic diseases, the concept of a complex genetic susceptibility has been introduced. This refers to the fact that a particular genetic make up can contribute to the development of a disease in conjunction with other risk factors. This is the case of many chronic diseases in which the interaction between environmental risk factors with a specific genetic make up increases or decreases the risk of developing a disease.

8.5.2 Genetic susceptibility

Mutations are rare events (conventionally they are considered to affect less than 1 percent of the population), while polymorphisms are frequent variants (allele frequencies greater than 1 percent). The human genome contains approximately 3 500 000 000 base pairs; of these, more than 10 000 000 are likely to differ among different individuals. Such variants in single base pairs are called single nucleotide polymorphisms (SNPs) and are potentially responsible for susceptibility to disease. They can be either dominant or recessive, and subjects could be either homozygotic (AA, aa) or heterozygotic (Aa), resulting in different risk patterns (see Figure 8.7). It is becoming clear that only a minority of diseases, however, have a frank genetic origin, in the sense that they are due to a highly penetrant gene. For example, about 5–10 percent of breast cancers occur in women carrying mutations of the *BRCA1* gene. At the other extreme of the gradient, there are diseases that are entirely due to the environment with no role for genetic predisposition. This is the case, e.g., of 15 workers who were exposed to beta-naphthylamine in the British chemical industry in the 1950s. All of them developed transitional-cell bladder cancer with no role for individual susceptibility [171]. The vast majority of diseases, however, are likely to be due to an interaction between external exposure and genetic susceptibility caused by 'low penetrance' gene variants (see Figure 8.8) [172]. One type of such susceptibility is related to the metabolism of carcinogens. Individuals with a SNP at

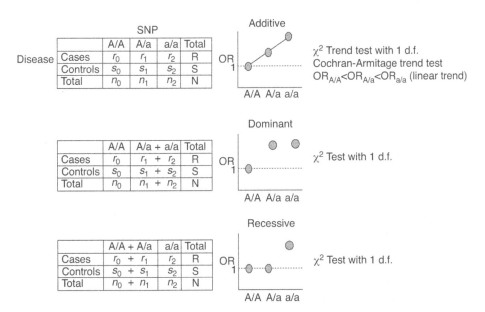

Fig. 8.7 Assessing associations between single SNPs and disease. Figure courtesy of Juan R. Gonzalez.

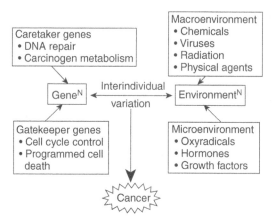

Fig. 8.8 Many genes and environmental exposures contribute to the carcinogenic process. The effects can be additive or multiplicative, which are modifiable by inter-individual variation in genetic function. Adapted by permission from the American Society of Clinical Oncology [172].

a particular gene locus have a defect in the enzyme involved in the metabolism of a carcinogen and, therefore, develop cancer more easily if they are exposed to the substance.

The study of SNPs in epidemiological investigations has become common under the assumption that the identification of highly susceptible subgroups in the population can contribute also to an easier identification of environmental hazards. This assumption is at the basis, for example, of the popularity of 'Mendelian randomization' (see below). However, the study of gene–environment interactions is not easy and can even be misleading if the methods are not accurate.

8.5.3 Human genome epidemiology

With the increasing amount of knowledge about genetic susceptibility to diseases and interaction between genes and the environment, a new discipline is being delineated: Human Genome Epidemiology (HuGE) [173]. HuGE encompasses all the epidemiological aspects that are involved in this field, from gene discovery to health policy. This process has different steps, the majority of which involve epidemiological methods (see Figure 8.9 and Table 8.5). In the initial disease characterization process (often starting from a family manifesting a higher frequency of a disease compared to the rest of the population), a genetic epidemiology approach is needed in order to confirm the contribution of a genetic component to the disease and to establish the model of transmission. Linkage-based approaches are set up in families and the genealogic information is crucial for evaluating the co-segregation of the genetic marker (proxy for the disease gene) and the phenotype. Moreover, these studies are very powerful for detecting or excluding candidate DNA regions in families where the phenotype shows a high hereditability.

After a genetic component has been hypothesized, studies are developed to localize the responsible gene or genes so that molecular biologists and biochemists can attempt to

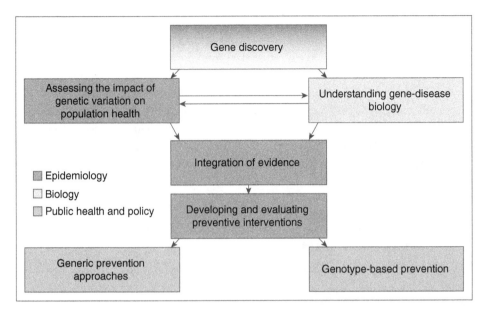

Figure 8.9 The role of epidemiology in the continuum from gene discovery to disease prevention. Adapted with permission from [173], Khoury MJ, Little J, Burke W. *Human genome epidemiology: a scientific foundation for using genetic information to improve health and prevent disease.* Oxford and New York: Oxford University Press 2004.

Table 8.5 The role of various branches of epidemiology in studying diseases with a genetic component

Type of study	Study design	Branch of epidemiology
Gene discovery and characterization	Several methods (see Table 8.6)	Genetic epidemiology
Gene characterization at population level	Population prevalence Genotype-disease association Gene–gene interaction Gene–environment interaction	Molecular epidemiology
Application of genetic information	Evaluating validity and usefulness of genetic tests in clinical use	Clinical epidemiology
	Evaluating usefulness of genetic tests for population screening	Public health epidemiology

clarify the pathophysiology of the disease in which the gene(s) is involved. After the identification of the relevant gene and its functions, a further process encompasses the estimation of the allele prevalence in different populations, the study of the association between gene variants and disease at the population level, and the evaluation of the interactions of the gene in question with other genes and with environmental factors (molecular epidemiology). Finally, epidemiological methods are required in order to evaluate the validity and the usefulness of genetic tests in clinical use (clinical epidemiology), and to estimate the usefulness of genetic tests for population screening (public health epidemiology). Data coming from these studies will eventually address health policies for genetic preventive approaches. The next section of the chapter will address the epidemiological methods that are required in the process.

8.5.4 Genetic epidemiology: identification of the genetic component of a disease

The first question an epidemiologist should ask him or herself about a disease that affects some members of the same family is: 'Is this disease genetic? Or, at least, does it have a heritable component?' The answer to this question is less straightforward than it seems. Members of the same family share not only part of their genetic makeup, but also many environmental and behavioral factors which may contribute to specific diseases. The epidemiological approach to find out to what extent a disease has a genetic component and which model of inheritance the genetic component follows encompasses studies of familial aggregation, heritability and segregation analysis (see Table 8.5). These studies are carried out without actually looking at the DNA of individuals.

Table 8.6 Stepwise approach of genetic and molecular epidemiology in studying gene–environment interactions

Question	Study design	Level of assessment
Has this disease a genetic component?	Familial aggregation analysis	Pedigree and phenotypes
Which genetic model does the disease follow?	Segregation analysis	Pedigree and phenotypes
Which is the responsible gene?		
Broader mapping	Linkage analysis	DNA and phenotypes
Finer mapping	Linkage disequilibrium	DNA and phenotypes
Gene identification	Candidate gene association studies	Genotypes and phenotypes
Identification of the mutation	Experimental	DNA
Gene characterization	Population-based or family-based studies	Genotypes and phenotypes

Familial aggregation studies are done to demonstrate that the disease tends to occur in families more than would be expected by chance. Usually they are family studies in which the proportion of the effect of the shared environment and of the genetic influences is estimated. In addition to testing the hypothesis of familial aggregation, these studies provide estimates of the relative contribution of genes (heritability) and of unmeasured environmental factors (environmentality) using variance component models for continuous traits and liability models for binary traits. These studies can also be done by investigations on twins and on adopted children. See [174] for more detailed information on these studies.

In the case of Parkinson's disease, a recent family aggregation study conducted in Iceland seems to confirm a genetic component contributing to all forms of the disease. The population-based familial aggregation study reported that patients with Parkinson's disease were significantly more related to each other than were the controls, and that the risk ratio for Parkinson's disease was 6.7 (95% CI 4.3, 9.6) for siblings, 3.2 (95% CI 1.2, 7.8) for offspring, and 2.7 (95% CI 1.6, 3.9) for nephews and nieces of patients with late-onset Parkinson's disease. In addition, the spouses of the patients were not at increased risk for developing the disease [175]. These data suggest a familial component for the disease, and by demonstrating that the familial clustering of Parkinson's disease extends beyond the nuclear family, focus attention more on genetic factors than on the environmental ones which are usually shared closely by nuclear families.

Once a disease has been found to have a genetic component, *segregation analysis studies* are used to identify the genetic model of the disease, usually by applying a maximum likelihood approach. This approach is based on the trait penetrance, the phenotype distribution in the population, and the probability of transmission within families. Some adjustments are needed because the families under study are more likely to have more affected members and to present a higher penetrance (referral bias), thus leading to over-estimating gene frequency and penetrance. Moreover in these studies particular attention must be paid to phenotype assessment: age at onset of the disease and increasing gradient of severity of the disease with age must be taken into consideration. As an example, a segregation analysis of Parkinson's disease among more than 1000 individuals clustered in 199 nuclear families was conducted in 1998. This analysis anticipated what later was confirmed in the familial aggregation study in Iceland. In fact, the general conclusion was that Parkinson's disease was best explained by a rare familiar factor transmitted in a non-Mendelian fashion, which influences the age at onset of the disease [176].

Once the genetic component has been verified and a hypothesis on the way of transmission has been tested, the actual responsible gene(s) must be identified, allowing different scenarios: from a major-effect gene and few small-effect genes; to small-effect genes alone, to the presence of few major-effect genes combined with some small-effect genes. The process of *gene identification* follows a stepwise approach in which each step narrows down the genomic search. As a first step, it is possible to broadly identify chromosomal location through linkage analysis. This method is based on the principle that two genes located on different chromosomes, at the moment of meiosis, segregate independently. During meiosis, the phenomenon of crossing-over takes place, i.e., homologous chromosomes exchange parts of their genetic material before splitting into gametes. During crossing-over, the further apart two DNA sequences are located, the more likely they are to be separated. The observation of recombination between generations provides crucial information which is used to localize susceptibility genes. Based on this principle, it is possible to identify one or more genetic 'markers' (which co-segregate with the phenotype or the disease within the family) for a particular phenotype. These markers may have nothing to do with the responsible gene, other than the physical location on the chromosomes (they are located nearby, i.e., are in linkage disequilibrium—LD—with the causative genetic variant). A difficulty often faced in linkage analysis is that genotype is not a good proxy for phenotype in incompletely penetrant traits. To overcome these problems, linkage analysis uses various techniques from *lod score methods* and *affected sib methods*, to nonparametric linkage methods. These analyses are considered the most powerful for studying low-penetrance phenotypes or traits whose genetic model is unknown. It is beyond the scope of this chapter to describe these methods in detail.

Together with the gene identification, it is possible to outline the main characteristics of the responsible gene through association studies. Different association study designs can be used in order to obtain a finer genomic mapping through linkage disequilibrium techniques, to test a candidate gene hypothesis, or to characterize a cloned gene. The main distinction between association studies concerns whether they are population- or family-based. The particular issues of study design of association studies are dealt with in the next section.

8.5.5 Molecular epidemiology: gene characterization at population level

Molecular epidemiological studies aim at gene discovery (by finer mapping using linkage disequilibrium techniques or testing an association with a candidate gene), gene characterization, or gene interactions with other genes and with environmental factors. They can be population- or family-based. The population-based study designs could be both case-control and cohort studies. The design itself is not affected by the fact that one of the exposures being evaluated is genetic rather than environmental.

8.5.5.1 Case-control studies

The case-control study design is usually considered when the traits under investigation are not too rare. The usual limits and strengths of case-control design in classical epidemiology apply to these studies (see Chapter 6). One advantage of measuring a genetic exposure is that it is not affected by recall bias, which eliminates a main source of bias in case-control studies. Moreover, the fact that genetic exposures are transmitted randomly by parents to the offspring is thought to be responsible for significant reduction in selection bias and residual confounding and has been compared to what happens in randomized controlled trials. This has been referred to as 'Mendelian randomization'. On the other hand, genetic exposure assessment itself is not completely error-free as it is based on laboratory analyses.

Table 8.7 The relation between CYP2D6*4, exposure to pesticides and Parkinson's disease

Model	None		Gardening Use		Professional Use	
	OR (95% CI)	p	OR (95% CI)	p	OR (95% CI)	p
Model 1 (–2 log likelihood = 406.288)						
0 CYP2D6*4 allele	1.00	–	1.73 (0.86–3.48)	0.12	1.85 (0.96–3.55)	0.06
1 CYP2D6*4 allele	1.39 (0.70–2.76)	0.35	1.17 (0.49–2.77)	0.72	1.83 (0.84–3.95)	0.13
2 CYP2D6*4 allele (PMs)	0.41 (0.04–3.99)	0.44	2.75 (0.55–13.74)	0.22	4.74 (1.29–17.45)	0.02
Model 2 (–2 log likelihood = 407.859)						
0 or 1 CYP2D6*4 allele	1.00	–	1.34 (0.76–2.35)	0.31	1.65 (0.91–2.98)	0.10
2 CYP2D6*4 alleles (PMs)	0.35 (0.04–3.46)	0.37	2.45 (0.50–11.98)	0.27	4.18 (1.17–14.96)	0.03
Model 3 (–2 log likelihood = 409.604)						
0 or 1 CYP2D6*4 allele	1.00	–	1.50 (0.92–2.43)	0.10		
2 CYP2D6*4 alleles (PMs)	1.00	–	3.28 (1.16–9.27)	0.02		
Model 4 (–2 log likelihood = 412.298)						
0 or 1 CYP2D6*4 allele	1.00	–	1.00	–		
2 CYP2D6*4 alleles (PMs)	1.00	–	2.39 (0.92–6.24)	0.07		

From [177]. Reproduced with permission from Elbaz A, Levecque C, Clavel J, Vidal JS, Richard F, Amouyel P, et al. CYP2D6 polymorphism, pesticide exposure, and Parkinson's disease. Annals of Neurology. 2004 55(3):430–4.

As an example, Elbaz *et al.* [177] performed a case-control study of Parkinson's disease in a population characterized by a high prevalence of pesticides exposure and studied the joint effect of pesticides exposure and CYP2D6. Although the study was based on a small group of subjects, the findings are consistent with a gene–environment interaction disease model according to which

1. pesticides have a modest effect in subjects who are not CYP2D6 poor metabolizers,

2. pesticides' effect is increased in poor metabolizers (approximately twofold) and

3. poor metabolizers are not at increased risk in the absence of pesticides exposure (see Table 8.7).

8.5.5.2 Cohort studies

Cohort studies are usually involved in investigating gene–gene or gene–environment interactions, taking advantage of existing large cohorts in which DNA has already been collected. Due to the fact that genotyping is still expensive and, therefore, genotyping entire cohorts would be prohibitive, generally investigators conduct nested case-control studies and case-cohort studies within the cohorts. The strengths and limits of classical epidemiology apply to these study designs as well. In particular, selection biases can arise from incomplete case ascertainment within the cohort that could be due to an inappropriate follow-up of cohort members. As regards control selection for nested case–control studies, a number of sampling techniques are available in order to optimize the study design, such as multi-stage sampling. In multi-stage sampling, selection of controls is done starting from a pool of individuals chosen on the basis of a surrogate for the risk factor under consideration (using, for example, family history as a surrogate of a particular genotype).

In general, when a genetic trait is investigated as exposure, in both case-control and cohort studies a particular confounding effect of ethnicity needs to be taken into consideration. Ethnicity can represent, in fact, not only a surrogate for unaccounted risk factors, but can also be strongly associated with the genetic exposure, as allele frequencies within a population can vary greatly; this phenomenon is referred to as 'population stratification'. There is wide debate on the extent of concern that should be attributed to this effect, and some elaborate techniques to correctly classify ethnic backgrounds, when accounting for ethnicity, have been proposed.

8.5.5.3 Family-based studies

Family-based studies have the great advantage of overcoming concerns about population stratification. The most important and most commonly used designs are the 'case-sibling', and the 'case-parent-trio' studies. However, as these study designs are quite specialized, they will not be reviewed here.

8.5.6 Specific issues in studying gene–environment interactions

One issue that is relevant to all epidemiological investigations aimed at gene–environment interactions is statistical power (sample size). Statistical power is usually inadequate in most studies on this subject, and appropriate *a priori* calculations of the size required to detect an interaction are needed. A second, related issue is subgroup analysis: statistically significant associations may arise by chance when multiple comparisons are made within a single study. An additional problem is publication bias, i.e., the fact that, among many comparisons that are made in a dataset, only those which turn out positive are published. The overall effect is a large number of false positive results. Small studies tend to suggest, for many gene-disease associations, much larger odds ratios than those found in following larger studies. The best way to avoid the pitfalls associated with subgroup analysis, multiple comparisons and publication bias is to define sound scientific hypothesis *a priori*. This goal can be accomplished by assuring a strong cooperation among all the involved investigators, i.e., geneticists, biochemists, molecular biologists, epidemiologists and biostatisticians. In the case of gene–environment interactions in cancer, for example, a sound *a priori* hypothesis implies (a) that evidence has been provided that a genetic polymorphism is implicated in the metabolism of a given carcinogen; (b) that the polymorphism can be measured with a reasonably small degree of misclassification; (c) that epidemiological tools allow the investigators to identify the exposed subjects with sufficient accuracy (i.e., exposure assessment is sound). Once a convincing association between a particular genetic trait and an environmental factor is found, the evidence on gene–environment interactions needs causal assessment before being fully accepted adapting the Bradford-Hill criteria for causality assessment in epidemiology (see Chapter 2).

Many investigations on gene–environment interactions are underway in different parts of the world. All of them employ similar methods for genotyping (e.g., Taqman, and now high-throughput methods such as Illumina), while methods used for exposure assessment are extremely variable. Gene–environment interactions imply studying both environmental exposures (e.g., to pesticides or environmental tobacco smoke) and genetic variants that are supposed to modulate the effects of the former. However, there is an asymmetry between the two. Genotyping is much more accurate than the vast majority of methods used to measure environmental exposures. This implies a lower degree of classification error, which in turn means an easier identification of associations with disease. Let us suppose that classification error is expressed by the correlation coefficient between each exposure 'assessor' and a reference standard (r = 1 means no error, r = 0.9 means a 10 percent classification error). For different expected relative risks that associate exposure with disease, one can compute the observed relative risks under different conditions of classification error. For example, a classification error of 10 percent implies the drop of a relative risk of 2.5 to 2.3, i.e., little change. With a classification error of 90 percent, however, even a relative risk of 2.5 becomes 1.1, i.e., undetectable with common epidemiological methods. Things become even more complex if one wants to study interaction, e.g., between a frequent exposure (prevalence 25 percent) and a frequent genotype (prevalence 50 percent). Let us suppose that classification error is 20 percent for the environmental exposure (sensitivity = 80 percent), a value likely to be smaller than in reality for most exposures. Classification error could be around 7 percent for genotyping (sensitivity 93 percent). This is realistic, since genotyping techniques are currently validated and extremely accurate. The consequence of this situation is that one would need approximately 1800 cases to observe main effects (but no statistical interaction between exposure and genes), if no classification error occurs; 2700 if exposure is incorrectly classified 20 percent of the times; and 3200 if also the genotype is mistaken 7 percent of the times. (Sensitivity is considered in the example; with specificity lower than 100 percent numbers increase further.)

A further difficulty is related to the rarity of many environmental exposures (that, however, may have an important impact on human health), while several of the polymorphic alleles that are investigated are common (e.g., 40–50 percent for NAT2 or GSTM1). This, again, increases the probability of detecting an association with genotypes if this is real, but not with environmental exposures.

8.5.7 Emerging issues in studying gene–environment interactions

Whole genome scanning (WGS) for the search of genetic variants predisposing to disease has become a reality thanks to technological developments such as the Affymetrix and Illumina platforms. WGS have been already conducted, e.g., in the context of the US National Cancer Institute Consortia on breast and prostate cancers, and for Parkinson's disease.

Strategies for WGS are mainly aimed at avoiding false positive results, due to the large number of comparisons (typically, 300 000 to 500 000 SNPs in a run). False positives arise simply as a consequence of the multiple comparisons: in 500 000 comparisons, with a nominal level of 0.01 for type-I error, 5000 'statistically significant' results will arise. For this reason multi-stage approaches are used, e.g., the first 5000 SNP are tested in a second stage in a separate dataset. Up to four or five stages have been proposed.

However, false negatives are also a serious problem. False negatives do not arise principally from type-II error, i.e., from setting a high threshold (say, 0.01 or lower) for type-I error in the first or the following stages. A much more important and underestimated source of false negative results is the testing of main genetic effects without considering the existence of gene–environment interactions (GEI). It has been repeatedly stressed that GEIs are the norm and not the exception in the etiology of chronic diseases. Let us consider an example. Let us suppose that the absolute risk of lung cancer in smokers with a functioning metabolic enzyme (compared to nonsmokers) is 2.0/1000 per year, while it is 4.0 in those with enzyme deficiency (a relative risk of 2.0, a conservative assumption). Let us suppose that the prevalence of smoking is 50 percent. For the sake of simplicity we assume that the absolute risk in nonsmokers is 2/1000 irrespective of enzyme status (a complete GEI interaction). The (average) main effect of the genetic deficiency in the population will be estimated as a relative risk of $((4.0 \times 0.5)+(2.0 \times 0.5))/2.0$, i.e., 1.5. Now, let us suppose that the prevalence of the relevant exposure is not 0.5 but 0.1 (say, an environmental exposure). In this case the main genetic effect will be estimated as $((4.0 \times 0.1) + (2.0 \times 0.9))/2.0 = 2.2./2.0 = 1.1$, i.e., a very small and practically undetectable increase.

8.5.8 **Conclusions**

In the past, there have been great expectations from the study of gene–environment interactions in chronic diseases. The advantages that were foreseen included at least (a) the possibility of studying subgroups at high risk of chronic diseases in the population, thus increasing the power of epidemiological studies in detecting environmental risks; (b) the possibility of increasing the biological plausibility of environmental associations by identifying gene variants that modulate the risk of disease; (c) the possibility of getting rid of confounding (e.g., by social class) by showing that a certain disease is increased among the carriers of a gene variant involved in the metabolism of a certain exposure (genes are randomly allocated from parents to the offspring, they are not confounded by social class and the other usual confounders: Mendelian randomization). The situation today is much more complex than originally foreseen. Most associations are weak or very weak, and thus difficult to detect with epidemiological methods, and many associations are extremely heterogeneous or inconsistent in different investigations. However, this is currently one of the main avenues of etiologic research and the current paradigm – in spite of sporadic failures – is still that the vast majority of diseases arise because of gene–environment interactions.

8.6 **References**

[1] Rossi G, Schindler C, Schwartz J, Katsouyanni K, Touloumi G, Atkinson R, *et al*. Analysis of health outcome time series data in epidemiological studies. *Environmetrics*. 2004 15(2):101–17.

[2] Schwartz J, Marcus A. Mortality and air pollution in London: a time series analysis. *Am J Epidemiol*. 1990 131(1):185–94.

[3] Mazumdar S, Schimmel H, Higgins IT. Relation of daily mortality to air pollution: an analysis of 14 London winters, 1958/59–1971/72. *Archives of Environmental Health*. 1982 37(4):213–20.

[4] Ostro B. A search for a threshold in the relationship of air pollution to mortality: a reanalysis of data on London winters. *Environmental Health Perspectives*. 1984 58:397–9.

[5] Hatzakis A, Katsouyanni K, Kalandidi A, Day N, Trichopoulos D. Short-term effects of air pollution on mortality in Athens. *Int J Epidemiol*. 1986 15(1):73–81.

[6] Katsouyanni K, Touloumi G, Spix C, Schwartz J, Balducci F, Medina S, *et al*. Short-term effects of ambient sulphur dioxide and particulate matter on mortality in 12 European cities: results from time series data from the APHEA project. Air Pollution and Health: a European Approach. *BMJ (Clinical research edn)*. 1997 314(7095):1658–63.

[7] Katsouyanni K, Zmirou D, Spix C, Sunyer J, Schouten J, Pönkä A, *et al*. Short-term effects of air pollution on health: a European approach using epidemiological time-series data. The APHEA project: background, objectives, design. *Eur Respir J*. 1995 8:1030–38.

[8] Katsouyanni K, Touloumi G, Samoli E, Gryparis A, Le Tertre A, Monopolis Y, *et al*. Confounding and effect modification in the short-term effects of ambient particles on total mortality: results from 29 European cities within the APHEA2 project. *Epidemiology (Cambridge, MA)*. 2001 12(5):521–31.

[9] Samoli E, Touloumi G, Zanobetti A, Le Tertre A, Schindler C, Atkinson R, *et al*. Investigating the dose–response relation between air pollution and total mortality in the APHEA-2 multicity project. *Occup Environ Med*. 2003 60(12):977–82.

[10] Schwartz J, Spix C, Touloumi G, Bacharova L, Barumamdzadeh T, le Tertre A, *et al*. Methodological issues in studies of air pollution and daily counts of deaths or hospital admissions. *J Epidemiol Community Health*. 1996 50(Suppl 1):S3–11.

[11] Health Effects Institute. *Revised analyses of time-series studies of air pollution and health*. Boston: Health Effects Institute 2003.

[12] Zanobetti A, Schwartz J, Samoli E, Gryparis A, Touloumi G, Peacock J, *et al*. The temporal pattern of respiratory and heart disease mortality in response to air pollution. *Environmental Health Perspectives*. 2003 111(9):1188–93.

[13] Sunyer J, Spix C, Quenel P, Ponce-de-Leon A, Ponka A, Barumandzadeh T, *et al*. Urban air pollution and emergency admissions for asthma in four European cities: the APHEA Project. *Thorax*. 1997 52(9):760–5.

[14] Samoli E, Aga E, Touloumi G, Nisiotis K, Forsberg B, Lefranc A, *et al*. Short-term effects of nitrogen dioxide on mortality: an analysis within the APHEA project. *Eur Respir J*. 2006 27(6):1129–38.

[15] Burnett RT, Stieb D, Brook JR, Cakmak S, Dales R, Raizenne M, *et al*. Associations between short-term changes in nitrogen dioxide and mortality in Canadian cities. *Archives of Environmental Health*. 2004 59(5):228–36.

[16] Bell ML, McDermott A, Zeger SL, Samet JM, Dominici F. Ozone and short-term mortality in 95 US urban communities, 1987–2000. *JAMA*. 2004 292(19):2372–8.

[17] Gryparis A, Forsberg B, Katsouyanni K, Analitis A, Touloumi G, Schwartz J, *et al*. Acute effects of ozone on mortality from the 'air pollution and health: a European approach' project. *Am J Respir Crit Care Med*. 2004 170(10):1080–7.

[18] Sunyer J, Ballester F, Tertre AL, Atkinson R, Ayres JG, Forastiere F, *et al*. The association of daily sulfur dioxide air pollution levels with hospital admissions for cardiovascular diseases in Europe (The Aphea-II study). *Eur Heart J*. 2003 24(8):752–60.

[19] Barnett AG, Williams GM, Schwartz J, Best TL, Neller AH, Petroeschevsky AL, *et al*. The effects of air pollution on hospitalizations for cardiovascular disease in elderly people in Australian and New Zealand cities. *Environmental Health Perspectives*. 2006 114(7):1018–23.

[20] Samet JM, Dominici F, Curriero FC, Coursac I, Zeger SL. Fine particulate air pollution and mortality in 20 U.S. cities, 1987–1994. *The New England Journal of Medicine*. 2000 343(24):1742–9.

[21] Dominici F, Peng RD, Bell ML, Pham L, McDermott A, Zeger SL, *et al*. Fine particulate air pollution and hospital admission for cardiovascular and respiratory diseases. *JAMA*. 2006 295(10):1127–34.

[22] Schwartz J, Dockery DW, Neas LM. Is daily mortality associated specifically with fine particles? *J Air Waste Manag Assoc*. 1996 46(10):927–39.

[23] Curriero FC, Heiner KS, Samet JM, Zeger SL, Strug L, Patz JA. Temperature and mortality in 11 cities of the eastern United States. *Am J Epidemiol*. 2002 155(1):80–7.

[24] Jamason PF, Kalkstein LS, Gergen PJ. A synoptic evaluation of asthma hospital admissions in New York City. *American Journal of Respiratory and Critical Care Medicine*. 1997 156(6):1781–8.

[25] Schwartz J, Levin R, Goldstein R. Drinking water turbidity and gastrointestinal illness in the elderly of Philadelphia. *J Epidemiol Community Health*. 2000 54(1):45–51.

[26] Egorov AI, Naumova EN, Tereschenko AA, Kislitsin VA, Ford TE. Daily variations in effluent water turbidity and diarrhoeal illness in a Russian city. *Int J Environ Health Res*. 2003 13(1):81–94.

[27] Welty LJ, Zeger SL. Are the acute effects of particulate matter on mortality in the National Morbidity, Mortality, and Air Pollution Study the result of inadequate control for weather and season? A sensitivity analysis using flexible distributed lag models. *Am J Epidemiol*. 2005 162(1):80–8.

[28] Rainham DG, Smoyer-Tomic KE. The role of air pollution in the relationship between a heat stress index and human mortality in Toronto. *Environ Res*. 2003 93(1):9–19.

[29] O'Neill MS, Hajat S, Zanobetti A, Ramirez-Aguilar M, Schwartz J. Impact of control for air pollution and respiratory epidemics on the estimated associations of temperature and daily mortality. *Int J Biometeorol*. 2005 50(2):121–9.

[30] Zanobetti A, Schwartz J. Are diabetics more susceptible to the health effects of airborne particles? *American Journal of Respiratory and Critical Care Medicine*. 2001 164(5):831–3.

[31] Gouveia N, Fletcher T. Time series analysis of air pollution and mortality: effects by cause, age and socioeconomic status. *J Epidemiol Community Health*. 2000 54(10):750–5.

[32] Levy JI, Chemerynski SM, Sarnat JA. Ozone exposure and mortality: an empiric bayes metaregression analysis. *Epidemiology (Cambridge, MA)*. 2005 16(4):458–68.

[33] Berhane K, Thomas DC. A two-stage model for multiple time series data of counts. *Biostatistics (Oxford, England)*. 2002 3(1):21–32.

[34] Higgins JP, Thompson SG, Deeks JJ, Altman DG. Measuring inconsistency in meta-analyses. *BMJ (Clinical Research edn)*. 2003 327(7414):557–60.

[35] Katsouyanni K, Zmirou D, Spix C, Sunyer J, Schouten JP, Ponka A, *et al*. Short-term effects of air pollution on health: a European approach using epidemiological time-series data. The APHEA project: background, objectives, design. *Eur Respir J*. 1995 8(6):1030–8.

[36] Daniels MJ, Dominici F, Samet JM, Zeger SL. Estimating particulate matter–mortality dose–response curves and threshold levels: an analysis of daily time-series for the 20 largest US cities. *Am J Epidemiol*. 2000 152(5):397–406.

[37] Analitis A, Katsouyanni K, Dimakopoulou K, Samoli E, Nikoloulopoulos AK, Petasakis Y, *et al*. Short-term effects of ambient particles on cardiovascular and respiratory mortality. *Epidemiology (Cambridge, MA)*. 2006 17(2):230–3.

[38] Gamble JF, Lewis RJ. Health and respirable particulate (PM10) air pollution: a causal or statistical association? *Environmental Health Perspectives*. 1996 104(8):838–50.

[39] Phalen RF. Uncertainties relating to the health effects of particulate air pollution: the US EPA's particle standard. *Toxicol Lett*. 1998 96–97:263–7.

[40] Rothman KJ. *Epidemiology: an introduction*. New York: Oxford University Press 2002.

[41] Kelsall JE, Samet JM, Zeger SL, Xu J. Air pollution and mortality in Philadelphia, 1974–1988. *Am J Epidemiol*. 1997 146(9):750–62.

[42] Dominici F, Samet JM, Zeger SL. Combining evidence on air pollution and daily mortality from the 20 largest US cities: a hierarchical modeling strategy. *Journal of the Royal Statistical Society: Series A (Statistics in Society)*. 2000 163(3):263–302.

[43] McCullagh P, Nelder JA. *Generalized linear models, 2nd edn*. London: Chapman and Hall 1989.

[44] Dominici F, McDermott A, Zeger SL, Samet JM. On the use of generalized additive models in time-series studies of air pollution and health. *Am J Epidemiol*. 2002 156(3):193–203.

[45] Ramsay TO, Burnett RT, Krewski D. The effect of concurvity in generalized additive models linking mortality to ambient particulate matter. *Epidemiology (Cambridge, MA)*. 2003 14(1):18–23.

[46] Chambers JM, Hastie T. *Statistical models*. Wadsworth & Brooks/Cole Advanced Books & Software 1992. Pacific Grove, California.

[47] Efron B, Tibshirani R. *An introduction to the bootstrap*. New York: Chapman & Hall 1993.

[48] Marx BD, Eilers PHC. Direct generalized additive modeling with penalized likelihood. *Computational Statistics and Data Analysis*. 1998 28(2):193–209.

[49] Wood SN, Augustin NH. GAMs with integrated model selection using penalized regression splines and applications to environmental modeling. *Ecological Modeling*. 2002 157(2–3):157–77.

[50] Currie ID. Flexible smoothing with P-splines: a unified approach. *Statistical Modeling*. 2002 2:333–49.

[51] Brumback BA, Ryan LM, Schwartz JD, Neas LM, Stark PC, Burg HA. Transitional regression models, with application to environmental time series. *JASA*. 2000 95:16–27.

[52] Smith R, Guttorp P, Sheppard L, Lumley T, Ishikama N. Comments on the criteria document for particulate matter air pollution. NRCSE *Technical report* 2001.

[53] Schwartz J. The distributed lag between air pollution and daily deaths. *Epidemiology (Cambridge, MA)*. 2000 11(3):320–6.

[54] Zanobetti A, Schwartz J, Samoli E, Gryparis A, Touloumi G, Atkinson R, *et al*. The temporal pattern of mortality responses to air pollution: a multicity assessment of mortality displacement. *Epidemiology (Cambridge, MA)*. 2002 13(1):87–93.

[55] Schwartz J, Zanobetti A. Using meta-smoothing to estimate dose-response trends across multiple studies, with application to air pollution and daily death. *Epidemiology (Cambridge, MA)*. 2000 11(6):666–72.

[56] Samoli E, Analitis A, Touloumi G, Schwartz J, Anderson HR, Sunyer J, *et al*. Estimating the exposure-response relationships between particulate matter and mortality within the APHEA multicity project. *Environmental Health Perspectives*. 2005 113(1):88–95.

[57] Green PJ. Reversible jump Markov chain Monte Carlo computation and Bayesian model determination. *Biometrika*. 1995 82(4):711–32.

[58] Dominici F, M D, L. ZS, M SJ. Air pollution and mortality: Estimating regional and national dose-response relationships. *JASA*. 2002 97(457):100–11.

[59] Draper D. Assessment and propagation of model uncertainty (Disc: P71–97). *J R Stat Soc, series B, Methodological*. 1995 57:45–70.

[60] Hodges JS. Uncertainty, policy analysis and statistics. *Statistical Science*. 1987 2(3):259–75.

[61] Dominici F, Sheppard L, Clyde M. Health effects of air pollution: a statistical review. *Internat Statist Rev*. 2003 71(2):243–76.

[62] Roemer W, Hoek G, Brunekreef B. Effect of ambient winter air pollution on respiratory health of children with chronic respiratory symptoms. *Am Rev Respir Dis*. 1993 147(1):118–24.

[63] Peters A, Goldstein IF, Beyer U, Franke K, Heinrich J, Dockery DW, *et al*. Acute health effects of exposure to high levels of air pollution in eastern Europe. *American Journal of Epidemiology*. 1996 144(6):570–81.

[64] Scarlett JF, Abbott KJ, Peacock JL, Strachan DP, Anderson HR. Acute effects of summer air pollution on respiratory function in primary school children in southern England. *Thorax*. 1996 51(11):1109–14.

[65] Peters A, Dockery DW, Heinrich J, Wichmann HE. Short-term effects of particulate air pollution on respiratory morbidity in asthmatic children. *Eur Respir J*. 1997 10(4):872–9.

[66] Aekplakorn W, Loomis D, Vichit-Vadakan N, Shy C, Plungchuchon S. Acute effects of SO2 and particles from a power plant on respiratory symptoms of children, Thailand. *Southeast Asian J Trop Med Public Health*. 2003 34(4):906–14.

[67] Ward DJ, Ayres JG. Particulate air pollution and panel studies in children: a systematic review. *Occupational and Environmental Medicine*. 2004 61(4):E13.

[68] Ranzi A, Gambini M, Spattini A, Galassi C, Sesti D, Bedeschi M, *et al*. Air pollution and respiratory status in asthmatic children: hints for a locally based preventive strategy. AIRE study. *Eur J Epidemiol*. 2004 19(6):567–76.

[69] Peled R, Friger M, Bolotin A, Bibi H, Epstein L, Pilpel D, *et al*. Fine particles and meteorological conditions are associated with lung function in children with asthma living near two power plants. *Public Health*. 2005 119(5):418–25.

[70] Forsberg B, Stjernberg N, Falk M, Lundback B, Wall S. Air pollution levels, meteorological conditions and asthma symptoms. *Eur Respir J*. 1993 6(8):1109–15.

[70] Pope CAR, Dockery DW, Kanner RE, Villegas GM, Schwartz J. Oxygen saturation, pulse rate, and particulate air pollution: A daily time-series panel study. *Am J Respir Crit Care Med*. 1999 159(2):365–72.

[72] Devlin RB, Ghio AJ, Kehrl H, Sanders G, Cascio W. Elderly humans exposed to concentrated air pollution particles have decreased heart rate variability. *Eur Respir J Suppl*. 2003 40:76S–80S.

[73] de Paula Santos U, Braga AL, Giorgi DM, Pereira LA, Grupi CJ, Lin CA, *et al*. Effects of air pollution on blood pressure and heart rate variability: a panel study of vehicular traffic controllers in the city of Sao Paulo, Brazil. *Eur Heart J*. 2005 26(2):193–200.

[74 Ruckerl R, Ibald-Mulli A, Koenig W, Schneider A, Woelke G, Cyrys J, *et al*. Air pollution and markers of inflammation and coagulation in patients with coronary heart disease. *Am J Respir Crit Care Med*. 2006 173(4):432–41.

[75] Lagorio S, Forastiere F, Pistelli R, Iavarone I, Michelozzi P, Fano V, *et al*. Air pollution and lung function among susceptible adult subjects: a panel study. *Environ Health*. 2006 5:11.

[76] Pope CAR, Hansen ML, Long RW, Nielsen KR, Eatough NL, Wilson WE, *et al*. Ambient particulate air pollution, heart rate variability, and blood markers of inflammation in a panel of elderly subjects. *Environmental Health Perspectives*. 2004 112(3):339–45.

[77] Ostro B. A search for a threshold in the relationship of air pollution to mortality: a reanalysis of data on London winters. *Environmental Health Perspectives*. 1984 58:397–9.

[78] Schwartz J, Timonen KL, Pekkanen J. Respiratory effects of environmental tobacco smoke in a panel study of asthmatic and symptomatic children. *Am J Respir Crit Care Med*. 2000 161 (3 Pt 1):802–6.

[79] Ostro BD, Lipsett MJ, Mann JK, Wiener MB, Selner J. Indoor air pollution and asthma. Results from a panel study. *Am J Respir Crit Care Med*. 1994 149(6):1400–6.

[80] Hoek G, Dockery DW, Pope A, Neas L, Roemer W, Brunekreef B. Association between PM10 and decrements in peak expiratory flow rates in children: reanalysis of data from five panel studies. *Eur Respir J*. 1998 11(6):1307–11.

[81] Roemer W, Hoek G, Brunekreef B, Haluszka J, Kalandidi A, Pekkanen J. Daily variations in air pollution and respiratory health in a multicenter study: the PEACE project. Pollution Effects on Asthmatic Children in Europe. *Eur Respir J*. 1998 12(6):1354–61.

[82] Brunekreef B, Janssen NA, de Hartog JJ, Oldenwening M, Meliefste K, Hoek G, *et al*. Personal, indoor, and outdoor exposures to PM2.5 and its components for groups of cardiovascular patients in Amsterdam and Helsinki. *Res Rep Health Eff Inst*. 2005 (127):1–70; discussion 1–9.

[83] Janssen NA, Lanki T, Hoek G, Vallius M, de Hartog JJ, Van Grieken R, *et al*. Associations between ambient, personal, and indoor exposure to fine particulate matter constituents in Dutch and Finnish panels of cardiovascular patients. *Occupational and Environmental Medicine*. 2005 62(12):868–77.

[84] Peters A, Schneider A, Greven S, Bellander T, Forastiere F, Ibald, *et al*. Air pollution and inflammatory response in myocardial infarction survivors: gene-environment-interactions in a high-risk group study design of the airgene study. *Inhal Toxicol*. 2007 19(Suppl 1):161–75.

[85] Timonen KL, Vanninen E, de Hartog J, Ibald-Mulli A, Brunekreef B, Gold DR, *et al*. Effects of ultrafine and fine particulate and gaseous air pollution on cardiac autonomic control in subjects with coronary artery disease: the ULTRA study. *J Expo Sci Environ Epidemiol*. 2006 16(4):332–41.

[86] de Hartog JJ, Hoek G, Peters A, Timonen KL, Ibald-Mulli A, Brunekreef B, *et al*. Effects of fine and ultrafine particles on cardiorespiratory symptoms in elderly subjects with coronary heart disease: the ULTRA study. *American Journal of Epidemiology*. 2003 157(7):613–23.

[87] Delfino RJ, Zeiger RS, Seltzer JM, Street DH, McLaren CE. Association of asthma symptoms with peak particulate air pollution and effect modification by anti-inflammatory medication use. *Environ Health Perspect*. 2002 110(10):A607–17.

[88] Zeger SL, Liang KY, Albert PS. Models for longitudinal data: a generalized estimating equation approach. *Biometrics*. 1988 44(4):1049–60.

[89] Diggle P, Liang K-Y, Zeger SL. *Analysis of longitudinal data*. Repr. 1994, 1995 (with corrections). Oxford and New York: Clarendon Press, Oxford University Press 1995.

[90] Breslow NE, Clayton DG. Approximate inference in generalized linear mixed models. *JAMA*. 1993 88(421):9–25.

[91] Stiratelli R, Laird N, Ware JH. Random-effects models for serial observations with binary response. *Biometrics*. 1984 40(4):961–71.

[92] Schlink U, Fritz GJ, Herbarth O, Richter M. Longitudinal modeling of respiratory symptoms in children. *Int J Biometeorol*. 2002 47(1):35–48.

[93] Trenga CA, Sullivan JH, Schildcrout JS, Shepherd KP, Shapiro GG, Liu LJ, *et al*. Effect of particulate air pollution on lung function in adult and pediatric subjects in a Seattle panel study. *Chest*. 2006 129(6):1614–22.

[94] Fitzmaurice GM, Laird NM, Rotnitzky AG. Regression models for discrete longitudinal responses. *Statistical Science*. 1993 8(3):284–309.

[95] Korn EL, Whittemore AS. Methods for analyzing panel studies of acute health effects of air pollution. *Biometrics*. 1979 35:795–802.

[96] van der Zee SC, Hoek G, Boezen MH, Schouten JP, van Wijnen JH, Brunekreef B. Acute effects of air pollution on respiratory health of 50–70 yr old adults. *Eur Respir J*. 2000 15(4):700–9.

[97] Laird NM. Missing data in longitudinal studies. *Stat Med*. 1988 7(1–2):305–15.

[98] Touloumi G, Babiker AG, Pocock SJ, Darbyshire JH. Impact of missing data due to drop-outs on estimators for rates of change in longitudinal studies: a simulation study. *Stat Med*. 2001 20(24):3715–28.

[99] Wu MC, Bailey K. Analysing changes in the presence of informative right censoring caused by death and withdrawal. *Stat Med*. 1988 7(1–2):337–46.

[100] Schluchter MD. Methods for the analysis of informatively censored longitudinal data. *Stat Med*. 1992 11(14–15):1861–70.

[101] Touloumi G, Pocock SJ, Babiker AG, Darbyshire JH. Estimation and comparison of rates of change in longitudinal studies with informative drop-outs. *Stat Med.* 1999 18(10):1215–33.

[102] Little RJA. Modeling the drop-out mechansim in repeated-measures studies. *JASA.* 1995 Sep;90(431):1112–21.

[103] Robins J, Rotnitzky AG, Zhao LP. Analysis of semiparametric regression models for repeated outcomes in the presence of mission data. *JASA.* 1995 90(429):106–21.

[104] Elliott P, Wartenberg D. Spatial epidemiology: current approaches and future challenges. *Environmental Health Perspectives.* 2004 112(9):998–1006.

[105] Openshaw S. *The modifiable areal unit problem.* Norwich: Geobooks 1984.

[106] Mather FJ, White LE, Langlois EC, Shorter CF, Swalm CM, Shaffer JG, *et al.* Statistical methods for linking health, exposure, and hazards. *Environmental Health Perspectives.* 2004 112(14):1440–5.

[107] Jarup L, Best N, Toledano MB, Wakefield J, Elliott P. Geographical epidemiology of prostate cancer in Great Britain. *Int J Cancer.* 2002 97(5):695–9.

[108] Goldman DA, Brender JD. Are standardized mortality ratios valid for public health data analysis? *Stat Med.* 2000 19(8):1081–8.

[109] Jarup L, Best N. Editorial comment on 'Geographical differences in cancer incidence in the Belgian province of Limburg' by Bruntinx and colleagues. *Eur J Cancer.* 2003 39(14):1973–5.

[110] Besag J, Newell J. The detection of clusters in rare diseases. *Journal of the Royal Statistical Society Series A.* 1991 32676(154 part 1):143–55.

[111] Best N, Richardson S, Thomson A. A comparison of Bayesian spatial models for disease mapping. *Statistical Methods in Medical Research.* 2005 14(1):35–59.

[112] Richardson S, Thomson A, Best N, Elliott P. Interpreting posterior relative risk estimates in disease-mapping studies. *Environmental Health Perspectives.* 2004 112(9):1016–25.

[113] Monmonier M. *How to lie with maps, 2nd edn.* Chicago, IL: University of Chicago Press 1996.

[114] Best N, Wakefield J. Accounting for inaccuracies in population counts and case registration in cancer mapping studies. *Journal of the Royal Statistical Society: Series A (Statistics in Society).* 1999 162(3):363–82.

[115] Knorr-Held L, Best N. A shared component model for detecting joint and selective clustering of two diseases. *J Roy Stat Soc A Sta.* 2001 164:73–85.

[116] Feltbower RG, Manda SO, Gilthorpe MS, Greaves MF, Parslow RC, Kinsey SE, *et al.* Detecting small-area similarities in the epidemiology of childhood acute lymphoblastic leukemia and diabetes mellitus, type 1: a Bayesian approach. *American Journal of Epidemiology.* 2005 161(12):1168–80.

[117] Hansell A, Best N, Aylin P. Spatial variations in chronic obstructive respiratory disease mortality in the UK. *Epidemiology.* 2004 15:S105–S6.

[118] Greenland S. Divergent biases in ecologic and individual-level studies. *Stat Med.* 1992 11(9):1209–23.

[119] Elliott P, Briggs D, Morris S, de Hoogh C, Hurt C, Jensen TK, *et al.* Risk of adverse birth outcomes in populations living near landfill sites. *BMJ.* 2001 323(7309):363–8.

[120] Jarup L, Briggs D, de Hoogh C, Morris S, Hurt C, Lewin A, *et al.* Cancer risks in populations living near landfill sites in Great Britain. *British Journal of Cancer.* 2002 86(11):1732–6.

[121] Richardson S, Stucker I, Hemon D. Comparison of relative risks obtained in ecological and individual studies: some methodological considerations. *Int J Epidemiol.* 1987 16(1):111–20.

[122] Prentice RL, Sheppard L. Aggregate data studies of disease risk factors. *Biometrika.* 1995 82(1):113–25.

[123] Whitaker H, Best N, Nieuwenhuijsen MJ, Wakefield J, Fawell J, Elliott P. Modeling exposure to disinfection by-products in drinking water for an epidemiological study of adverse birth outcomes. *J Expo Anal Environ Epidemiol.* 2005 15(2):138–46.

[124] Jackson C, Best N, Richardson S. Improving ecological inference using individual-level data. *Stat Med*. 2006 25(12):2136–59.

[125] Hodgson S, Nieuwenhuijsen MJ, Colvile R, Jarup L. Assessment of exposure to mercury from industrial emissions: comparing 'distance as a proxy' and dispersion modeling approaches. *Occupational and Environmental Medicine*. 2007 64(6):380–8.

[126] Warner S, Aldrich TE. The status of cancer cluster investigations undertaken by state health departments. *American Journal of Public Health*. 1988 32676(78):306–7.

[127] Greenberg M, Wartenberg D. Communicating to an alarmed community about cancer clusters: a fifty state survey. *Journal of Community Health*. 1991 32676(16 2):71–82.

[128] Trumbo CW. Public health requests for cancer cluster investigations: a survey of state health departments. *American Journal of Public Health*. 2000 8:1300–2.

[129] Bender AP, Williams N, Johnson RA, Jagger HG. Appropriate health responses to clusters: the art of being responsibly responsive. *American Journal of Epidemiology*. 1990 32676(132 Suppl):S48–S52.

[130] Struewing JP, Hartge P, Wacholder S, Baker SM, Berlin M, McAdams M, *et al*. The risk of cancer associated with specific mutations of BRCA1 and BRCA2 among Ashkenazi Jews. *New England Journal of Medicine*. 1997 336(20):1401–8.

[131] Berry M. Mesothelioma incidence and community asbestos exposure. *Environmental Research*. 1997 75(1):34–40.

[132] McBride WG. Thalidomide and congenital abnormalities [letter]. *Lancet*. 1961 32676(2):1358.

[133] Herbst A, Ulfelder H, Poskanzer D. Adenocarcinoma of the vagina. Association with maternal stilbestrol therapy with tumor appearance in young women. *New England Journal of Medicine*. 1971 32676(284):878–81.

[134] Creech JL, Jr., Johnson MN. Angiosarcoma of the liver in the manufacture of polyvinyl chloride. *Journal of Occupational Medicine*. 1974 32676(16):150–1.

[135] Whorton D, Krauss R, Marshal S, Milby T. Infertility in male pesticide workers. *Lancet*. 1977 32676(2):1259–60.

[136] Steere AC, Malawista SE, Snydman DR, Shope RE, Andiman WA, Ross MR, *et al*. Lyme arthritis: an epidemic of oligoarticular arthritis in children and adults in three connecticut communities. *Arthritis & Rheumatism*. 1977 20(1):7–17.

[137] Fraser DW, Tsai TR, Orenstein W, Parkin WE, Beecham J, Sharrar RG, *et al*. Legionnaires' disease. *New England Journal of Medicine*. 1977 297(22):1189–97.

[138] Friedman-Kien A, *et al*. Kaposi's sarcoma and pneumocystis pneumonia among homosexual men – New York City and California. *Morbidity and Mortality Weekly Report*. 1981 30:305–8.

[139] Schulte P, Ehrenberg R, Singal M. Investigation of occupational cancer clusters: Theory and practice. *American Journal of Public Health*. 1987 32676(77 1):52–6.

[140] Caldwell GG. Twenty-two years of cancer cluster investigations at the Centers for Disease Control. *American Journal of Epidemiology*. 1990 32676(132 Suppl):S43–S7.

[141] Quataert PKM, Armstrong B, Berghold A, Bianchi F, Kelly A, Marchi M, *et al*. Methodological problems and the role of statistics in cluster response studies: A framework. *European Journal of Epidemiology*. 1999 15:821–31.

[142] Wartenberg D, Greenberg M. Solving the cluster puzzle: clues to follow and pitfalls to avoid. *Statistics in Medicine*. 1993 32676(12):1763–70.

[143] Fiore BJ, Hanrahan LP, Anderson HA. State health department response to disease cluster reports: A protocol of investigation. *American Journal of Epidemiology*. 1990 32676(132 Suppl):S14–S22.

[144] Fleming L, Ducatman A, Shalat S. Disease clusters in occupational medicine: A protocol for their investigation in the workplace. *American Journal of Industrial Medicine*. 1992 32676(22):33–47.

[145] Alexander FE, Boyle P. *Methods for investigating localized clustering of disease.* Lyon, France: International Agency for Research on Cancer 1996.

[146] Centers for Disease Control. *Guidelines for investigating clusters of health events.* Atlanta, Georgia: Centers for Disease Control 1990.

[147] Kingsley BS, Schmeichel KL, Rubin CH. An update on cancer cluster activities at the Centers for Disease Control and Prevention. *Enviromental Health Perspectives.* 2007 115(1):165–71.

[148] Kulldorff M. Tests for spatial randomness adjusting for an underlying inhomogeneity: A general framework. *Journal of the American Statistical Association.* 2006 101:1289–305.

[149] Pinkel D, Nefzger D. Some epidemiologic features of childhood leukemia in the Buffalo, New York area. *Cancer.* 1959 32676(12):351–7.

[150] Ederer F, Myers MH, Mantel N. A statistical problem in space and time: do leukemia cases come in clusters? *Biometrics.* 1964 32676(20):626–38.

[151] Knox G. The detection of space–time interaction. *Applied Statistics.* 1964 32676(13):25–9.

[152] Mantel N. The detection of disease clustering and a generalized regression approach. *Cancer Research.* 1967 32676(27):209–20.

[153] Cuzick J, Edwards R. Methods for investigating localized clustering of disease. Cuzick–Edwards one-sample and inverse two-sampling statistics. *IARC Scientific Publications.* 1996 135:200–2.

[154] Jacquez GM. A k-nearest neighbor test for space-time interaction. *Statistics in Medicine.* 1995 15:1934–49.

[155] Cliff AD, Ord JK. *Spatial processes: models and applications.* London: Pion Ltd. 1981.

[156] Stone RA. Investigations of excess environmental risks around putative sources: statistical problems and a proposed test. *Statistics in Medicine.* 1988 32676(7):649–60.

[157] Waller LA, Lawson AB. The power of focused tests to detect disease clustering. *Statistics in Medicine.* 1995 32676(14):2291–308.

[158] Naus JI. The distribution of the size of the maximum cluster of points on a line. *Journal of the American Statistical Association.* 1965 32676(60):532–8.

[159] Openshaw S, Charlton M, Wymer C, Craft A. A Mark 1 geographical analysis machine for the automated analysis of point data sets. *International Journal of Geographical Informations Systems.* 1987 1(4):335–58.

[160] Openshaw S, Craft AW, Charlton M, Birch JM. Investigation of leukaemia clusters by use of a geographical analysis machine. *Lancet.* 1988 32676(1):272–3.

[161] Rushton G, Lolonis P. Exploratory spatial analysis of birth defect rates in an urban population. *Statistics in Medicine.* 1996 15:717–26.

[162] Kulldorff M, Athas WF, Feurer EJ, Miller BA, Key CR. Evaluating cluster alarms: a space–time scan statistic and brain cancer in Los Alamos, New Mexico. *American Journal of Public Health.* 1998 88(9):1377–80.

[163] Kulldorff M, Fang Z, Walsh SJ. A tree-based scan statistic for database disease surveillance. **Biometrics.** 2003 59(2):323–31.

[164] Kulldorff M, Heffernan R, Hartman J, Assuncao R, Mostashari F. A space–time permutation scan statistic for disease outbreak detection. *PLoS Medicine.* 2005 2(3):E59.

[165] Kulldorff M, Huang L, Pickle L, Duczmal L. An elliptic spatial scan statistic. *Statistics in Medicine.* 2006 25(22):3929–43.

[166] Kulldorff M, Mostashari F, Duczmal L, Katherine Yih W, Kleinman K, Platt R. Multivariate scan statistics for disease surveillance. *Statistics in Medicine.* 2007 26(8):1824–33.

[167] Puett RC, Lawson AB, Clark AB, Aldrich TK, M., Porter DE, Feigley CE, *et al.* Scale and shape in focused cluster power tests for count dataspatial randomness adjusting for an underlying inhomogeneity: A general framework. *International Journal of Health Geographics the American Statistical Association.* 2005/2006 4101(16):1289–305.

[168] Besag J, Newell J. The detection of clusters in rare diseases. *Journal of the Royal Statistical Society Series A*. 1991 32676(154 part 1):143–55.

[169] Neutra R. Counterpoint from a cluster buster. *American Journal of Epidemiology*. 1990 32676(132 1):1–8.

[170] Wartenberg D. Should we boost or bust cluster investigations (Editorial). *Epidemiology*. 1995 6:575–6.

[171] Case RA, Hosker ME, Mc DD, Pearson JT. Tumours of the urinary bladder in workmen engaged in the manufacture and use of certain dyestuff intermediates in the British chemical industry. I. The role of aniline, benzidine, alpha-naphthylamine, and beta-naphthylamine. *Br J Ind Med*. 1954 11(2):75–104.

[172] Shields PG, Harris CC. Cancer risk and low-penetrance susceptibility genes in gene–environment interactions. *J Clin Oncol*. 2000 18(11):2309–15.

[173] Khoury MJ, Little J, Burke W. *Human genome epidemiology: a scientific foundation for using genetic information to improve health and prevent disease*. Oxford and New York: Oxford University Press 2004.

[174] Thomas D. *Statistical methods in genetic epidemiology*. New York: Oxford University Press 2004.

[175] Sveinbjornsdottir S, Hicks AA, Jonsson T, Petursson H, Gugmundsson G, Frigge ML, *et al*. Familial aggregation of Parkinson's disease in Iceland. *The New England Journal of Medicine*. 2000 343(24):1765–70.

[176] Zareparsi S, Taylor TD, Harris EL, Payami H. Segregation analysis of Parkinson disease. *Am J Med Genet*. 1998 80(4):410–17.

[177] Elbaz A, Levecque C, Clavel J, Vidal JS, Richard F, Amouyel P, *et al*. CYP2D6 polymorphism, pesticide exposure, and Parkinson's disease. *Annals of Neurology*. 2004 55(3):430–4.

Chapter 9

The epidemiology of chemical incidents and natural disasters

Paul Cullinan and Anna Hansell

9.1 Introduction

Disasters—of human or natural origin—share much in their epidemiological investigation and management. To illustrate some of the principles involved, this chapter focuses on chemical incidents related to industrial accidents and natural disasters arising from volcanoes. Other disasters generated by humans such as complex emergencies (war, civil strife, political conflict), technological disasters, transportation disasters, dam breaks, energy supply interruption and those due to other natural forces are covered elsewhere (e.g., see [1]).

9.1.1 Definitions

A *chemical incident* is the unexpected release of industrial or other toxic material that is potentially hazardous either to humans, other animals or the environment [2]. A common synonym is the term 'accident' but this presupposes an unanticipated failure of control, while 'incidents' include also unanticipated events resulting from mechanical or organizational failures and occasionally even sabotage such as terrorist releases of toxic materials. Although the principles of management are very similar, it does not generally include toxic releases contained entirely within an occupational setting where only employees are affected. Major chemical incidents are those which pose a threat to a large number of people—dependent on the size of the release, its area of distribution and the magnitude of the population at risk.

A *natural disaster* relates to an event or change in the physical environment caused by natural forces that occurs on such a scale that it has a marked adverse impact on human beings or other life-forms. Some definitions of a disaster include the need for a relief effort involving outside help or international aid [3, 4]. Natural disasters include earthquakes, volcanic eruptions, hurricanes, floods, drought, fire, tornadoes and extremes of temperature; some definitions also include epidemics of disease [1]. Generally, such natural disasters occur suddenly, although there are exceptions (e.g., drought).

The essence of both chemical incidents and natural disasters is generally their unexpectedness and scale. The term 'disaster' is not used to describe, say, continuing, predictable and more-or-less regulated releases of toxic substances from industrial sources such as waste incinerators or ongoing degassing of hydrogen sulphide or sulphur dioxide in geothermal areas. However, while the timing may be unexpected and the details of the event may be unpredictable, risk assessment techniques can often be used in advance of the event to define and assess hazards and make general or specific management plans.

9.1.2 Nature of chemical incidents and natural disasters

Incidents may be either 'agent-' or 'event'-oriented or they may be 'effect-oriented' [5]. Agent- or event-oriented incidents arise from the unexpected release of a toxic agent or a large-scale natural event such as a volcanic eruption. Examples include chemical releases in Bhopal, Chernobyl and Meda (Seveso) or the eruptions of Mount St Helens in 1980 and Pinatubo in 1991, Tables 9.1, 9.2. Effect-oriented incidents are manifest initially by an outbreak of disease, often detected by its unusual nature; outbreaks of acute asthma in Barcelona and 'itai-itai' disease in Japan, for example, were eventually traced to repeated releases of soybean dust and cadmium, respectively. An outbreak of rare cardiomyopathy in Canada was eventually traced to the use of cobalt chloride as a foam-stabilizer in the brewing of beer [6].

Effect-oriented incidents rely almost entirely on epidemiological and, where available, toxicological investigation to demonstrate associations. In event-orientated situations, there is often some prior knowledge about the hazards involved. Volcanic eruptions can give rise to a wide range of health hazards [7] including volcanic ash, pyroclastic flows ('avalanches' of superheated ash and gas), lahars (mud flows) and, if large enough, secondary impacts on climate or food production. Toxicological information can be helpful for release of chemical agents, but for most chemicals in wide industrial use relevant information on human toxicity is simply unavailable [8]. Information relevant to exposure assessment in terms of exposure pathways (e.g., water, food, soil or air contamination) and amounts will be needed for epidemiological assessments. In some cases the health effects may be immediate; in others there may also be long-term adverse consequences. Where effects are not specific, attribution of cause to the released agent(s) may be difficult and will rely almost entirely on epidemiological techniques.

9.1.3 Impacts of chemical incidents and volcanic disasters

The Emergency Disasters Database (EM-DAT), a continuously updated database with information on occurrence and effects of >12 800 mass disasters from 1900 onwards, is maintained at the Center for Research on the Epidemiology of Disasters in Brussels. The database can be searched online at http://www.em-dat.net. However, there are issues about the accuracy and completeness of this database, so impacts should be treated as representative rather than precise [9].

Table 9.1 shows the scale of various human effects from the worst volcanic disasters in the twentieth century, from a database of 491 events compiled by Witham [9].

Table 9.1 Worst volcanic disasters in the twentieth century by type of effect (numbers of death, injuries, people made homeless, total numbers affected)

Rank	Killed		Injured		Homeless		Evacuated/affected	
	Event	People	Event	People	Event	People	Event	People
1	Pelée, 1902	29 000	Nevado del Ruiz, 1985	4470	Pinatubo, 1991	53 000	Guagua, Pichincha 1999	1 200 400
2	Nevado del Ruiz, 1985	23 080	Awu, 1966	2000	Kelut, 1919	45 000	Pinatubo, 1991	967 443
3	Santa Maria, 1902	8750	Ambrym, 1979	1000	Galunggung, 1982	22 000	Pinatubo, 1992	787 042
4	Kelut, 1919	5110	Dieng, 1979	1000	Pinatubo, 1992	15 700	Agung, 1963	332 234
5	Santa Maria, 1929	5000	Lake Nyos, 1986	845	Tokachi, 1926	15 000	Vesuvius, 1906	100 000
6	Lamington, 1951	2942	Taal, 1965	785	El Chichón, 1982	15 000	Popocatépetl, 1994	75 000
7	El Chichón, 1982	2000	El Chichón, 1982	500	Merapi, 1930	13 000	Soufrière Guadeloupe, 1976	73 500
8	Lake Nyos, 1986	1746	Merapi, 1994	500	Merapi, 1961	8000	Mayon, 1984	73 000
9	Soufrière St. Vincent, 1902	1565	Merapi, 1998	314	Soufrière Hills, 1995	7500	Arenal, 1976	70 000
10	Merapi, 1930	1369	Vesuvius, 1906	300	Colo (Una Una), 1983	7101	Galunggung, 1982	62 755
Sum		80 562		11 714		201 301		3 741 374
(% of total)		(87.8)		(73.2)		(69.1)		(70.8)

Adapted from [9]. Reproduced with permission from Witham C. Volcanic disasters and incidents: a new database. *Journal of Volcanology and Geothermal Research*. 2005 148(3–4):191–233. Elsevier.

Pyroclastic density currents and lahars accounted for the majority of deaths and injuries. Table 9.2 details notable industrial and technological disasters with estimates, where feasible, of their impacts.

9.2 Study design issues

9.2.1 Use of epidemiological methods in disasters

The purposes of epidemiological evaluation of a chemical incident or natural disaster are several and include:

- Measurement of the magnitude and dispersion of its health impact, if any.

Table 9.2 Selected major chemical incidents

Place	Year (start)	Agent(s)/contaminants	Impact (approximate)
Airborne			
Meuse Valley, Belgium	1930	Sulphur dioxide, sulphuric acid, soot	c. 60 dead >10 000 affected
Flixborough, England	1974	Cyclohexane, related combustion products	29 dead 100 injured >3000 affected
Meda (Seveso), Italy	1976	2,3,7,8-tetrachloro-dibenzodioxin	193 injured >700 affected >190 000 homeless
Bhopal, India	1984	Methylisocyanate, related combustion products	c. 3500 dead >100 000 injured >250 000 affected
Schweizerhalle, Switzerland	1986	Agrochemicals, related combustion products	Extensive environmental damage
Chernobyl, USSR	1986	Radioactive isotopes	c. 60 dead >150 000 affected >100 000 evacuated
Foodborne			
Morocco	1959	Cooking oil (triarylphosphate)	2000 injured
Minamata, Japan	1965	Seafood (methyl mercury)	c. 1800 dead >2500 affected
Yusho, Japan	1968	Rice oil (polychlorinated biphenyls)	>3000 affected
Spain	1981	Rapeseed oil (aniline?)	c. 2000 dead >20 000 affected
Canada, Belgium, USA		Cobalt chloride	>100 affected
Skin contamination			
France	1972	Baby powder (hexachlorophene)	c. 36 dead >200 affected

+ Distinction of cases of disease induced by the incident from the background frequency of disease.

+ Establishment—or otherwise—of a causative role for the incident.

+ Improved understanding of the human toxicology of the chemical or other released materials.

+ Provision of measures of risk across different levels of exposure.

+ Prediction of future health impacts and needs.

+ Planning of appropriate healthcare provision.

+ Prevention—primary or secondary—of future incidents.

Epidemiological evaluation is valuable in both the immediate ('response') and later ('follow-up') phases following an incident. The former is often the responsibility of public health professionals, while the assessment of later effects is generally coordinated by physicians and epidemiologists. While the priorities of early and subsequent epidemiological assessments are often different, their methods and approaches are common. It is important, in the often chaotic management of the immediate response to an incident, to bear in mind the likely requirements of subsequent, longer-term investigations.

In principle, epidemiological investigation should be both descriptive—'how many cases of which disease(s) in which populations?'—and analytical—'how do these cases of disease relate to the event or incident?' This requires delineation of the population at risk and of their exposures, the identification of cases within this population and the exploration of any relationships between these two. The place of epidemiological methods in different phases of an event or disaster is discussed below.

9.2.2 Pre-event: anticipating and planning for the unpredictable

In many situations, hazard identification and risk assessment (see Chapter 14) are possible and may already have been conducted prior to an event. In the industrial setting, risk assessment is a legal health and safety requirement in many countries. In the case of natural disasters, some form of risk assessment may be carried out by geologists in association with other agencies such as local government and health services.

A large range of information on potential hazards can be accessed online or from published research. For example, the US Centers for Disease Control and Prevention (http://www.cdc.gov) has a range of information on environmental health and on emergency preparedness and response. The Agency for Toxic Substances and Disease Registry (ATSDR, http://www.atsdr.cdc.gov) contains a toxicological profile database for over 250 hazardous substances (http://www.atsdr.cdc.gov/toxpro2.html#bookmark05). The US Geological Survey geology website (http://geology.usgs.gov/) has information and links to a wide range of information relating to natural hazards worldwide. Information on volcanic health hazards can be accessed via expert groups, e.g., the International Volcanic Health Hazard Network (http://www.ivhhn.org) or from published research [1, 10, 11].

Assessment of risk should be multidisciplinary and include an input into the planning and organization of relevant health services for any casualties. Previous preparations should ideally facilitate epidemiological investigation during an event, by providing information on likely hazards and establishing communication between agencies. However, the quality of risk assessment mitigation planning can be highly variable (or even absent), and some events or their consequences are difficult to predict, e.g., the Lake Nyos disaster described towards the end of this chapter.

9.2.3 During the event: good record–keeping

Recognizing an event has occurred may take some time, and labeling it as an incident or disaster is an art rather than a science—to some extent this will involve both local and political factors. However, in most situations, the immediate problems will generally be handled by existing health and emergency services. The situation may be chaotic, but good record-keeping should be encouraged and can be invaluable in investigating the event later on. Ideally public health and epidemiological considerations will be represented on any disaster management team—this will be fostered by involvement in any pre-event risk assessment and disaster planning.

9.2.4 After the event—the short to medium term

9.2.4.1 Exposure assessment

Testing the existence of an relationship between 'exposure' and the risk of an adverse health outcome is essential in attributing probable cause following a chemical or natural disaster—and especially so where the outcomes are not specific. Examples of the usefulness of this approach include studies that examined cancer incidence and the prevalence of chronic airflow obstruction following the disasters at Seveso [12] and Bhopal [13]. Understanding exposure–response relationships is helpful also in predicting anticipated health needs. Estimates of exposure may be made for all members of the at-risk population or for only a representative sample—a common approach where estimation is difficult or costly.

As in other areas of environmental epidemiology, population exposures may be assessed through assessment of individuals including biological sampling, inferred by geographical location or through a combination of both. Most assessments of individual exposure are expensive and difficult to apply to large populations. Much more commonly, 'ecological' approaches are used whereby estimates of exposure are related not to individuals but to subgroups of the at-risk population. In general they are based on the expected or measured geographical and temporal distribution of the agent(s) released during the incident. Techniques used might include plume dispersion modeling, using knowledge of type, speed and height of emission, meteorological factors and topography, or (with a volcanic eruption) mapping of the extent and size fractionation of an ashfall. Most experience is with air- or waterborne contaminations and the most sophisticated estimates combine toxicological, meteorological, engineering and geo-modeling approaches [14] for which multidisciplinary input is essential. Groups of individuals can then be allocated to different categories of exposure, based, for example, on their location at the time of the incident or, in longer-term studies, their place of residence or work during the relevant period afterwards. Such information is often collected by interview, and possible subjective reports should be corroborated with objective evidence, such as address of residence, and cross-referenced with biological sampling if possible.

Biomarkers may be of the index compound(s) or of its metabolites; even if there is no currently available assay for the agent(s) released in a chemical or natural incident, it is worth considering the collection of biological samples for the time when an appropriate assay may become available, or for when it subsequently transpires that other, testable, agents were also involved in the incident. Factors which are important to consider if biomarkers are to be used include the relevant timing of sample collections, the acceptability to target populations and the facilities for appropriate storage which may need to be lengthy. Samples from autopsies can also be helpful, e.g., thiosulphate detected in body tissues or blood can help to establish hydrogen sulphide exposures [15].

Other samples may also prove very helpful in assigning exposure estimates to the population under evaluation. Air, water, soil or food samples often provide valuable supportive information and have the advantage that they may be collected relatively easily and over extended periods following an incident. Examination of volcanic ash can yield useful information on levels of reactive metal species [11] and of silica [16] that affect toxicity. Chemical or molecular assessment in animals or plants within the exposure zone ('bioindicators') may also be useful.

As mentioned in Chapter 2, a distinction between 'exposure' and 'dose' is helpful, especially as 'dose' is generally impossible to estimate with any certainty because it is dependent on a large number of environmental and host factors that are difficult if not impossible to measure. These include:

◆ the distribution of the initial toxic release and any chemical transformations it may undergo

◆ the extent of any secondary route of exposure, such as groundwater or soil contaminated by chemical run-off

◆ the sum of mode(s) of personal exposure: inhalation, mucous membrane or skin contact, ingestion etc.

◆ modifying influences such as hyperventilation through exercise, the use of protective equipment or simply whether exposure took place outdoors or indoors

◆ the rate and efficacy of individual metabolism and excretion.

These factors among others determine the 'biologically effective dose' which is probably the closest determinant of any health effects. Unfortunately this information is universally unavailable and alternative surrogates—perhaps derived using features of the list above—are widely employed. In doing so, the potential gains in specificity derived from incorporating extra detail can readily be offset by an increase in misclassification, especially where the detail is derived indirectly and retrospectively. That is to say, complicated, inaccurately measured exposure estimates may be less useful than crude ones that are more broadly accurate. Exposure misclassification that is essentially random will tend to reduce subsequent risk estimates towards the null, making any epidemiologic evaluation inefficient. Misclassification that is systematic, on the other hand, will introduce bias, often suggesting an exposure–response effect that does not, in reality, exist [17] (see Chapter 5).

9.2.4.2 Case identification

Where health effects are specific—either by their nature or through the immediacy of their occurrence—the definition and ascertainment of cases of disease attributable to a disaster may be straightforward. Many of the acute effects of the Union Carbide explosion in Bhopal, for example, were obviously related to the intensely irritant effects of the released gases on the eyes and respiratory airways resulting in immediate symptoms and, frequently, death. More commonly, the adverse effects of a disaster are less specific or unknown. Even if specific, the scale of the effects may be harder to establish where they exacerbate pre-existing disease, e.g., volcanic ash and gases may exacerbate pre-existing asthma [18] or cause small or moderate increases in relatively common conditions such as cancer. In these instances it can be difficult to establish an appropriate definition of a 'case'. In the early, descriptive phase of investigation it is helpful to cast a wide net; in later, analytic phases, when particular hypotheses are being tested, tighter case definitions are necessary.

When deciding case status for analytical studies of exposure and response it is helpful to begin with what is biologically plausible. Airborne releases of irritant gases, for example, are likely to give rise to respiratory disease but will be less likely to cause, say, gastrointestinal disease. This is not to say that other outcomes are impossible, particularly when the identity and toxicology of the released substances—and their metabolites—are poorly understood. However, in such instances it is particularly important to establish a real increase in local disease frequency, above that which might be expected by natural fluctuation, before embarking on formal epidemiological study. It is also worth remembering that among other potential outcomes, the effects of stress—both in those with other demonstrable health effects and in those exposed but otherwise unaffected—may be both frequent and prominent. Anxiety may manifest as an array of minor symptoms but may also have more important long-term effects; it can also be difficult to distinguish from directly toxic disease.

Broadly, case-finding may be either 'reactive' or 'active'. The former approach relies for its ascertainment of cases through routinely used methods while the latter uses specifically designed instruments such as population-based surveys. Commonly used sources in reactive case finding include:

- attendances at local family practice medical services
- activity in other medical or paramedical facilities such as off-peak family practice services, ambulance services, pharmacies etc.
- attendances at hospital emergency services
- admissions to hospital
- mortality figures (all-cause and cause-specific). Autopsy-derived information may be available.

Active case-identification requires a special survey of the population at risk—or more often a representative sample—and sometimes, for the purposes of comparison, an unexposed population. Surveillance systems—often of routinely collected information—may be useful, particularly in long-term studies.

Whatever methods are used, two principles of case definition are particularly important. First, and essential, the definition should not include criteria of exposure or other facets of any etiological mechanism; where they do, the later interpretation of epidemiological studies is impossible. Second, where possible, it is valuable to include criteria that have some degree of 'objectivity' such as the results of laboratory, radiological or other clinical investigations.

In any case, depending on the specificity of any adverse health effects, the number of cases involved and the immediacy of the incident it is often difficult to distinguish cases arising from a disaster from the background frequency of disease. Comparisons with unexposed but otherwise similar populations or with 'non-incident' periods within the same population may be necessary—as may more or less sophisticated methods of assessing temporal or spatial clustering. In Barcelona repeated releases of soy-bean dust from a harbour silo caused repeated epidemics of hospital admission for a severe and abrupt, but otherwise unremarkable asthma; the identification of an epidemic pattern over and above the normal background experience of asthma in the city eventually led to the etiological agent being recognized—a process that took several years [19]. Classification matrices for disaster-related outcomes exist [20] and may be adaptable to a particular chemical incident.

9.2.4.3 Special studies: design issues

The usual types of epidemiological study are employed in investigations, and these have been discussed in Chapters 6 and 8. Studies are of most use if fed into future emergency planning [21].

Pragmatic and organizational issues relate to all study designs. For example, societal disruption as a result of the incident or disaster may make epidemiological research difficult or impossible. Local political factors may hinder research and the safety of researchers needs to be considered. Local resources may be extremely limited and epidemiological investigations may be resourced by a visiting team, who typically conduct a cross-sectional study some time after the event.

In some circumstances, for example, where the goal is to inform future emergency preparedness, a formal epidemiological study that may take months if not years to set up and analyze may not be appropriate. In these circumstances, rapid appraisal methods [22] may be more appropriate. These include both qualitative and quantitative methods, including interviews with key informants and limited surveys of representative areas, conducted by a multidisciplinary team.

9.2.4.4 Communication and coordination issues

It is, arguably and unfortunately, the case that in the epidemiological investigation of natural and chemical disasters, many opportunities have been lost and far less has been learned than was possible. To an extent this is inevitable; disasters tend to occur in settings where preparation is lacking and where resources are few. Other factors—including the emotional and political heat naturally generated by tragedy and the involvement of many different, poorly communicating agencies—also play their part. In any coordinated or other response to a disaster, the epidemiologist is likely to be only one of many involved professionals. In the immediate aftermath, others will include emergency services, those responsible for the source of an industrial release, hospital and other clinical medical staff, toxicologists and environmental health experts, public health specialists and local community and government representatives. Leadership of the response and its coordination will be disputed but is often provided from within the public health service that employs the epidemiologist(s). Acute effects are best studied quickly, for any delay frustrates epidemiological assessments of both exposures and outcomes [23].

In the longer term the epidemiologist may play a more prominent role but other interested parties will include, importantly, politicians, activists, the media and legal experts. Some countries have an epidemiological service dedicated to the investigation of chemical or natural incidents but the task may fall to university-based academics for whom funding is frequently an issue, as is timeliness. Political difficulties frequently arise where investigations are carried out by external—especially foreign—agencies.

A strategy for the regular communication of accurate information between interested agencies, both in the short and longer terms, is vital. This is as true for smaller incidents as it is for large [24], and especially where there remains considerable uncertainty over the impact of an incident. The communication of risk to lay bodies, including the media, is best handled by an expert.

9.2.5 After the event—the long term: surveillance and long-term follow-up

Many if not most incidents and natural disasters have long-term sequelae—social, psychological and physical, e.g., Bhopal. Some effects, e.g., cancers, may be seen a long time after the event and ongoing surveillance or follow-up studies are often desirable. However, the nature of follow-up, who does it, who pays, research funding mechanisms [25] and political and legal issues may make this difficult. Follow-up may end up with local health and public health services that may not be adequately prepared for this type of work. These issues are illustrated in the examples below.

9.3 Examples

Four examples—two chemical incidents and two volcanic disaster events—are described below. They are well-known and illustrate the types of epidemiological investigations conducted and some of the typical problems encountered. Learning points are highlighted at the end of each description.

9.3.1 Bhopal

In 1969 Union Carbide (India) set up a pesticide formulation plant on the north edge of Bhopal, the state capital of Madya Pradesh (Figure 9.1). The original plant imported, mixed and packaged pesticides manufactured in the United States. Ten years later, a 5000 tonne methyl isocyanate (MIC) production unit was installed, primarily to manufacture an effective and inexpensive pesticide marketed as 'Sevin'.

MIC is colorless, with a low boiling point (39°C) and high vapour pressure; chemically unstable, it is stored under refrigeration in dry, stainless steel vessels. For reasons that remain unclear, early in the morning of 3 December 1984, a violent, exothermic reaction caused the largest storage tank to rupture. Over the next hours approximately 27 tonnes of vapour were discharged. Although most of this was probably pure MIC,

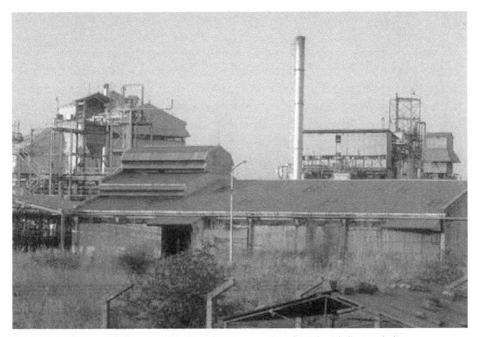

Fig. 9.1 The Union Carbide plant in Bhopal. It is now abandoned and dismantled.

products of hydrolysis and pyrolysis—including CO_2, CO, nitrous oxides, hydrogen cyanide and various ureas—may also have been released in smaller quantities. The exact constitution of the discharged gases remains unclear to this day.

The scarce information on meteorological conditions that night suggest an air temperature of about 10°C and a slow, northerly wind. At this temperature the discharged MIC rapidly condensed and fell to the ground, the plume passing over the northern edge of the city and towards its center. Up to 400 000 people were exposed.

The timing of the explosion was such that most of those exposed were asleep. Survivors report being awakened by an acrid ('chilli-like') stinging of the eyes and throat. The low boiling point of MIC caused it to be re-vaporized at body temperature and inhaled deeply into the lungs. As a result, damage to the bronchial system was extensive; post-mortem findings in those who died immediately after the leak reported widespread airway necrosis with pulmonary edema and hemorrhage. It has not been possible to enumerate such deaths exactly since public health resources in the city were rapidly overwhelmed, a large part of the population fled the city and most bodies were cremated before they and their cause of death could be officially documented. Within 24 hours of the explosion it is estimated that 1700 people died and a similar number within the next three weeks. Given the pathological findings described above, most early deaths were believed to be due to acute pulmonary toxicity.

The literature on the subsequent health effects is surprisingly scanty and largely comprises case series, or crudely designed population studies. Most have concentrated on respiratory disease and have been based on the clinical experience of cases hospitalized in the immediate period after the leak. In almost all instances subjects were drawn from a potentially unrepresentative section of the population and it is questionable how far their findings can be generalized. A particular weakness has been the question of attribution. Few studies have examined to what extent abnormal findings can be causally attributed to gas exposure. Admittedly, this is difficult where most of the proposed (respiratory) outcomes are barely distinguishable, if at all, from other, more frequent disease states only by elaborate and invasive investigation—and where individual and community data on respiratory disease rates prior to the disaster are not available. These deficiencies are not unique to Bhopal—though arguably were exacerbated by the scale of the disaster—and indeed are common problems in the assessment of industrial disasters, where specific outcomes are rare. The difficulties in this case are compounded by the continuing uncertainty over exactly which gases were discharged and the lack of previous human toxicological data on MIC.

A common approach to this problem is the comparison of disease frequencies across two or more groups with differing levels of estimated exposure and the establishment, in this way, of an exposure–response relationship. A number of the studies cited above have employed this technique. Naik *et al.* [26] described a higher prevalence of respiratory symptoms among those resident <2 km from the factory at the time of the disaster and reported an increased frequency of obstructive changes on spirometry in this group—although this is not consistent with their published figures. Gupta *et al.* [27] categorized their subjects into three groups of estimated exposure, again based on distance of residence from the plant, but failed to correlate this with morbidity. On the other hand, Andersson *et al.* [28] reported findings from an unusually elaborate and carefully followed cohort of survivors, sampled using a cluster technique and comprising eight exposed and two nonexposed groups. Although they aimed primarily to examine ophthalmic outcomes, some information on respiratory disease three years after the disaster is available. Reported symptoms of breathlessness, cough and chest pain were each more common across three categories of estimated exposure, though only for the first of these was the trend statistically significant. The gradients were not explained by differences in cigarette smoking. No measurements of lung function were made, and it remains possible that the findings were influenced by differential reporting across the exposure gradient. Irritant eye symptoms and reported frequency of eye infections showed similar findings. Vijayan *et al.*[29] carried out bronchoalveolar lavage in 36 exposed survivors and demonstrated a trend of increasing (macrophage) cellularity across three categories of self-reported exposure intensity. Again, no functional measurements were made and the clinical implications of their findings are unclear.

In 1994 an international group of physicians was invited to undertake investigations into the medium-term morbidity of those who had survived the disaster ten years previously. On the basis of the likely toxicity of the discharged fume, particular attention was paid to respiratory disease. Through cross-sectional survey of city residents, stratified by the distance of their current home from the factory site, a gradient of increasing subjective and objective respiratory morbidity with estimated exposure was identified [13].

The findings were consistent with the development of obliterative disease in the small airways consequent on inhalation of a respiratory irritant fume. This study demonstrated that valuable information can be obtained using simple but carefully conducted epidemiological methods.

Learning points

◆ A potentially dangerous factory was sited on the edge of heavily populated city

◆ The likely health effects of the hazard were unknown

◆ There was inadequate emergency preparedness

◆ A very simple emergency action—putting a wet cloth over the nose and mouth— would probably have greatly reduced health impacts

◆ Political infighting hampered responses to the emergency

◆ A large proportion of the long-term studies set up soon after the disaster have inexplicably failed to reach publication.

9.3.2 **Chernobyl**

On 26 April 1986 two steam explosions in the core of the Chernobyl nuclear power station in Ukraine destroyed the reactor core, blew off the roof of the building and set fire to much of the remaining plant. Ironically the disaster followed a failed safety experiment designed to test the effects of losing power to an emergency cooling system, such as might occur during a major power supply failure. Over the subsequent ten days very large quantities of radioactive gases, aerosols and particles were released from the damaged reactor. Local meteorological conditions including frequent changes in wind speed and direction and intermittent rainfall caused widespread contamination; in total an estimated 1019 Bq of radioisotopes—most importantly ^{131}I and ^{137}Cs— were deposited across large areas of Ukraine, Belarus and, to a lesser extent, the Russian Federation. Nearby countries—Sweden, Finland, Austria and Norway—also experienced extensive (>5000 km^2) contamination. Within a month of the incident almost every country in the northern hemisphere had registered some level of ground contamination.

Little is certain about events immediately after the explosion. Indeed the first recognition outside the country that anything untoward had happened came from routine measurements made at a Swedish nuclear power plant two days later, and for some time afterwards, the Soviet government pursued a policy of providing only incomplete and sometimes misleading information. What seems clear is that around 600 emergency workers were immediately dispatched to the area to assist in putting out the fires. An estimated 100 000 local residents were evacuated over the following fortnight. Over the next three years approximately 600 000 'clean-up workers' helped to reduce further contamination. In addition around 150 000 people of all ages continued to live in heavily contaminated (>555 kBq/m^2) surrounding areas and a further 5 000 000 in less contaminated areas (>37 kBq/m^2).

The immediate effects of heavy radiation exposure are sometimes described as 'deterministic' and are strongly dose-related. Following the Chernobyl fire, 134 emergency workers were reported to have been treated for radiation sickness including (in all cases) bone marrow failure and intestinal, pulmonary, ophthalmic and other organ damage. Exposures for the emergency worker cohort were expected to be measured using radiation dosimeters; unfortunately all of these were overexposed and estimates of exposure using biological measures of irradiation were available only from those who underwent treatment for radiation sickness. Mortality in those with very high exposures (estimated >6 Gy) was almost universal; a third of those with estimated exposures of >4 Gy died. Survival was much higher in those with exposures <4 Gy.

Others with direct exposure to radioactive contaminants—including the cohorts of clean-up workers and local residents—received doses too low to induce radiation sickness. However they were liable to the longer-term ('stochastic') adverse health effects of radiation poisoning. Important among these effects are cancers, particularly thyroid cancer and leukemia, which have a relatively short latency.

For the clean-up workers the main route of exposure was external, but some internal exposure—concentrated in the thyroid—probably occurred too. Direct estimates of external exposure are available for a proportion of the cohort although there are concerns over their accuracy; attempts have been made to model estimates for the remainder [30]. Clean-up workers were registered and offered annual health surveillance; these registries, together with the accompanying exposure estimates, have been used to study the incidence of malignant disease. Very large cohort and, less often, nested case-control studies have suggested an increase in the risk of leukemia and, less clearly, thyroid cancer. The findings have not, however, been consistent, dose–response relationships have not always been clear and there remain concerns over ascertainment bias.

Exposures for residents of the contaminated lands were primarily internal (through drinking contaminated milk and other foods) with some external exposure through contaminated ground deposits. Hundreds of thousands of measurements of thyroid doses were made among the populations of Belarus, Ukraine and parts of Russia; where direct measurements were not made, personal estimates have been made by geostatistical extrapolation. Similarly bone-marrow doses—equivalent to whole-body doses—have been estimated for 5 000 000 local residents [31]. An increase in reports of childhood thyroid cancer was apparent within five years of the disaster [32]. This finding has since been replicated many times with clear evidence of a (linear) exposure–response relationship [33]. The risk decreases with increasing age; indeed it is questionable whether there has been any increase in risk among adults. Nonetheless it is estimated that the total excess of (childhood) thyroid cancers attributable to the disaster will eventually lie between 17 000 and 66 000 cases [34]. In contrast there is, as yet, no definite evidence of an increase in leukemia among the residents—of any age—of the contaminated areas. Nor is there any clear evidence of an increase in risk of other tumors such as breast cancer or of other nonmalignant effects such as birth defects, cataracts, mental illness or cardiovascular disease.

Learning points

♦ Emergency planning and emergency responses were inadequate or absent, particularly with respect to regional and international alerts.

♦ National data—particularly in a period of great economic and political upheaval—can be difficult to interpret. Case registries are especially valuable in such situations.

♦ It was possible to attain relatively good information on exposure to an agent with which there was considerable prior experience.

♦ Radiation is a relatively well understood (and highly feared) agent, but even here the long-term effects on local cancer rates other than thyroid cancers have been difficult to predict.

♦ Where there is comparatively poor local epidemiological expertise there may need to be reliance on international efforts.

♦ Even carefully conducted scientific research can be highly controversial.

9.3.3 Lake Nyos

On the night of 21 August 1986 several thousand individuals living near a volcanic crater lake, Lake Nyos, in a remote area of Cameroon in West Africa lost consciousness. Those who survived woke 6–36 hours later, finding that oil lamps had gone out despite having oil in them, family members and domestic animals had died and there were no birds, insects or small mammals in the area (these were first seen 48 hours later) although plant-life was unaffected [35]. Because the area was so remote, a rescue team did not arrive until two days after the event [35, 36].

Geological investigations pieced together a sequence of events to suggest that a cloud of gas, principally carbon dioxide, had been released from Lake Nyos. The origin of the gas was large volumes of degassing magma which had slowly accumulated and been held under pressure at depths in the lake—temperature profiles and sedimentation patterns suggested this was not a volcanic injection of hot gas and lava. Some event, possibly a small landslip, had caused a disturbance in the lake equilibrium and a release of around 1.2 km^3 of CO_2, resulting in an observed drop in lake level of 110 cm [35]. The gas cloud flowed downhill under gravity, suffocating many in its path.

Initial epidemiological investigations were descriptive and used reports of survivors: an estimated 1700 people died. A review of hospital records showed 548 of an estimated 5000 survivors living in the affected area were admitted to local hospitals and a further 297 attended over the following weeks [36]. Detailed history taking was difficult, but victims reported hearing noises of wind or of animals being disturbed and, for some, a smell of gunpowder or rotten eggs before they suddenly lost consciousness. The commonest symptom was cough, seen in 31 percent, but only 5 percent had difficulty breathing. The commonest physical abnormalities were erythema and skin changes resembling burns seen in 19 percent of those attending hospital. There were no reports of thermal injuries to people, animals or plants, nor were injuries consistent with exposure to acidic or irritant gases, which would have been expected to give a high prevalence of severe irritation of the eyes and mucous membranes and pulmonary oedema. It was noted that 6 percent had weakness of arms or legs. Almost all patients improved within two weeks.

There were anecdotal reports that many of those who did not survive had prominent skin bullae, but investigation of those who had died was extremely limited due to the remoteness of the area, lack of facilities and tropical climate. Very few necropsies were performed—four are recorded in Baxter et al. [36], all of which were performed some days after death. Three of the necropsies were consistent with asphyxiation [36]. The main gases emitted in volcanic areas that are capable of this are carbon dioxide, carbon monoxide and hydrogen sulphide. Forensic tests ruled out major exposures to cyanide, ammonia, carbon monoxide, gaseous halides and sulphur compounds [37], suggesting that the gas responsible was carbon dioxide.

There was no good geological or forensic evidence that the gas cloud had been hot, so the blister and burn-like appearances on those exposed were attributed to pressure sores, dependent changes or post-mortem changes, although this was hindered by lack of information as such events had not been well described before. The smell of rotten eggs was attributed to olfactory hallucinations, which have been reported with CO_2 exposure.

Baxter et al. [36] commented on the absence of reports of any gross neurological or psychological sequelae in survivors two weeks and one year after the event. A follow-up cross-sectional study of survivors was conducted with support of a French team four-and-a-half years after the event, but this focused on respiratory effects. No evidence of respiratory symptoms or reduced peak flow was seen in a population comprising approximately a quarter of Lake Nyos survivors. However, those potentially most susceptible—the elderly, children and those with pre-existing respiratory disease—were excluded from the study. Long-term effects, particularly on non-regenerating tissue such as the brain and nervous system, were not investigated.

In fact, a similar situation had occurred at Lake Monoun, about 100 km south of Lake Nyos, in 1984 when 37 people were killed by a cloud of gas also thought to be CO_2 [38]. The skin of victims were reported to have the appearance of burns and blistering. However, formal investigation in the Lake Monoun event took place six months afterwards; no autopsies had been performed, and no tissue samples were available. While the literature contains a number of reports of small numbers of CO_2-related deaths in many other volcanic areas [39] (Table 9.2), including southern Italy [40, 41] Japan [42], and Nicaragua [43], these chiefly relate to CO_2 accumulations in low-lying areas, basements or wells, and the Lake Nyos disaster arguably established the recognition of risks from large-scale effects from CO_2 clouds.

Learning points

- Establishing the sequence of events required multidisciplinary input making use of all available evidence including eyewitness reports and local hospital records.
- Little toxicological information was available for large-scale population exposures to CO_2—previous events were small-scale and reports were scattered throughout different branches of scientific literature [10].

◆ The event occurred in a remote area of a developing country with a lack of expertise and facilities and no emergency planning—outside experts were involved in investigation and efforts to prevent future exposures.

9.3.4 **Mount St Helens**

The eruption of Mount St Helens (Figure 9.2 A) in 1980 was an important event in establishing multidisciplinary research into the health effects of volcanoes [44]. As often with natural hazards, an event was expected, but the timing and exact impact could not be

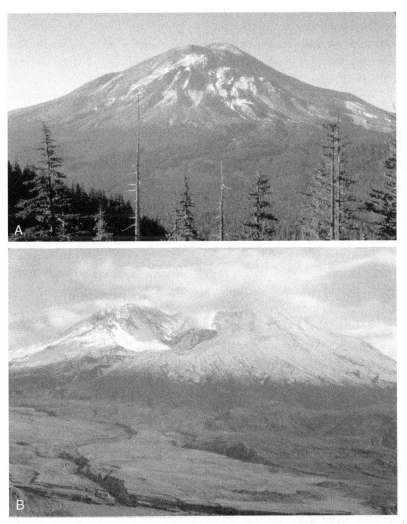

Fig. 9.2 Mount St Helens from Johnston ridges—pictures taken in 1980 one day pre-eruption and four years later. The blast from the 1980 eruption stripped the slopes of trees and vegetation. Image from USGS/Cascades Volcano Observatory (http://vulcan.wr.usgs.gov/Volcanoes/MSH/Images/before_after.html)

readily predicted: a risk assessment by the US Geological Survey published in 1978 had concluded further activity was likely before the end of the century [45]. However, even with detailed monitoring of minor volcanic activity in the preceding two months, the events of the major eruption were unpredictable [46]. In the morning of 18 May 1980 an earthquake triggered a collapse of the north flank of the volcano, immediately followed by a large, lateral blast and subsequent pyroclastic flow (a hot avalanche of gas, rock and ash travelling at 100s of km/hr). This was followed by an ash and gas eruption rising more than 20 km in under 10 minutes [45]. In all, around 2.5 km^3 of ash, lava and stone was displaced resulting in a huge crater on the north of the volcano (Figure 9.2 B). The eruption cloud blew north-eastward giving troublesome ashfall in four states—Washington, Idaho, Montana and North Dakota—with further ashfalls in Washington state on 25 May and 12 June. One of the most heavily affected cities in central Washington State, Yakima, experienced an average total suspended particulate concentrations of 13.3 mg/m^3 over the first week. The number of fatalities was relatively small—there were 35 deaths (only two of which occurred later in hospital) and 23 persons reported missing and presumed dead. However, 150 miles square miles of forest and recreational area was destroyed and in Washington State alone an estimated 1.25 million people lived in areas affected by the eruption (mainly the ashfall). Ash persisted in the environment for many months and was re-suspended in dry periods, causing increases in airborne particulates.

The eruption was extensively studied in terms of both exposure assessment and health effects. Physical scientists set up a sampling network for volcanic gases and ash and characterized the ash in terms elemental composition (e.g., free silica content), water-soluble constituents (e.g., fluoride, which can contaminate groundwater) acidity; and radioactivity of ash [47]. *In vitro* and *in vivo* studies were conducted to determine the toxicity of the ash [48–50]. The free silica of the respirable fraction of the ash (diameter <10μm) was relatively low at 3–7 percent (much less than the 10–24 percent seen in ash from pyroclastic flows in Montserrat [16] and toxicology studies suggested the ash, although not entirely inert, was only mildly toxic to lung cells. There was also judged to be little hazard from water or food contamination by heavy metals or fluorine, seen in some eruptions [51].

Health effects were studied in a variety of ways. A hospital surveillance system was set up within the first week [52] and this triggered further epidemiological studies [53]. Surveys relating to exposure and physical health-effects were conducted of those most heavily exposed to ash such as forest, agricultural or clean-up workers [52, 54] and psychiatric parameters were studied in the disaster area and a control community [55]. A survey of healthcare specialists—in this case, ophthalmologists—was conducted to investigate specific health problems [56, 57]. Use was made of a pre-existing ongoing cohort study measuring lung function in schoolchildren to compare lung function pre- and post-ash exposure [57]. A panel study was set up on children attending a summer camp in an area of ashfall shortly after the eruption [58]. A four year follow-up study of a cohort of loggers working in the area to investigate respiratory effects was conducted [59]—these were considered the most cost-effective group to study as they were the highest exposed [44, 54].

Conclusions of physical health effects of the eruption [51] were that extremely high concentrations of ash (either in a pyroclastic flow or near the volcanic vent) could lead to death from acute pulmonary injury or suffocation. Acute exposures to lower levels of ash caused nasal and bronchial irritation and acute irritation of the eye. Media warnings to stay indoors at periods of highest ashfall were generally heeded, but despite this a household survey in the heavily exposed city of Yakima [51] suggested a third of patients with known chronic respiratory disease experienced an exacerbation of their symptoms after the ashfalls, which continued for a least three months while ash was still in the environment. Chronic respiratory irritation and inflammation were seen and a slight decrease in FEV_1 were documented in the most heavily exposed loggers, but these changes were largely reversible over time [44]. However, there was no measurable effect on lung function in children at relatively low levels of exposure [58]. No long-term ocular effects were documented. Mental health effects including depression, generalised anxiety and post-traumatic stress were seen in a dose–response relationship among both the bereaved and those with property loss [60]. It was generally believed that the detailed evacuation plans, ongoing monitoring and surveillance and public education reduced the potential health effects of the eruption [52].

Learning points

- This is an example of an ongoing event with exposure to a number of agents. The hazards from the 18 May eruption included an explosive blast, pyroclastic flows, mud flows and ashfalls. Some eruptive activity, leading to ashfalls, was seen until 1986.

- Emergency management including evacuation, exclusion zones and public education reduced health impacts.

- A large number of studies were carried out and a huge amount was learnt about health effects of volcanoes. However, most volcanoes are in poorer areas of the world that cannot afford such extensive investigations.

- Studies were multidisciplinary, which allowed proper evaluation of the effects of exposures on health outcomes.

- There was opportunistic use of various information sources including other studies ongoing in the area and a fast response to set up simple but useful timely new studies, e.g., the panel study.

9.4 **References**

[1] Noji EK. *The public health consequences of disasters*. New York: Oxford University Press 1997.

[2] Govaerts-Lepicard M. Definition of a major incident involving chemicals. In: Murray V, ed. *Major chemical disasters—medical aspects of management*. London: Royal Society of Medicine 1990.

[3] Lechat M. Disasters and public health. *Bulletin of the World Health Organization*. 1979 **57**(1):11–7.

[4] Gunn S. Earthquakes. In: Baskett P, Weller R, eds. *Medicine for disasters*. London: Wright-Butterworth 2007: 285–90.

[5] Bakhshi SS. Framework of epidemiological principles underlying chemical incidents surveillance plans and training implications for public health practitioners. *J Public Health Med*. 1997 **19**(3):333–40.

[6] Kesteloot H, Roelandt J, Willems J, Claes JH, Joossens JV. An enquiry into the role of cobalt in the heart disease of chronic beer drinkers. *Circulation.* 1968 **37**(5):854–64.

[7] Hansell AL, Horwell CJ, Oppenheimer C. The health hazards of volcanoes and geothermal areas. *Occup Environ Med.* 2006 **63**(2):149–56, 25.

[8] Magos L. Thoughts on life with untested and adequately tested chemicals. *Br J Ind Med.* 1988 **45**(11):721–6.

[9] *Witham C.* Volcanic disasters and incidents: a new database. *Journal of Volcanology and Geothermal Research.* 2005 **148**(3–4):191–233.

[10] Hansell A, Oppenheimer C. Health hazards from volcanic gases: a systematic literature review. *Arch Environ Health.* 2004 **59**(12):628–39.

[11] Horwell CJ, Fenoglio I, Vala Ragnarsdottir K, Sparks RS, Fubini B. Surface reactivity of volcanic ash from the eruption of Soufriere Hills volcano, Montserrat, West Indies with implications for health hazards. *Environ Res.* 2003 **93**(2):202–15.

[12] Bertazzi PA, Zocchetti C, Pesatori AC, Guercilena S, Sanarico M, Radice L. Ten-year mortality study of the population involved in the Seveso incident in 1976. *Am J Epidemiol.* 1989 **129**(6):1187–200.

[13] Cullinan P, Acquilla S, Dhara VR. Respiratory morbidity 10 years after the Union Carbide gas leak at Bhopal: a cross sectional survey. The International Medical Commission on Bhopal. *BMJ.* 1997 **314**(7077):338–42.

[14] Colvile R, Briggs D, Nieuwenhuijsen M. Environmental measurement and modeling: introduction and source dispersion modeling. In: Nieuwenhuijsen MJ, ed. *Exposure assessment in occupational and environmental epidemiology.* Oxford and New York: Oxford University Press 2003: xiv.

[15] Kage S, Ito S, Kishida T, Kudo K, Ikeda N. A fatal case of hydrogen sulfide poisoning in a geothermal power plant. *Journal of Forensic Sciences.* 1998 **43**(4):908–10.

[16] Baxter P, Bonadonna C, Dupree R, Hards V, Kohn S, Murphy M, *et al.*Cristobalite in volcanic ash of the Soufriere Hills Volcano, Montserrat, British West Indies. *Science.* 1999 **283**:1142–5.

[17] Armstrong BK, White E, Saracci R. *Principles of exposure measurement in epidemiology.* Oxford and New York: Oxford University Press 1995.

[18] Naumova E, Yepes H, Griffiths JK, Sempértegui F, Khurana G, Jagai JS, et al. Emergency room visits for respiratory conditions in children increased after Guagua Pichincha volcanic eruptions in April 2000 in Quito, Ecuador. *Environ Health.* 2007 6:21.

[19] Antó JM, Sunyer J, Rodriguez-Roisin R, Suarez-Cervera M, Vazquez L. Community outbreaks of asthma associated with inhalation of soybean dust. Toxicoepidemiological Committee. *The New England Journal of Medicine.* 1989 **320**(17):1097–102.

[20] Combs DL, Quenemoen LE, Parrish RG, Davis JH. Assessing disaster-attributed mortality: development and application of a definition and classification matrix. *Int J Epidemiol.* 1999 **28**(6):1124–9.

[21] Baxter PJ, Bernstein RS, Buist AS. Preventive health measures in volcanic eruptions. *Am J Public Health.* 1986 **76**(3 Suppl):84–90.

[22] Murray SA. Experiences with "rapid appraisal" in primary care: involving the public in assessing health needs, orientating staff, and educating medical students. *BMJ.* 1999 **318**(7181):440–4.

[23] Young W, Lacey R, Coggon D, Fawell JK. *Assessing the value of epidemiological studies of acute chemical contamination incidents affecting drinking water: Report to the Department of the Environment.* London: HMSO 1996.

[24] MacLehose R, Pitt G, Will S, Jones A, Duane L, Flaherty S, *et al.* Mercury contamination incident. *J Public Health Med.* 2001 **23**(1):18–22.

[25] Buist AS, Martin TR, Shore JH, Butler J, Lybarger JA. The development of a multidisciplinary plan for evaluation of the long-term health effects of the Mount St. Helens eruptions. *Am J Public Health.* 1986 **76**(3 Suppl):39–44.

[26] Naik SR, Acharya VN, Bhalerao RA, Kowli SS, Nazareth H, Mahashur AA, *et al*. Medical survey of methyl isocyanate gas affected population of Bhopal. Part II. Pulmonary effects in Bhopal victims as seen 15 weeks after M.I.C. exposure. *J Postgrad Med*. 1986 **32**(4):185–91.

[27] Gupta BN, Rastogi SK, Chandra H, Mathur AK, Mathur N, Mahendra PN, *et al*. Effect of exposure to toxic gas on the population of Bhopal: Part I–Epidemiological, clinical, radiological and behavioral studies. *Indian J Exp Biol*. 1988 **26**(3):149–60.

[28] Andersson N, Ajwani MK, Mahashabde S, Tiwari MK, Muir MK, Mehra V, *et al*. Delayed eye and other consequences from exposure to methyl isocyanate: 93% follow up of exposed and unexposed cohorts in Bhopal. *Br J Ind Med*. 1990 **47**(8):553–8.

[29] Vijayan VK, Pandey VP, Sankaran K, Mehrotra Y, Darbari BS, Misra NP. Bronchoalveolar lavage study in victims of toxic gas leak at Bhopal. *Indian J Med Res*. 1989 **90**:407–14.

[30] Bouville A, Chumak VV, Inskip PD, Kryuchkov V, Luckyanov N. The Chernobyl accident: estimation of radiation doses received by the Baltic and Ukrainian cleanup workers. **Radiat Res**. 2006 **166**(1 Pt 2):158–67.

[31] Bennett B, Bouville A, Hall P, Savkin M, Storm H. *Chernobyl accident exposures and effects*. The proceedings of the 10th International Congress of the International Radiation Protection Association; 2000; Hiroshima, Japan International Congress of the International Radiation Protection Association; 2000. p. Paper T-12–1.

[32] Prisyazhiuk A, Pjatak OA, Buzanov VA, Reeves GK, Beral V. Cancer in the Ukraine, post-Chernobyl. *Lancet*. 1991 **338**(8778):1334–5.

[33] Jacob P, Goulko G, Heidenreich W, Likhtarev I, Kairo I, Tronko N, *et al*. Thyroid cancer risk to children calculated. *Nature*. 1998 **392**(6671):31–2.

[34] Cardis E, Amoros E, Kesminiene A. Cardis E, Amoros E, Kesminiene A. Observed and predicted thyroid cancer incidence following the Chernobyl accident: evidence for factors influencing susceptibility to radiation induced thyroid cancer. In: Thomas G, Karaoglou A, Williams E, eds. *Radiation and thyroid cancer*. Singapore: World Scientific Publishing Co 1999: 395–404.

[35] Kling G, Clark M, Wagner G, Compton H, Humphrey A, Devine J, *et al*. The 1986 Lake Nyos gas disaster in Cameroon, West Africa. *Science*. 1987 **236**:169–75.

[36] Baxter PJ, Kapila M, Mfonfu D. Lake Nyos disaster, Cameroon, 1986: the medical effects of large scale emission of carbon dioxide? *BMJ*. 1989 **298**(6685):1437–41.

[37] Wagner G, Clark M, Koenigsberg E, Decata S. Medical evaluation of the victims of the 1986 Lake Nyos disaster. *Journal of Forensic Sciences*. 1988 **33**(4):899–909.

[38] Sigurdsson H, Devine J, Tchoua F, Presser T, Pringle M, Evans W. Origin of the lethal gas burst from Lake Monoun, Cameroon. *Journal of Volcanology and Geothermal Research*. 1987 b:1–16.

[39] Stupfel M, Le Guern F. Are there bioimedical criteria to assess an acute carbon dioxide intoxications by a volcanic emission? *Journal of Volcanology and Geothermal Research*. 1989 **39**:247–64.

[40] Beaubien S, Ciotoli G, Lucchese R. Carbon dioxide and radon gas hazard in the Alban Hills area (central Italy). **Journal of Volcanology and Geothermal Research**. 2003 **123**:63–80.

[41] Baubron J, Allard P, Toutain J. Diffuse volcanic emissions of carbon dioxide from Vulcano Island, Italy. *Nature*. 1990 **344**:51–3.

[42] Perez P, Notsu K, Tsurumi M, Mori T, Ohno M, Shimoike Y, *et al*. Carbon dioxide emissions from soils at Hakkoda, north Japan. *Journal of Geophysical Research*. 2003 **108**(B4):2210, doi:10.1029/2002JB001847.

[43] Romero B, Tomas F. Hermanos perecen envenenados en pozo. *El Nuevo Diario*. 1998 5.

[44] Buist AS, Bernstein RS. Health effects of volcanoes: an approach to evaluating the health effects of an environmental hazard. *Am J Public Health*. 1986 **76**(3 Suppl):1–2.

[45] Baxter PJ, Ing R, Falk H, French J, Stein GF, Bernstein RS, *et al*. Mount St Helens eruptions, May 18 to June 12, 1980. An overview of the acute health impact. *JAMA*. 1981 **246**(22):2585–9.

[46] Bernstein RS, Baxter PJ, Buist AS. Introduction to the epidemiological aspects of explosive volcanism. *Am J Public Health*. 1986 **76**(3 Suppl):3–9.

[47] Olsen KB, Fruchter JS. Identification of the physical and chemical characteristics of volcanic hazards. *Am J Public Health*. 1986 **76**(3 Suppl):45–52.

[48] Green FH, Bowman L, Castranova V, Dollberg DD, Elliot JA, Fedan JS, *et al*.Health implications of the Mount St. Helen's eruption: laboratory investigations. *Ann Occup Hyg*. 1982 **26**(1–4):921–33.

[49] Grose EC, Grady MA, Illing JW, Daniels MJ, Selgrade MK, Hatch GE. Inhalation studies of Mt. St. Helens volcanic ash in animals. III. Host defense mechanisms. *Environ Res*. 1985 **37**(1):84–92.

[50] Martin TR, Wehner AP, Butler J. Evaluation of physical health effects due to volcanic hazards: the use of experimental systems to estimate the pulmonary toxicity of volcanic ash. *American Journal of Public Health*. 1986 **76**(3 Suppl):59–65.

[51] Baxter PJ. Volcanoes and occupational health. *Br J Ind Med*. 1986 **43**(5):289–90.

[52] Merchant JA, Baxter P, Bernstein R, McCawley M, Falk H, Stein G, *et al*.Health implications of the Mount St. Helen's eruption: epidemiological considerations. *Ann Occup Hyg*. 1982 **26**(1–4):911–9.

[53] Bernstein RS, Baxter PJ, Falk H, Ing R, Foster L, Frost F. Immediate public health concerns and actions in volcanic eruptions: lessons from the Mount St. Helens eruptions, May 18–October **18**, 1980. *Am J Public Health*. 1986 **76**(3 Suppl):25–37.

[54] Buist AS, Bernstein RS, Johnson LR, Vollmer WM. Evaluation of physical health effects due to volcanic hazards: human studies. *American Journal of Public Health*. 1986 **76**(3 Suppl):66–75.

[55] Shore JH, Tatum EL, Vollmer WM. Evaluation of mental effects of disaster, Mount St. Helens eruption. *Am J Public Health*. 1986 **76**(3 Suppl):76–83.

[56] Fraunfelder FT, Kalina RE, Buist AS, Bernstein RS, Johnson DS. Ocular effects following the volcanic eruptions of Mount St Helens. *Arch Ophthalmol*. 1983 **101**(3):376–8.

[57] Johnson KG, Loftsgaarden DO, Gideon RA. The effects of Mount St. Helens volcanic ash on the pulmonary function of 120 elementary school children. *Am Rev Respir Dis*. 1982 **126**(6):1066–9.

[58] Buist AS, Johnson LR, Vollmer WM, Sexton GJ, Kanarek PH. Acute effects of volcanic ash from Mount Saint Helens on lung function in children. *Am Rev Respir Dis*. 1983 **127**(6):714–9.

[59] Buist AS, Vollmer WM, Johnson LR, Bernstein RS, McCamant LE. A four-year prospective study of the respiratory effects of volcanic ash from Mt. St. Helens. *Am Rev Respir Dis*. 1986 **133**(4):526–34.

[60] Shore JH, Tatum EL, Vollmer WM. Psychiatric reactions to disaster: the Mount St. Helens experience. *Am J Psychiatry*. 1986 **143**(5):590–5.

Chapter 10

Environmental epidemiology in developing countries

Isabel Romieu and Horacio Riojas Rodríguez

10.1 Environmental health problems in developing countries

In developing countries, as in other parts of the world, the burden of disease due to environmental exposure is close to 24 percent [1]. However, in developing countries, this burden is a mixture of old problems, mainly related to poor sanitation and hygiene and lack of infrastructure, and new ones related to mass urbanization and the increase of industrial production without strict environmental control, leading to an increase in exposure to chemicals such as air pollutants, heavy metals, pesticides and other toxic substances.

Among the major environmental threats, poor water quality and sanitation, indoor and outdoor air pollution, exposure to heavy metals and pesticides, and malaria are the most prevalent. In addition, factors such as poor nutrition and co-exposure to different pollutants increase the susceptibility to adverse health effects of environmental exposure.

10.1.1 Water and sanitation

Poor water quality continues to pose a major threat to human health. Diarrheal disease alone amounts to an estimated 4.1 percent of the total disability-adjusted life years (DALY) global burden of disease and is responsible for the deaths of 1.8 million people every year [2, 3] (see Chapter 14 for more information on DALY and related measures). It is estimated that 88 percent of that burden is attributable to unsafe water supply and poor sanitation and hygiene. The population that is most likely to be threatened by waterborne diseases is children, in particular those in poor rural communities [4]. Young children (<5 years) are at higher risk than older children because of behavior that increases their contact with the environment, and diarrheal diseases are an important contributor to malnutrition. A significant amount of disease could be prevented through better access to safe water supply, adequate sanitation facilities and better hygiene practices [3]. The WHO has assessed the cost-effectiveness of different interventions in 14 WHO subregions. However, transitional research (i.e., research applying scientific discovery to provide solutions to society) is still needed.

10.1.2 **Indoor air pollution**

More than three billion people worldwide continue to depend on solid fuels for their energy needs, including biomass fuels (wood, dung, agricultural residues) and coal. Cooking and heating with solid fuels on open fires or traditional stoves results in high levels of indoor air pollution. Indoor smoke contains a range of health-damaging pollutants, such as small particles and carbon monoxide, and particulate pollution levels may be 20 times higher than accepted guideline values. According to the World Health Report of 2002 [5], indoor air pollution is responsible for 2.7 percent of the global burden of disease. Most at risk are women and young children who spend a large amount of time exposed to open fire on a daily basis.

10.1.3 **Outdoor air pollution**

Outdoor air pollution is a major problem in cities in the developing world mainly because of vehicular exhaust, although fixed sources also contribute substantially to particulate and sulphur dioxide emissions [6, 7]. Several studies that have been conducted among healthy and asthmatic children and the elderly have reported an increase in morbidity including emergency visits, hospitalization, respiratory illnesses and symptoms, and change in lung functions associated with air pollution levels, in particular small particulates and ozone [8]. Of major concern is the health impact observed among children at levels that do not exceed current standards and the fact that fine particulates, in particular from diesel emissions, may increase sensitization to allergens. Although there is a growing body of studies conducted in developing countries that document the adverse effect of outdoor air pollution on children's health, many countries are still postponing the implementation of legislation and control measures.

10.1.4 **Heavy metals**

Heavy metal exposure is highly prevalent in developing countries. The major sources of lead exposure include fixed industrial sources, including smelting, petrochemical processing, and mining. For example, Latin America and the Caribbean contribute 14 percent of the world production of lead, Peru and Mexico being the leading producers in the hemisphere. Lead in different forms and compounds is also used in numerous industries and activities, but numbers and intensity of lead use are not well known. In countries such as Mexico, Peru, and Honduras, for example, lead varnishes are commonly used as glazes for ceramic ware, although the extent of production and distribution of lead-glazed ceramics is not precisely known. Some countries such as Venezuela are still using gasoline with a high lead content. The reutilization and recycling of batteries is also a major source of lead exposure. Only sparse information is available on other sources of exposure in developing countries such as paint, food contamination, and water contamination.

Lead pollution levels have been rising in the urban areas of many developing countries, with more than 90 percent of the children in some African cities suffering from lead poisoning [9]. Concern over the prevalence of lead exposure has focused on young children because of their susceptibility to its adverse health effect on growth and neurobehavioral development. Lead is not the only heavy metal of concern in developing countries; according to the United Nations, high concentrations of arsenic, mercury and cadmium are found in drinking water in countries like Bangladesh, Pakistan, China, Chile, Argentina and different countries in Africa [10].

10.1.5 Pesticides

Pesticides are used throughout the developing world, primarily for agricultural purposes and for malaria control. Many areas in developing countries rely on agricultural production as a major source of economic and social development through the exportation of products such as coffee, cotton, sugar, fruits and vegetables, and flowers among others. Latin America's pesticide market has grown at twice the world average. Brazil, Colombia and Costa Rica are the heaviest consumers, applying pesticides at a rate of 1.1 to 18.0 metric tons annually per 1000 hectares. Latin American countries both import and produce pesticides, including DDT, paraquat, and heptachlor, which have been banned from the US and European countries [11]. Pesticides are often incorrectly handled in agricultural and home use, producing acute intoxication among workers and their families and contaminating water, soil and foods.

Children are more vulnerable than adults to experiencing latent or delayed effects over the long course of their lifetime. To date, there is little available data on the incidence of acute pesticide intoxication in developing countries, in part because of the lack of surveillance systems. Chronic exposure is also of major concern because of its potential association with cancer, developmental neurotoxicity, teratogenesis, and endocrine disruption.

10.1.6 Other chemicals

Other chemicals of concern include persistent organic pollutants that are emitted into the petrochemicals and other industries in developing countries. Most of the time there is not enough information to estimate the exposure to these contaminants. However, new studies show that this is an important issue that should be addressed. For example, in Asian developing countries, significant amounts of persistent organic pollutants (POPs) have been found in dumping sites [12].

10.1.7 Malaria and other parasitic diseases

The emergence of vector-borne diseases (VBD) like dengue and dengue hemorrhagic fever (DHF), along with the endemic transmission of malaria, Chagas diseases, and oncocercosis in many developing countries is intimately associated with the complex social and economic transition faced by these countries. The growth of population, especially in urban centers, the unplanned urbanization, the lack of provision of public services like potable water, sewage and garbage collection systems, and the ecological disruption caused by global warming, agricultural practices and deforestation, are major determinants in the transmission dynamics of VBDs in the region. These economic and social forces are facilitating the routes of contagion. The threats to the health of children are a major concern, since this age group is the most affected by VBD. There are no vaccines available to prevent transmission, and the severity of infection and lethality are higher in children, especially in the undernourished. In many VBDs like Chagas, onco-cercosis and DHF, the risk of infection at an early age predisposes children to suffer the severe manifestations of the infection later in life. According to WHO data (http://www.who.int/healthinfo), infectious and parasitic diseases account for 23 percent of the world's DALYs acute respiratory infections in accounting for 6 percent, followed by diarrheas (5 percent), AIDS (5 percent), and malaria and tropical diseases (3.6 percent).

10.1.8 Susceptibility factors

Poverty, global malnutrition, micronutrient deficiency, crowding and poor living condi-tions, and co-exposure to various pollutants are prevalent in developing countries and are likely to increase the susceptibility to the environmental exposure, particularly among children. Several factors are responsible for the high susceptibility of children to illness related to environmental exposure. Behavior characteristics of early childhood strongly affect a child's exposure to toxicants by being in closer contact with the ground and through hand-to-mouth behavior. Children also spend more time outdoors than do most adults, often engaged in vigorous play, and may ingest more contaminated food and drink in proportion to their body weight than adults. Thus, children have a greater likelihood of exposure. Children are in general less able to metabolize, detoxify, and excrete toxic chemicals, and thus are more vulnerable. They also undergo extensive growth and development throughout gestation and the first years of life, and their delicate developmental process are easily disrupted [13].

Based on the burden of disease developed by the WHO [14], the per capita number of healthy life years lost to environmental risk factors is five times greater in children under five years of age than in the total population. In developing countries, diarrhea, malaria and respiratory infections account for an average of 26 percent of all deaths in children under five years old.

10.2 Methodological challenges of environmental epidemiology studies in developing countries

10.2.1 General context of environmental health research in developing countries

The general context related to the economic and health situation in developing countries has an important impact on the development of environmental health research, for which lack of government support and poor institutional capacity are the most limiting factors (see Table 10.1).

Most developing countries assign low budgets for research in health and particularly for environmental health. Developed countries spend an average of 2.5 percent of their income on research and development, while developing countries spend less than 0.5 percent. Competing priorities are the main reason.

Table 10.1 Major challenges to develop environmental epidemiological studies in developing countries

Challenge	Alternative solution
Persistence of sanitary risks with presence of new chemical risks	Increase research projects to evaluate mixed risks
Lack of governmental support for environmental health research	Place environmental health problems as priorities in the agenda of the government
Lack of human resources for research in environmental health	Support postgraduate programs in environmental epidemiology
Lack of laboratory infrastructure	Networking within and between countries to invest in laboratory and infrastructure
Lack of international support	Increase the international cooperation in the area of environmental epidemiology
Lack of established networks	Strengthen networks in environmental health society such as ISEE and obtain support from WHO and international organizations
Lack of routinely collected data on mortality and morbidity	Invest in environmental surveillance programs in order to prevent risk and to collect reliable information
Rapid demographic change migration and high percentage of children in the population	Increase research and prevention programs aimed at children and pregnant women
Lack of complete case ascertainment	Improve the coverage and quality of surveillance systems and establish active vigilance
Lack of complete sampling frame	Improve data on census in study area prior to sampling
Exposure data	Use validated field methods and adapt the type of sampling to the local conditions and feasibility. Equipment for specific tests. Importance of portable instruments.

In most developing countries, there is a lack of well-trained researchers in environmental health. Few medical students are attracted to public health, which is not as highly regarded as other medical specialties and provides comparatively much lower income. In addition, few superior education institutions in developing countries provide training in this area. For example, at the National Institute of Public Health in Mexico, during the last 15 years only 52 students received training in environmental health, while in developed countries such as the US or Europe, a much larger number of students were trained in this area. This contrasts with the number and magnitude of environmental problems in developed and developing countries.

The limitation in research budgets affects strategic issues for the development of environmental epidemiology research, such as access to good-quality laboratories with certified technicians. Researchers have to make an extra effort to guarantee that the results are valid according to the accepted quality assurance and quality control (QA/QC) criteria. More often than not, the environmental and biological samples have to be sent to laboratories abroad for analysis. The development of the laboratory infrastructure is therefore a key necessity for the development of environmental epidemiology in developing countries.

In general, there is a lack of international support to investigate specific problems related to environmental exposure in developing countries given that the research agenda is, in general, focused on the environmental issues of developed countries. Networks are an efficient way to support research in environmental epidemiology through human resource development and knowledge and equipment exchange. Unfortunately, while such networks have been developed in Europe and the US, there are few participating institutions from developing countries.

10.2.2 Conducting environmental epidemiological research in developing countries

The availability of accurate, routinely collected environmental and health data are important to determine the potential adverse health effects of environmental exposure. In developing countries, the lack of systematic and standardized collection of such data limit their use. When data are available, they often suffer from lack of reliability and are not usually available over long periods of time. For example routine collection of national mortality data is usually carried out in all developing countries. In many countries, a death certificate is needed to obtain the legal authorization to bury a person. However, in some cases, death may not be registered, particularly for infants, young children or the elderly. Inadequate registration varies between countries. For example, the sub-registration of mortality is estimated to be 0.4 percent in Canada, but it reaches 40 percent in Nicaragua [15]. In developing countries, the accuracy of the death certificate is often poor, particularly regarding the specific cause of death, and only the primary cause of death is recorded. Autopsies are rarely conducted, and rates vary between countries and periods. For example, in a study to determine the impact of air pollution on health in three major Latin American cities from Brazil, Chile and Mexico, cities were chosen based on the availability of large series of air pollution monitoring data with good quality control and mortality data. Several cities were excluded because of the poor reliability of air pollution monitoring or the absence of a series of continuous monitoring over at least two years. Air pollution data were obtained from the city monitoring networks and mortality data from national statistics databases. Death certificates were obtained from official sources. However, careful revision of these data was necessary, including use of different codes to enter variables such as gender, scholarship, place of death and different ways to enter missing data. Different ICD codes (9 or 10) were used to classify specific causes of death; therefore a validation study needed to be carried out. In addition, there was discrepancy in the format of data captured electronically between the three countries. Mexico recorded only the primary cause of death and did not provide socio-economic status (SES) indicators for infant and children deaths, while in Brazil two causes of death were captured and the education of the mother was included on death certificates of infants and children.

While a wide range of routine morbidity statistics are available in developed countries (such as abortion, cancer, congenital abnormalities, hospital inpatients, infectious diseases, school health and sickness absence, accidents at work and occupational diseases), these types of statistics are seldom collected in a systematic and standardized manner in most developing countries. This has impaired the use of these data in environmental epidemiology. The records are usually incomplete, provide poor coverage of the population and may be biased, particularly in relation to socioeconomic status. Additionally, the source population is often not well-specified. For example, in a study on Mexican children's air pollution-related emergency visits, Hernandez-Cadena *et al.* [16] used data collected from all social security clinics of Ciudad Juárez, Mexico. Some of the data for several time periods had not been captured, and the investigators had to refer to the original records to complete the database. In addition, due to migration, the source population changed over time and had to be adjusted to the total daily number of emergency visits in order to study the variation in the proportion of respiratory-related emergency visits in conjunction with daily air pollution variation. In a study conducted in Santiago, Chile, Llabaca *et al.* [17] used hospital records to study the relation of air pollution and emergency visits for pneumonia in children. To validate the diagnosis of pneumonia reported in the chart, they had to evaluate the standardization of physician diagnosis during the study with clinical examination reports and prescription records.

International comparison is often difficult due to diagnostic practice and coverage of the population, among other reasons. The WHO is playing a major role in the standardization of the collection of environmental health indicators to be used by all countries, an initiative that is of major importance in order to determine countries and areas with major environmental health problems (Figure 10.1).

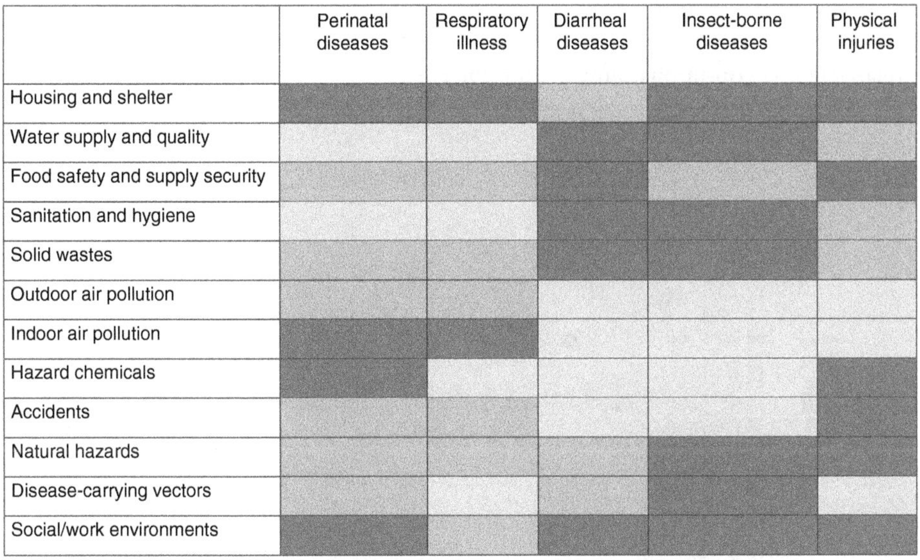

	Perinatal diseases	Respiratory illness	Diarrheal diseases	Insect-borne diseases	Physical injuries
Housing and shelter					
Water supply and quality					
Food safety and supply security					
Sanitation and hygiene					
Solid wastes					
Outdoor air pollution					
Indoor air pollution					
Hazard chemicals					
Accidents					
Natural hazards					
Disease-carrying vectors					
Social/work environments					

Fig. 10.1 Environmental indicators for children in environmental health: prioritizing environmental health risks at the global level. Source: http://www.who.int/ceh/indicators/en/indicatorsoverview.pdf

Migration is an issue in developing countries because a high percentage of the rural population leave their original communities due to poverty and environmental degradation. Currently, there is wide interest in comparing the health of a migrant population with the health of a similar population in the receiving country and with the health of a similar population in the country of origin. These comparisons are likely to provide information on potential environmental factors related to specific diseases. However, it is very important to compare the quality of the data obtained on the different population subgroups regarding access to healthcare, diagnostic practice, lifestyle environment, age distribution, and genetic susceptibility as well as considering the 'healthy migrant effect'. Examples of these include studies on pesticides effects and asthma in migrants [18, 19].

In general, geographical contrasts between areas within countries are likely to be less than those between countries but might be more revealing in relation to environmental influence on urban and rural prevalence of diseases, keeping in mind that rural health statistics might be of poorer quality than urban statistics. Long-term trends of mortality and morbidity rates for specific diseases can be of value in indicating possible effects of the environmental factors. However, over time, the absence of the standardized collection of incidence data limits the use of data. In developing countries, cancer registries are usually very limited with poor population coverage. For example, in Mexico, mortality data for breast cancer have been used to show an increase in incidence of the disease in the last decade. However, mortality data for breast cancer is a combination of incidences of breast cancer, access to care, therapeutic treatment, age structure of the population, and competing risk of death (due to other causes). Although these factors are unlikely to change drastically over the short term, they can create problems when interpreting long-term trends (Figure 10.2).

It is sometimes possible to identify environmental agents related to the development of relatively rare conditions, simply from the clustering of a few cases in local areas or in

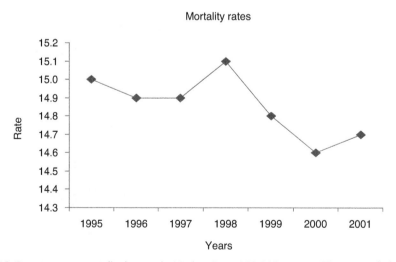

Fig. 10.2 Breast cancer mortality by year in Mexico. Rate: 100 000 women 25 years and older.

particular occupations. However, interpretation is often difficult because of incomplete ascertainment of cases. When an active surveillance system is implemented in an area where cases of rare outcomes have been observed, comparison with regional or national statistics can be misleading because of the difference in case diagnosis and ascertainment due to the poor quality of mandatory disease reporting systems in many developing countries [20].

General surveys are periodically conducted in some developing countries in order to determine the prevalence of diseases and other characteristics of the population and support health program development. In Mexico, chronic disease surveys and nutrition surveys are conducted every five years. Probabilistic sample frames are developed in order to obtain good population representation by regions, urban and rural areas, age groups and gender. These data, collected in a standardized manner, allow comparison within the country and specific groups. However, health-related questions rely on participants' answers and knowledge about their own health. While in some cases, biological samples are obtained in subsamples, health data and biological samples rarely include environmental health questions or any measure of specific chemicals in biological samples.

The majority of illnesses are multifactorial, and environmental factors are likely to interact. One of the difficulties of studying environmental exposure in developing countries is that subjects are often exposed to several pollutants and are more likely to be susceptible due to poor nutrition, poor housing conditions and lifestyle in general. Conditions where one single environmental factor may be tested are sparse, and, therefore, it is difficult to assess the specific effect of one single pollutant.

Intervention studies and natural experimental situations provide strong design and are the most likely to support causal association between exposure and outcome. For example, in Xuanwei, China, residents traditionally burned 'smoky' coal in unvented indoor fire pits that generated very high levels of air pollution. Since the 1970s, most residents have changed from fire pits to stoves with chimneys. This study assessed whether lung cancer incidence decreased after this stove improvement. A cohort of 21 232 farmers, born from 1917 to 1951, was followed retrospectively from 1976 to 1992. All subjects were users of smoky coal who had been born into homes with unvented fire pits. During their lifetime, 80.9 percent subjects changed permanently to stoves with chimneys. A hospital record search detected 1384 cases of lung cancer (6.5 percent) during follow-up. A long-term reduction in lung cancer incidence was noted after stove improvement. Levels of indoor air pollution during burning with chimneys were less than 35 percent of levels during unvented burning [21].

One of the major problems to designing a sampling frame in developing countries is the quality of census data. Census data are frequently incomplete and not up to date due to the rapid growth of the urban population. This implies that, in many cases, a census of the population to be studied needs to be carried out, particularly in rural areas and in the surrounding areas of large cities where the population tends to migrate. For example, in order to develop a health survey in the area of rural Michoacán, Mexico, investigators carried out a census of six villages from door to door and selected a random sample after the census was established. Several types of sampling can be used: a probabilistic sampling (i.e., simple random sampling, systematic random sampling, stratified random sampling, conglomerate sampling, multilevel sampling or mixed sampling), and nonprobabilistic sampling when randomization is not possible or too expensive [22]. In Mexico, there is an official source of population and cartographic data (National Institute of Statistics, Geography and Data Processing) that facilitates population sampling. However, these data need to be verified when conducting a study because of the scales on the maps, incomplete data on migration, and topographical characteristics. In other developing countries, the situation may be scarcer and will also depend on the frequency of the census populations.

When conducting case-control studies, it is very important to obtain a census of the cases in the area of study. However, given that disease registry is sparse or incomplete, it is often difficult to assume that the cases included in the study are representative of all cases from the area under study. For example, in a study of neural tube defect, investigators established an active vigilance system in all hospitals from the northern part of Mexico to identify all newborns with neural tube defect because the registry is largely incomplete. This allowed the recruitment of all newborns with NTD for a case-control study in which cases were matched by hospital of birth and date of birth [20].

10.2.3 Data gathering

The quality of exposure data is a major factor in the validity of epidemiological studies. Instruments for exposure assessment include:

1. interviews and questionnaires, activity pattern diaries;
2. measurement of external media (air monitoring network);
3. concentration in the microenvironment (CO in indoor air);
4. individual doses (personal monitoring);
5. concentration in human tissue (e.g., blood lead);
6. physiologic effects markers (e.g., DNA adducts).

Table 10.2 presents some examples is of available data on environmental exposure in most developing countries and potential health effects. The main issues with exposure assessment to which researchers are confronted in developing countries are the following:

- Questionnaires need to be adapted to local conditions and languages and tested in pilot studies. Also, depending on the cultural background, some questions might not be applicable.

- Routine environmental sampling is uncommon in developing countries. Air pollutant and water monitoring are conducted mainly in large cities but data are not systematically reported and are poorly standardized. Data are not available in rural areas. Therefore, environmental sampling needs to be part of the study protocol. It is important to use validated field methods and adapt the type of sampling to the local conditions and feasibility. The development of field methods for exposure assessment using portable instruments has facilitated research, e.g., lead assessment of water and

Table 10.2 Some examples of available data on environmental exposure and associated effects

Exposure assessment	Limitation	Health effects	Limitation
Air pollutants monitoring	Only in major cities of developing countries Do not measure all pollutants Limited quality control Lack of long series of measurements	Respiratory diseases: all causes	Poorly registered and lack of standardization of diagnosis
		Mortality: all causes, respiratory, cardiovascular	Validity of specific causes of death In some countries only primary cause is recorded
Data on production, importation, distribution and use of pesticides	Aggregate data and difficulty to obtain use in a specific area Lack of data on specific products	Emergency visits for acute intoxication	Large underestimation of pesticide poisoning and other chemicals
Water quality	Poor quality of routinely collected data	Diarrheal diseases.	Poorly registered and lack of standardization of diagnosis
Natural disasters	Lack of registers on number and intensity	Deaths, diarrheal, respiratory and vector-borne diseases	Poorly registered and lack of standardization of diagnosis
Socio economic level (at small administrative units)	Difficult to obtain	Environmental related diseases	Need active surveillance system
Description of production process in industry	Industry might not cooperate to provide this information	Cancer registry	Incomplete
Emission inventory from industry	Aggregate data Poor accuracy	Morbidity	Difficulty for confirmation and standardization

soil content [23], measurement of blood lead level using the 'lead care' instrument, or passive monitoring of CO in indoor air.

◆ Exposure to complex mixtures of two or more toxic substances is frequent in developing countries. In addition to the difficulties of identifying specific agents in the environmental or biological samples, this increases the difficulty of interpretation of the relation between exposure and health effects.

◆ Finally, due to lack of data, it is often necessary to rely on aggregate information such as national use of pesticides and importation and exportation of chemicals.

In addition, some industries are reluctant to provide information on the products used in their production process.

The lack of laboratories enrolled in QA/QC programmes in the developing country is a strong limitation for obtaining accurate data. Although the laboratory networks enrolled in the QA/QC program for blood lead has grown extensively, this is not the case for other chemicals such as pesticides. This affects the comparison of results between studies and may add a level of misclassification that might mask adverse effects. Similarly, for biological samples such as blood, urine, and epithelial cells, the condition of preparation and conservation requirement of the samples is frequently not compatible with local conditions. It is often difficult to find a national laboratory that can process the samples, and international cooperation is the only possibility. This adds difficulties because of the shipment and conservation of the sample, which most of the time needs to be kept at $-70°C$.

Health effects should be defined and measured in a standardized manner. Information can be obtained by questionnaire (e.g., symptoms), functional tests, or based on medical diagnosis. Criteria to insure comparability are of great importance. For clinical symptoms questionnaires, it is important to test the understanding of the questions in the study population, and to use questions tested in international settings as much as possible. This facilitates comparison of results. For example, in the International Study on Asthma and Allergies in Childhood (ISAAC) a set of questions on respiratory symptoms were developed and special attention was given to their adaptation to different cultures and languages. Functional tests need to be conducted in accordance with guidelines. The advantages and disadvantages of techniques and instruments have to be judged on the basis of acceptability by the study population, the accuracy and reliability of the results, and the availability of technicians. For example, the validation of spirometric tests using portable instruments with more established instruments has allowed larger field research in respiratory epidemiology and better knowledge of the prevalence of chronic obstructive pulmonary disease (COPD), as in the PLATINO study conducted in Latin America [24].

Although criteria for medical diagnosis are usually standardized and include objective measures, it is important to review the criteria used for disease definition, in particular for international comparisons. In some circumstances, laboratory tests might not be feasible and diagnosis might be based only on clinical symptoms. Validation of the diagnosis in a subsample of the cases is important. For example, in the ISAAC study, case definition was further validated in a subsample with the bronchial hyperreactivity test with saline solution and skin prick test [25].

10.2.4 Logistics and other issues

The language diversity in developing countries reflects the challenge of cultural diversity in epidemiological studies. The understanding of health, illness and environmental concepts has to be taken into account in the questionnaire design as well as in the participation during the research process. It is important to explain the study in a language that participants will understand and to avoid long consent forms. All forms need to be translated to the local language. Cultural characteristics and perceptions of health problems and the environment differ between population and areas. It is important to be aware of the cultural differences and take them into account when planning the study. Some questions and biological samples might be acceptable in a certain culture but not in others. For example, having a child with a 'runny nose' would be considered normal in some rural areas; therefore, this symptom will not be reported if not specifically asked for.

It is important to involve local personnel who will have easier contact with the population. Differences in the concepts of health, exposure, diseases and environmental risk need to be considered. Literacy might be a major problem in some areas, particularly in rural populations. Interviewers are needed in order to apply questionnaires. Using community health workers will facilitate the contact and increase confidence in the study. The support of health authorities is of major importance in the various studies within rural and urban areas. In a place where health services are scarce, agreement with community leaders might be the key to a successful study.

It is difficult to access some remote areas, which causes problems for the research project. Time is lost in transportation, the insecurity of the road and the fact that homes are usually dispersed and without electricity. For example, a study was conducted in rural

Table 10.3 Characteristics of research settings and alternatives to conduct epidemiological research in developing countries

Setting	Difficulties	Alternatives
Mega cities, (Mexico, São Paulo, Bombay, etc.)	Insecurity Lack of sufficient secondary data for contaminants and/or health effects (e.g., databases in hospitals)	Gather information from different sources Extrapolation of data Validation of questionnaires for local population Spend more time in the data-gathering phase
Large cities (Buenos Aires, Bogotá, Lima, Monterrey)	Lack of sufficient data, for example, in air and water quality	Information and infrastructure need to be generated by the research team in collaboration with universities and other government or private institutions
Rural zones	Dispersion of the population Lack of communication, cultural diversity Lack of information on socioeconomic conditions and exposure and health data Logistical problems in carrying out research, such as lack of electricity	Implement local census strategies Participatory discussion to explain research objectives Use of alternative techniques for exposure modeling, satellite images Use of validated field techniques that are easy to use (nephelometers, CO and NO exhaled, portable spirometers, acetyl cholinesterase measurers, etc.) Larger investment in vehicles and means of transporting samples

Mexico in the high plateau of Purapecha. In order to study the impact of biomass burning, households were recruited in six villages with large distances between them. Many of these households did not have electricity, and the monitoring equipment to assess exposure to pollutants required batteries to be recharged. Therefore, they were recharged periodically at the regional health center or other sites with electricity. Similarly, in different studies related to the effect of pollutants in small mining villages in South America, the research team spent a large amount of time traveling through thick jungles and the rigid Sierra Mountains to reach the dispersed communities. In some poor areas with large metropolises, growing insecurity renders research unsafe for the study personnel. Strategies to enter such populations might be through schools or resident associations. In addition, social inequality and conflicts limit access to study populations in some regions of developing countries. Table 10.3 presents some characteristics of research settings in developing countries and alternatives to conduct epidemiological research.

10.3 The impact of local research in promoting prevention and control of environmental threats

Major difficulties exist in developing countries with regard to converting research results into environmental health policies or intervention programs. Several factors are responsible for the lack of translation between research results and policy making. Among them, the following play an important role:

◆ Disengagement of the academic sector with the decision makers.

◆ Pressure on the researchers to publish abroad but not to communicate results locally.

◆ Absence of personnel in the research centers dedicated to translating the results to the decision makers.

◆ Incapacity to develop long-term policies linked to research due to constant changes of authorities on state and federal levels.

It is important that, besides publishing in high-impact journals at the international level, results from research be published in local languages and summarized for health decision makers to enable the governments, the community and other stakeholders to use the results in an efficient way.

10.4 References

[1] Ginebra S. *Preventing disease through healthy environments*. Geneva, Switzerland: World Health Organization 2006.

[2] Prüss-Üstün A, Corvalan C. *Preventing disease through healthly environments: towards an estimate of the environmental burden of disease*. Geneva: World Health Organization 2006.

[3] Prüss-Üstün A, Kay D, Fewtrell L, Bartram J. Unsafe water, sanitation and hygiene: comparative quantification of health risk. *Global and regional burden of disease attributable to selected major risk factors*. Geneva: World Health Organization 2004: 1321–52.

[4] Reid R. *Status of water disinfection in Latin America and the Caribbean*. Proceedings of Regional symposium on Water Quality: Effective disinfection; 1998 27–29, October; Lima, Peru: Pan American Health Organization; 1998.

[5] **World Health Organization**. *The World Health Report 2002 – reducing risk, promoting healthy life.* Geneva, Switzerland: World Health Organization 2002.

[6] Romieu I, Weitzenfeld H, Finkelman J. Urban air pollution in Latin America and the Caribbean. *J Air Waste Managem Assoc.* 1991 **41**:1166–71.

[7] Lacasaña-Navarro M, Aguilar-Garduño C, Romieu I. Evolución de la contaminación del aire e impacto de los programas de control en tres megaciudades de América Latinna. *Salud Publica Mex.* 1999 **41**:203–15.

[8] Romieu I, Meneses F, Ramirez M, Ruiz S, Perez Padilla R, Sienra JJ, *et al.* Antioxidant supplementation and respiratory functions among workers exposed to high levels of ozone. *Am J Respir Crit Care Med.* 1998 **158**(1):226–32.

[9] Nriagu J. Cited in Motluk A, ed. Lead blights the future of Africa's children. *New Scientist.* 23 March 1996:6.

[10] **World Health Organization**. *Health and environment in sustainable development.* Geneva, Switzerland: World Health Organization 1997.

[11] Joyce S. Growing pains in South America. *Environmental Health Perspectives.* 1997 **105**(8):794–9.

[12] Minh NH, Minh TB, Kajiwara N, Kunisue T, Subramanian A, Iwata H, *et al.* Contamination by persistent organic pollutants in dumping sites of Asian developing countries: implication of emerging pollution sources. *Archives of Environmental Contamination and Toxicology.* 2006 **50**(4):474–81.

[13] Landrigan PJ, Carlson JE, Bearer CF, Cranmer JS, Bullard RD, Etzel RA, *et al.* Children's health and the environment: a new agenda for prevention research. *Environmental Health Perspectives.* 1998 **106**(Suppl 3):787–94.

[14] Ezzati M, Lopez AD, Rodgers A, Vander Hoorn S, Murray CJ. Selected major risk factors and global and regional burden of disease. *Lancet.* 2002 **360**(9343):1347–60.

[15] **Organización Panamericana de la Salud**. *Análisis de salud y sistemas de información. Atlas de indicadores básicos, 2001.* Washington DC: Iniciativa Regional de Datos Básicos en Salud; 2002.

[16] Hernández-Cadena L, Téllez-Rojo M, Sanín-Aguirre L, Lacasaña-Navarro M, Campos A, Romieu I. RelaciÓn entre consultas a ugencias por enfermedad respiratoria y contaminaciÓn atmosférica en Ciudad Juárez, Chihuahua. *Salud Publica Mex.* 2000 **42**:288–97.

[17] Ilabaca M, Olaeta I, Campos E, Villaire J, Romieu I. Association between levels of fine particulate and emergency visits for pneumonia and other respiratory illnesses among children in Santiago, Chile. *J Air & Waste Manag Assoc.* 1999 **49**:154–63.

[18] Holland N, Furlong C, Bastaki M, Richter R, Bradman A, Huen K, *et al.* Paraoxonase polymorphisms, haplotypes, and enzyme activity in Latino mothers and newborns. *Environmental Health Perspectives.* 2006 **114**(7):985–91.

[19] Cooper PJ, Chico ME, Vaca MG, Rodriguez A, Alcantara-Neves NM, Genser B, *et al.* Risk factors for asthma and allergy associated with urban migration: background and methodology of a cross-sectional study in Afro-Ecuadorian school children in Northeastern Ecuador (Esmeraldas-SCAALA Study). *BMC Pulm Med.* 2006 **6**:24.

[20] Howard SC, Metzger ML, Williams JA, Quintana Y, Pui CH, Robison LL, Ribeiro RC. Childhood cancer epidemiology in low-income countries. *Cancer.* 2008. Feb 1; **112**(3): 461–72.

[21] Chapman RS, He X, Blair AE, Lan Q. Improvement in household stoves and risk of chronic obstructive pulmonary disease in Xuanwei, China: retrospective cohort study. *BMJ.* 2005 **331**(7524):1050.

[22] Kageyama M, Sanin L, Romieu I. *Manual de muestreo poblacional. Aplicaciones en salud ambiental.* Metepec, Edo. de Mexico: Centro Panamericano de Ecología Humana y Salud; 1995.

[23] Parson P, Cummins S, Chaudhary-Webb M, Matson W, Saxena D, Parr R, *et al.* How to measure lead in humans, and to organize and conducto large-scale screening. Lead poisoning prevention &

treatment: implementing a national program in developing countries. Bangalore, India: The George Foundation, 1999, 109–10.

[24] Perez-Padilla R, Vazquez-Garcia JC, Marquez MN, Jardim JR, Pertuze J, Lisboa C, *et al*. The long-term stability of portable spirometers used in a multinational study of the prevalence of chronic obstructive pulmonary disease. *Respir Care*. 2006 **51**(10):1167–71.

[25] **ISAAC.** *Phase II modules*. Munster, Germany: International Study of Asthma and Allergies in Childhood 1998.

Chapter 11

Practical issues in study implementation

Dean Baker

The implementation of epidemiological studies can be quite different depending on whether the investigators plan to use existing data sources, or whether they will collect new exposure or health outcome data specifically for the investigation. However the same principles of study design and quality assurance apply to both types of studies. Furthermore, all studies require the development of a study protocol, consideration of the ethical implications, and similar approaches to data management, data analysis, and reporting.

For studies based on existing data, the primary tasks of study implementation are to obtain access to the databases, ensure quality of the primary data, develop methods to link the various databases, and conduct the appropriate data analysis. Although based on existing data, these studies can still be quite complex, depending on the nature of the databases and the steps needed to obtain, link, and analyze the data.

Epidemiological studies that require the collection of new environmental or health outcome data typically involve tasks to identify the sampling frame, recruit participants, collect environmental and biological data, process and analyze specimens, enter the data, and conduct the data analysis. This chapter will present guidelines for implementing studies that mainly involve new data collection, but the guidelines are also relevant to studies based on existing data. Of course, some studies use a combination of the two.

11.1 Steps in study implementation

Before undertaking an environmental epidemiology study, the investigator must have a clear understanding of the nature of the problem to be addressed and the motivation for resolving it. The investigator should therefore review available scientific literature and documents and discuss the problem with community representatives and government officials. A literature review should not be limited to published epidemiological research. Environmental, clinical, or toxicological research can provide useful information. Similarly, studies conducted by governmental agencies may be relevant to the proposed study. These latter studies are often reported only in governmental publications and are not listed in the scientific literature databases.

After reviewing existing data and the state of knowledge regarding potential exposures and health outcomes, the investigator should formulate hypotheses to be addressed by the study. The final preliminary step is to choose the study design that appears to be most feasible and efficient in terms of addressing these hypotheses. A key decision is whether the study can be conducted using existing data or whether the investigators will need to collect new data.

After choosing a study design, the first step in study implementation is to develop a protocol describing the study's purpose and methods. The protocol identifies the personnel and resources needed to conduct the study and serves as a guide for its implementation. With some modification, the study protocol can also be used to seek additional funding.

Before initiating a study, it is important to evaluate the feasibility of conducting the intended study. For example, if environmental exposure data or hospital admission data for a certain disease of interest are unavailable or incomplete, the proposed study may need a different approach. The same issue applies in studies that will collect new data. For example, if approval from relevant authorities or cooperation from communities is likely to be withheld, there would not be access to the study participants.

For studies that will involve new data collection, a preparatory stage should be carried out during which the field study methods are finalized. This generally includes training staff, pretesting study instruments, and planning field survey logistics. A 'pilot' study may be undertaken in order to gain insight about potential problems in implementing the proposed study. This may involve collecting data on a small number of subjects to evaluate the feasibility of accessing the population and collecting the desired information. The main study consists of collecting data on the exposures and health outcomes, followed by laboratory analysis of environmental or biological specimens, data management and statistical analysis. A study is not complete until the findings have been reported to the individual participants, the involved community, study sponsors, and if relevant, the general scientific community. Table 11.1 summarizes the steps in study implementation.

For a study using existing (routinely collected or registry) data, the preparatory stage should include staff training and an examination of available data. Where possible, a sample of the data should be obtained and evaluated to see if it is appropriate for use in the study.

11.2 Study protocol

A protocol should be prepared for every epidemiological study. The details of a protocol will depend on the precise nature of the study. For example, the protocol for a straightforward descriptive analysis of existing data may require only a few pages of explanation and justification. However, the protocol for an expensive, multicenter research study of several years duration could run to several hundred pages, containing detailed descriptions of all aspects of the study methods and organization. Whatever its length, the protocol should provide sufficient information to serve as complete documentation for the study. The recommended components of a study protocol are shown in Table 11.2.

Table 11.1 Steps in study implementation

1. Conduct background research
   - Nature of problem
   - Relevant prior studies
   - Study approaches and data collection methods
2. Develop study design and methods
   - Objectives and hypotheses
   - Study protocol
   - Statement concerning ethical use of human subjects ethics approval
   - Feasibility assessment
3. Assemble study team
4. Prepare for study.
   - Contact with community and government officials
   - Plan logistics and make arrangements for field studies
   - Study material and instruments
   - Staff training
   - Pilot study, if necessary
5. Conduct main study
6. Complete data management and analysis
7. Report study findings:
   - Individuals
   - Community and funding agency
   - Scientific community

Objectives and hypothesis formulation

The protocol should begin by clearly stating the study's objectives. These will vary according to the nature of the study. For example, the objective of a descriptive study may be to determine the distribution of blood lead levels among children living in densely populated cities. The objective of an analytical study of lead in children, however, might be to determine whether living within a 0.5 km radius of a lead smelting facility is associated with an increase in blood lead level among children between one and five years of age. The specific aims of this study may be to use a household survey to randomly select an age-stratified sample of 100 children in the identified study area, in order to administer a questionnaire, perform a physical examination, and obtain a blood specimen for analysis of blood lead concentration. If possible, investigators should state study objectives in specific and quantitative terms. For example, the hypothesis of the blood lead study just mentioned may be that mean blood lead concentration among

Table 11.2 Components of a study protocol

◆ Summary (usually not to exceed a few hundred words)

◆ Study objectives and hypotheses

◆ Statement of the problem, background, and significance

◆ Previous research and qualifications of investigators

Study design and methods:

  ◆ description of source population and statement of study design

  ◆ characteristics and size of study population(s)

  ◆ methods for selecting study samples, including inclusion/exclusion criteria

  ◆ data sources and data to be collected

  ◆ methods for measuring exposure and effects including specifications of measurements to be performed and instruments to be used

  ◆ list of anticipated activities and specifications of members of the study team; recruitment plan and training of field workers

  ◆ quality assurance plan for monitoring staff, instruments and procedures

  ◆ analytical strategy and methods, including plans for data entry and data management, and estimation of statistical power or precision

  ◆ plan for archiving data and procedures for future review

◆ Timetable of the study

◆ Required resources including premises, equipment, materials, administrative services

◆ Ethical considerations, especially procedures for studying human subjects

◆ Appendices, containing letters of agreement from participating colleagues and agencies

children living within a 0.5 km radius of the lead smelting facility is twice as high as that of children of similar age living in communities beyond this radius.

Background and significance

A protocol should provide sufficient information for a reader to understand the objectives and proposed study methods. The background section should describe the problem to be examined, review previous studies of the problem, and describe previous relevant work that has been carried out by the investigators. Another purpose of this background section is to explain why the proposed study is to be undertaken. The purpose of the study may be to answer a specific question about environmental exposures or health effects in a particular community. If so, the protocol should indicate how possible study findings will be used to make decisions regarding management of the problem. Alternatively, if the study is intended to address broader scientific issues, the protocol should explain the significance of the possible findings. It should be clear how the study relates to or differs from prior research identified in the literature review.

The background section should also provide information on the possible environmental exposures and disease association, and address issues such as the nature of the source population, potential confounding factors, and effect modifiers. The options for exposure and disease measurement should also be reviewed in order to document that the selected study methods are appropriate to the problem and hypotheses to be addressed.

Description of study design and methods

The methods section should describe the variables that are to be assessed. It should also provide an overview of the study design, methods for population selection, measurement of exposure and outcome variables, and preparation of data and data management. The type and size of study samples, including references to the sampling scheme and questionnaires and instruments to be used, and methods for the laboratory analysis of specimens should be described in detail. Procedures to monitor the quality of the study activities and data should also be mentioned. The protocol should describe the analytical strategy and statistical methods, including a statement about the statistical precision (power) based on the proposed size of the study population [1]. See Table 11.3.

The format and manner in which the study results will be reported to individual participants, and how they will be published, should be described. Reference should be made to the clearances that must be sought before data can be released. If any of the participants are discovered to be suffering adverse health effects, they should be referred to their healthcare providers for further clinical observation, examination or treatment. Agreements concerning these arrangements should be described in the protocol.

Table 11.3 Reasons for considering data analysis at the design stage

♦ Specific consideration of the data analysis plan will indicate whether the core objectives have been clearly identified.

♦ The data analysis plan may identify essential variables—determinants, confounders, or effect modifiers—that are not addressed adequately in the data collection plan. Conversely, it may be possible to identify data collection efforts that, as currently designed, would not contribute to meeting the study's objectives.

♦ The study team's data analysts are encouraged to participate at the planning stage, and to examine the entire study critically from a statistical point of view.

♦ Consideration of the data analysis plan and the nature of the variables to be evaluated is essential for determining whether the planned study size is adequate.

Adapted from Miettinen [1].

Timetable for study

A detailed timetable should be presented in the protocol. This timetable can:

♦ help the team leader to organize and assign the study tasks;

♦ serve as a combined calendar and checklist enabling the team leader to evaluate whether or not the various activities are proceeding as planned;

- enable the team leader to identify the optimal sequence of events—i.e., the sequence in which all tasks will be performed at maximum efficiency—which will determine the overall timing of the study;
- help the team leader identify points of obstruction in advance, so schedules can be modified or assignments redistributed.

The timetable usually consists of a table listing the specific beginning times and duration for each major study activity or a figure showing the activities according to a timeline.

Human subjects and ethical consideration

The human subjects section describes the participation of persons in the study, making clear the potential benefits and harm—from the participants' point of view—that could arise from their participation. The protocol should describe the methods for identifying and recruiting the study populations, the data collection procedures, and the procedures for ensuring the confidentiality of the participants. It should also indicate how informed consent will be obtained and describe how the participants will be notified of study findings.

A separate human subjects protocol is usually prepared for review by the investigators' institution or an ethics committee. The human subjects protocol describes the study methods and gives detailed information about the involvement and protection of the study participants. Preparation of an application for approval by a human subjects or ethics committee is described in Section 11.3.

Resources required

Detailed estimates of the personnel, equipment and financial resources required should be presented in the protocol. Such information is necessary for internal planning and for presentation to funding agencies. A budget typically includes the following components:

- salary support for personnel, with an indication of the amount of effort each person will devote to the project;
- support for consultants and advisors;
- travel costs;
- purchase or hiring of equipment; if equipment is to be shared among investigators or studies, it is appropriate to indicate what proportion of the equipment and costs are to be allocated to this particular study;
- supplies, e.g., office supplies, and consumable supplies such as blood test tubes;
- office and laboratory space, and clinical testing facilities;
- dissemination of study findings (e.g., page costs for publication in the literature);
- charges for maintenance of equipment, telephone calls, etc.

Besides listing specific budget items, the protocol should provide a statement explaining the costs. Such a statement is usually necessary if the protocol is to be submitted to authorities for approval or funding. If not, it will still be useful as an internal document and assist the investigators with adjusting the budget if the total anticipated funds do not materialize.

Personnel and resources
The protocol should list the key personnel and staff (see Section 11.4). The qualifications of the key study personnel should be documented if the protocol has to be submitted for the approval of a funding agency or external institution. However, even if this is not so, such documentation may be useful, helping to familiarize new collaborators with the qualifications of study team members, and serving as a source of documentation about the investigators' expertise should the study be evaluated at a later stage.

Existing institutional resources and equipment that are available for the study should be described, particularly if external funding is being sought. Funding agencies generally want evidence that the investigators have the necessary facilities to undertake the proposed research. Obtaining written approval for use of resources may not be necessary if the protocol is for internal use only. Nevertheless, it is advisable. This written approval should indicate precisely for how long the equipment will be available and who will be responsible for expenses such as supplies and repair. In the event of collaboration, the protocol should also include statements of collaboration from key collaborating personnel and institutions.

11.3 **Ethics review and informed consent**

Investigators must obtain approval of a study protocol from an appropriate ethics committee before starting a study. Committees and boards, such as ethics committees, institutional review boards, human subjects committees, research ethics boards, or ethics review committees, are established in many medical institutions and public health agencies to ensure that the public interest is protected whenever any medical investigation is proposed. These committees generally comprise a lay person and members from a variety of disciplines such as medicine, science, law, and philosophy. Broader ethical considerations in conducting epidemiological research are discussed in Chapter 13, while this section describes the completion of a human subjects application.

Completing a human subjects application form requires the investigator to describe clearly the aims of the proposed research and consider its potential consequences. The emphasis is on respecting the rights of study participants. Thus, not only must the scientific intent of the proposal be described, but also why the participation of human subjects is needed. If participating in the study could harm a subject (e.g., through venipuncture or by providing personal information on a questionnaire which could be misused), the proposed informed consent documents should be included for review by the ethics committee. Even for environmental epidemiological studies that are based exclusively on existing archived data, obtaining the approval of an ethics committee may be necessary. In this situation, ensuring confidentiality would be the most important ethical issue.

Each institution has its own application form for ethics review, but the required elements are similar in most institutions.

Questions about the investigator and sponsorship

The human subjects application form for most institutions requires the applicant to specify the names of the study investigators, the institution(s) where the research will be carried out, and the hypotheses of the proposed study. The form highlights the potential for conflicts of interest concerning funding and financial interests of the investigators.

Questions about the proposed procedures

Subsequent questions on the form concern the type of study design to be used and any proposed intervention(s). Background information on the study helps ethics reviewers understand why participants are required. The application should specify the inclusion and exclusion criteria for study participation, as well as the recruitment procedures. It should describe any proposed data collection that would involve the participants. If the proposed study is based solely on existing records and no direct human participation will be needed, this must be clearly stated.

At some institutions an expedited review process can be followed if the proposed study requires only the examination of medical records, use of a questionnaire, use of specimens collected non-invasively or of materials normally discarded such as hair, or if the project is a previously approved routine clinical protocol.

Questions about potential harms and benefits

Assurance must be given by the investigator that the participants' privacy will be protected and that participants will not be exposed to hazardous substances such as radiation, if these form part of any of the investigative procedures. The investigator must also explain clearly what will be gained by the study.

Informed consent

A written consent form, though not an absolute requirement, is commonly used to convey information about the study to each participant. It should be written in language that can be readily understood by any person who may be eligible to participate in the study. In the case of an illiterate participant, the information on the form should be read aloud. If the study population comprises several ethnic groups, it may be necessary to print the consent form in several languages. A copy of the document should be retained by the participant after signature. Informed consent requires that each potential participant:

- is fully informed about the nature of the study and each of its component procedures;
- is not pressured in any way to participate;
- is given every opportunity to ask questions about the study;
- is provided with answers to those questions;
- is given the opportunity to withdraw their participation, at any point, without prejudice.

11.4 **Composition of the study team**

The composition of an environmental epidemiological study team will depend on the design, objectives and scope of the study. For some preliminary studies, the aim of which is simply to generate a hypothesis, a principal investigator alone may be sufficient. A small study team would include between three and five persons, but for more complex studies, requiring collection of extensive field and laboratory data, a core team of several specialists with a large number of technicians and field staff may be necessary.

11.4.1 **Team leadership**

Generally, each study must have a team leader (also called a 'principal investigator' or 'project director') who is ultimately responsible for directing the investigation. The team leader is responsible for the overall planning and conduct of the study; for standardization of study procedures and maintenance of quality assurance; and for the accurate analysis, interpretation and reporting of data. For epidemiological studies that are large and complex, involving the collaboration of specialists from multiple disciplines, the team leader must have the skill and experience to manage the complex organization and operations. This person is not necessarily the one with the greatest seniority or the most overall impressive resume among the investigators. Some care should be taken in deciding on the team leader, with consideration to the person's ability to manage the personnel and project. This person could be from any of the collaborating specialties.

Many epidemiological studies are implemented as multicenter collaborations. Such studies tend to have a team leader or principal investigator for each center with an overall study director. Often, the center team leaders participate in an overall study planning or steering committee to ensure appropriate coordination among the centers.

11.4.2 **Principal collaborators and specialists**

11.4.2.1 Epidemiologists

Epidemiologists are often the team leaders of epidemiological studies because they typically have the best overall understanding of the study design and logistics and are familiar with the other relevant disciplines. However, epidemiologists also can serve as collaborators to focus on the study design and issues related to defining the sampling frame and conducting the population sampling, planning the logistics for the data collection, designing study questionnaires and data collection instruments, staff training, and developing and monitoring procedures for quality assurance.

11.4.2.2 Clinical specialists

Studies incorporating medical examinations or clinical measurements may require the services of a clinical specialist, even if the epidemiologist on the study team is a medical doctor. Clinical specialists may participate in environmental epidemiological studies as co-investigators or as expert clinical evaluators. If a clinical specialist is being considered as a study co-investigator, the team leader should carefully evaluate his or her qualifications.

This is important because, as study co-investigator, the clinical specialist may be assigned responsibility for all the clinical aspects of the study.

The role of a clinical evaluator is different from that of a co-investigator in that the clinical evaluator's role is primarily to measure clinical outcome variables. For example, he or she may serve as a member of a clinical review panel that is responsible for independently evaluating medical records, X-ray films and other clinical materials. The clinical evaluator need not be highly trained in research techniques, but must have strong clinical qualifications and must understand the importance of adhering to the study protocol.

11.4.2.3 Exposure assessment specialists or technicians

In environmental epidemiological studies, assessment of exposure to environmental pollutants is as important as assessment of the health outcomes. Thus, the role of environmental scientists in ambient air monitoring and modeling, for example, is crucial to establishing exposure–response relationships for air pollution. An exposure assessment specialist should help the team leader establish an exposure assessment protocol, including reference to environmental sampling and monitoring, transport and handling of samples, laboratory analysis and interpretation of results. Such a specialist should also be assigned responsibility for implementing quality assurance procedures related to collection of environmental exposure data.

If a study requires the use of sophisticated equipment, employing a repair and maintenance specialist may be worthwhile. Even if a study relies on simple equipment, such as air samplers, a specialist may be necessary during field work so that environmental monitoring is not disrupted unduly in the event of a breakdown of equipment. Alternatively, if a specialist is not available full-time, field workers should be trained in basic repair and troubleshooting techniques. This training is especially important for studies in developing countries where there may be no local facilities for equipment repair.

11.4.2.4 Laboratory scientists

Environmental epidemiological studies may involve collection of environmental samples or biological specimens, so laboratory scientists are needed to analyze these specimens. Indeed, considerations of the quality of laboratory analysis and of cost and feasibility may be major determinants of the overall study design. Consequently, the relevant laboratory scientists should be included at the earliest stages in planning a study. In many instances, environmental samples and biological specimens can be collected in the field and then transported to the laboratory for analysis, even if this requires special handling procedures. Therefore, in this situation, it is important to evaluate the ability of the field office to process and store specimens prior to shipment to the analytical laboratories. It is also important to evaluate the feasibility of shipping specimens that may require special handling, such as frozen biological specimens.

11.4.2.5 Statistician

A statistician's advice is generally sought even for small-scale studies. The statistician should be involved in the initial planning for a study. The statistician can help the team leader select and finalize the study design, including the proposed size of the study population based on considerations of statistical precision. The statistician should help the team leader to formulate the study hypotheses quantitatively to ensure that the anticipated statistical analyses will address the hypotheses.

During the study, the statistician should review the original data and computer files, indicating any omissions, inconsistencies, or errors. The statistician should also assess the quality of the data by comparing the data collected by different observers and coders, and collaborate with the team leader for the data analysis and interpretation.

11.4.2.6 Computer specialists and data management

With the widespread availability of relatively low-cost computers and development of the Internet for worldwide communication, virtually all epidemiological studies now rely on the availability of computers for study management, communications, development of study instruments, data tracking and management, statistical analysis, and report preparation. Many studies establish websites to communicate within the study team and with the public. Therefore, a computer specialist who can develop and manage the computer system (often called an information technology or information systems manager) for a study has become an essential member of most study teams.

The computer specialist will collaborate with the team leader and statistical specialist to design the data management system, which is used to track data collection and enter and store all of the study data. Depending on the volume of data to be collected, the study may need a dedicated data manager to design and implement the data management systems. Section 11.6 discusses data management procedures.

11.4.3 Interviewers and technicians

Interviewers and technicians often play as important a role in a study as the key staff. The task of interviewers is to obtain questionnaire data and that of technicians to carry out environmental sampling and perform clinical examinations. If adequately trained personnel are not available, less experienced personnel must be trained in the specific tasks.

If administering the questionnaire requires in-depth medical knowledge, the interviewers should be recruited from among nurses or others who have received medical training and possess appropriate experience. This will help ensure the accuracy of interview results. Nurses and medical technologists are also commonly recruited as interviewers because of their experience in dealing with people or patients. Likewise, sociologists and mass communication professionals are often recruited to work on a study because of their communication skills. Specially trained interviewers must be hired if any of the study subjects are disabled (e.g., blind or deaf) or illiterate.

Technicians who are to be responsible for carrying out personal monitoring or examination of study participants must also possess good communication skills. For example, they must be able to motivate study subjects to participate actively and cooperate in the performance of their tasks. The number of interviewers and technicians required will depend on the study design and the study's objectives and scope. However, the optimal number must be maintained to minimize observer bias and inter-observer differences. Random allocation of interviewers and technicians to study participants will make assessment and further reduction of interviewer bias possible.

Senior interviewers and technicians may be necessary for a large-scale field study, to supervise the work of other interviewers and technicians. One of their principal tasks is to ensure that questionnaires and other interview forms are completed properly, returned and edited, and that tests or environmental sampling are carried out correctly.

11.4.4 Other team members

Other professionals may be helpful in developing questionnaires and interview schedules (e.g., sociologists, psychologists), tests (e.g., physiologists, toxicologists, biochemists), and environmental sampling procedures (e.g., industrial hygienists, chemists). Their participation may be only part-time but is still crucial to the development of an appropriate sampling method.

Vital community information for the planning of the study can often be obtained from local health staff nurses, medical technologists, nursing aides, social workers and community volunteers, all of whom will be familiar with the study area and its social customs, and with the health status and other important characteristics of the community being investigated. They might also be very effective recruiters of potential study subjects, although care would have to be taken to ensure that selection bias did not occur.

11.5 Study organization

For all but the smallest of epidemiological investigations, it is important to define clearly the organizational structure of the study team. The lines of authority and reporting relationships should be clear. A well-defined organizational structure will facilitate communication among the collaborating specialists and between the study team and interested stakeholders, such as community organizations, science advisory boards, and funding agencies. Many tasks in an epidemiological study are related to other tasks, such as coordination between environmental sampling and clinical evaluations conducted at a participant's home in a field study, so the team leader and study managers will have to pay careful attention to logistics. Collaborating specialists and study staff will need to understand their roles and appreciate how their tasks relate to those of others in the project.

Figure 11.1 illustrates the basic organization of a typical epidemiological study team. The team leader is responsible for the overall project, while he or she receives advice from a stakeholder (or community advisory) board and often a science advisory board. The team leader would generally establish an executive committee (also called a steering committee), which consists of the key collaborating scientists or team members and the chief project coordinator. This executive committee should meet regularly throughout the course of the study to review progress and facilitate coordination across the study teams.

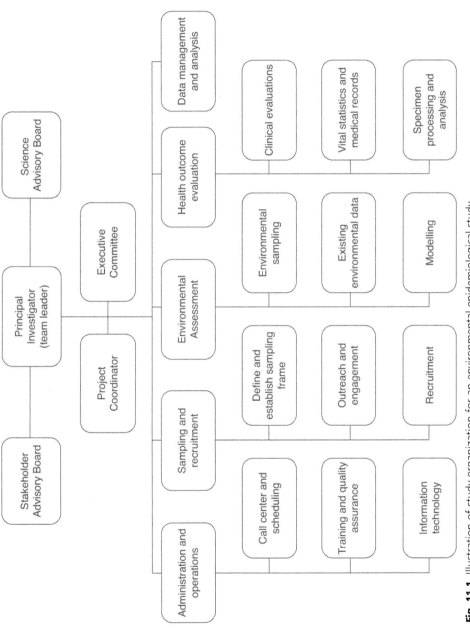

Fig. 11.1 Illustration of study organization for an environmental epidemiological study.

The study operations are then typically divided into teams that are responsible for the various facets of the study implementation. Sometimes these teams are organized by discipline, such as environmental assessment, clinical evaluation, and statistical analysis. However, teams may also be organized across disciplines to focus on different aspects of a study, such as field operations and collection of existing data (both environmental and clinical). Regardless of the specific organization of teams, it is essential to ensure good communication among the teams. Often technicians and staff are cross-trained for tasks both within a team and across teams for efficiency and for redundancy in the case of staff holidays or absences.

11.6 Study implementation

The quality of the study findings depends greatly on how carefully the investigators plan and prepare for the data collection. Therefore, prior to collecting the data—referred to as the main study—a preparatory phrase must be undertaken during which details of the study plans are finalized, the study instruments pretested, the study team members trained, and the logistics of any field or community-based data collection planned.

11.6.1 Preparatory phase

If a study is to be based on existing data, permission to access the data must be obtained from local authorities or relevant institutions. Enquiries should also be made concerning the completeness of the data, coverage (e.g., the geographical areas covered by a population census), and whether the data can be subdivided into smaller study areas which differ from municipal administrative areas. It should also be determined if the existing data have been collected in such a way that they can be used for study objectives.

If the study will require contact with study participants, the preparatory phase should include the following steps:

- negotiations with local authorities, community leaders, professional associations, etc.;
- purchase or rental of equipment and other materials;
- preparation of instructions for field workers, including specifications for completing forms (including coding instructions);
- recruitment and training of members of the field study team;
- pretesting of questionnaires;
- pretesting of instruments and observers;
- pretesting of examination procedures and content on a few of the study subjects;
- rental of space and facilities for field study and equipment;
- setting up of computer programs or software for analyzing data.

11.6.1.1 Arrangements with local authorities, study population and other interest groups

The cooperation and approval of local authorities should always be sought. Indeed, in some countries, an environmental epidemiology investigation cannot proceed unless the approval of the relevant local authorities has been obtained. The local authorities should be informed of the study's objectives and its organizational aspects. This information should convince them that the proposed study is in the community's interest. The investigators must be able to assure the local authorities that the study methods are safe.

Before embarking on a study, meetings should also be held with community leaders and representatives of interest groups or professional societies—often called stakeholders. They too should be provided with information about the study and their cooperation sought. The value of the study should be described, but the anticipated outcomes should not be exaggerated; otherwise the stakeholders and study participants may be disappointed if findings are not as substantial as expected.

The way in which the study participants are informed about the nature and purpose of the study will depend on the study design. If a high proportion of the population is to be asked to participate, community meetings or communication via mass media (radio, newspapers, or television if available) would be the most efficient. However, if the sampling fraction is small, individual contact, by telephone, letter, or home visits, would be more appropriate.

11.6.1.2 Training of staff

Training of the study team staff should be undertaken by professional training experts or experienced senior staff, according to a well-prepared program. At the beginning of the training, all staff should be given complete sets of instructions and forms to be used in the study. The objectives and organization of the study and the proposed investigative methods should then be described. Ideally, study staff should be trained and recruited at the start of a research project. If study staff remain with a project until its completion, observer variation will be minimized and training costs kept to a minimum.

Training interviewers should enable them to gain a good understanding of the study, so they can explain the study's objectives to participants in an unbiased manner. Additionally, study questionnaires should be explained to interviewers in depth and detailed written instructions provided concerning how to administer them. Instruction as to how to avoid bias during interviews will also be crucial. Administering of questionnaires should be practiced several times under simulated conditions so that potential interviewer bias can be identified and interview techniques modified as necessary.

Training should also enable interviewers to develop the necessary interpersonal skills, including how to motivate and win the trust of respondents, and how to convince them of their important contribution to the study. Role playing, in which interviewers alternately play the role of study subject and interviewer, using the study questionnaire, is a particularly useful method for training interviewers. Interviewers must also be instructed about the significant effects that their behavior, language and attire can have on participants, and of the need to be aware of participants' social customs.

Plans should be established in advance for training of new staff in the case of turnover in personnel during the study. It is a common error to provide less or more informal training to new staff brought into a study after the initial training has been completed. One approach toward this problem is to keep records and use the identical agenda, schedule, and materials for all training. In some larger studies, investigators have made video recordings of training sessions so that new staff can observe these tapes later on.

11.6.1.3 Designing and pretesting recording forms and questionnaires

The preparatory phase is used to design and pretest all recording and questionnaire forms to ensure that they facilitate accurate and efficient collection and recording of the data required. The ease with which data can be extracted from the form, for tabulation, coding, or direct entry into a computer, should be pretested before finalizing the form's format. The need for extracting or copying information from forms completed in the field or in the laboratory should be minimized. Such copying may be inevitable, however, if data is to be extracted from existing records, or if a number of clinical examinations are to be performed at different clinical sites. In the latter case, the study participant's ID number should be placed in a conspicuous position on each form and used consistently. In many instances, investigators may have the resources to use portable computers for the interviewers to administer the study questionnaire. This approach is efficient and reduces the potential for error by allowing direct entry of participants' responses and other data.

Questionnaires are some of the most important forms used in environmental epidemiological fieldwork. Questionnaires should be as precise and easy to complete as possible. They should be designed so as to facilitate checking (of completeness and accuracy) and data processing. Standardized questionnaires such as the ATS-DLD (American Thoracic Society and the Division of Lung Diseases of the United States National Heart and Lung Institute) questionnaire for respiratory symptoms [2] provide useful starting points when designing a questionnaire because they have been field-tested successfully in a number of countries. Use of standardized questionnaires also facilitates comparison of data generated by different studies. Thus, the ATS-DLD questionnaire has been translated into a number of languages. Translation of questionnaires can be problematic because literal translation of the words still may not convey the same meaning in different languages and cultures. The International Study of Asthma and Allergies in Childhood (ISAAC), for example, spent considerable effort to develop standardized questionnaires and videos that were used in more than 150 centers in 56 countries to describe the worldwide prevalence and severity of asthma [3].

Pretesting the questionnaire and forms before the main study is undertaken is especially important if the study team has not used them before, or if the questionnaire was previously used in a different socio-cultural setting. Questionnaires should be standardized to ensure accuracy and comparability, but they should also be relevant and specific to local situations.

11.6.1.4 Establishing laboratory analysis and data management procedures

If laboratory tests are to form part of a study, laboratory procedures should be established in advance of the study. All measurement methods should be evaluated during the preparatory phase to verify that valid results will be obtained from all instruments and all observers when the main study is carried out. This is usually done by measuring the reliability of the measurements. If specific reference measurement methods (e.g., a biological specimen with a known concentration of lead) are available, the accuracy of measurements should be evaluated by performing analyses on the reference material. The accuracy, precision, sensitivity and specificity of instruments should be evaluated, too.

During the course of a study, data may be generated from a variety of source points (e.g., interviewers, laboratories, hospitals, vital statistics departments) and over various periods of time. The flow of the data from the source to the location where they are to be stored and analyzed should therefore be planned and controlled. The methods for storing and computing the data should be determined during the preparatory phase. Plans should be made as to how the data are to be entered, edited and checked, and how data reports are to be generated. It is worthwhile to prepare computer programs for file creation and manipulation, for checking errors, and for checking the consistency of information within each subject in the study, before the field study starts.

11.6.1.5 Feasibility assessment

Feasibility assessment of the proposed study should be undertaken before or at the same time as the pilot study. Table 11.4 lists the principal items that should be evaluated to assess feasibility. A decision can then be made either to proceed with the study design as it is, or to modify it. Further clarification of feasibility issues will be possible after the pilot study.

11.6.1.6 Pilot study

A pilot study is undertaken to evaluate the overall adequacy, feasibility and appropriateness of the proposed study. It also enables the accuracy of cost and time estimates to

Table 11.4 Feasibility assessment of a field epidemiological study

- Obtain the approval of the relevant authorities
- Seek the cooperation of relevant communities and stakeholders
- Assess the availability, completeness, and usefulness of environmental exposure data
- Assess the availability and completeness of existing health effects data contained in existing vital statistics or medical records
- Ensure that an adequate population size exists, from which a suitable sample size can be drawn
- Secure sufficient resources, including funding, qualified personnel, time and equipment
- Check the availability of examination premises, equipment, power supply and facilities for storing biological specimens
- Check availability of facilities for the transportation of personnel and specimens
- Check the availability of laboratory facilities
- Check the availability of computing facilities and software for data storage, data analysis, and reporting

be checked. Although limited in duration and perhaps to a single location, the pilot study should nevertheless be a 'full-dress' operation and be designed so that the adequacy of each study component may be assessed. At the conclusion of the pilot study, the team leader should evaluate whether the study is feasible as planned or whether to modify it. A sufficient period of time should be allowed between the pilot study and the main study, so adjustments can be made.

The data analysis methods can be tested in the pilot study, if such a study is undertaken. However, a pilot study is not intended to address study hypotheses. The purpose of a pilot study is to obtain information on how the study methods could be refined to improve their application in the main study. Masurement instruments are often revised on the basis of the results of the pilot study; therefore, data from the pilot study generally should not be merged with data from the main study.

11.6.2 **Main study**

Once the study protocol has been finalized after the preparatory phase, it is essential that the main study interviews, examinations, and other data collection should be conducted strictly according to the study protocol. For studies that involve field data collection from study participants, a critical determinant of success is the ability of the field staff to schedule and coordinate the study participant visits to ensure high participation and retention in the study. It is also important to pay attention to the logistics of the field operations, so that the data collection activities are conducted for the comfort and at the convenience of the study participants, to the extent possible.

11.6.2.1 Advance contact

Issuing a letter in advance to the study participants is recommended for population studies. The letter should inform participants of the study objectives, the procedures, time schedules, and other details, as appropriate. An advance letter should motivate the participants and encourage them to cooperate with the interviewer, to attend the clinical evaluations, or to complete the questionnaires. It should be signed by the team leader or by a person who is trusted by the study participants. If the study population is illiterate or semi-illiterate, a community meeting, personal contact, or message sent via a primary healthcare worker can serve the same function as a letter. If students of a school are to be requested to participate in a study, contact with parents can be made via a teacher, the principal of the school, or the school's parent-teacher association.

11.6.2.2 Interview studies

Studies based exclusively on interviews may be done by staff in a project office, by staff in the participant's home, or through the mail. If an interviewer-administered questionnaire is to be used, interviewers should be allocated randomly among the study subjects or dwellings selected, as specified by the study protocol, and a schedule of visits drawn up for each interviewer. This random allocation will minimize the possibility of any bias due to systematic differences among the interviewers in how they interview. A letter requesting participation in the study should be delivered before the interviewer's visit, giving the time of the visit and the name of the interviewer.

If the questionnaires are to be self-administered, a check should be made to verify that all the study participants in the community to be studied are literate. The questionnaires can be sent with the advance contact letter, or separately, depending on the local situation. Records should be kept of questionnaires sent out and returned, and the accuracy of responses should be checked. Appropriate procedures for dealing with nonresponses should be worked out in advance. These may consist of sending one or more reminders, or making home visits or telephone calls. Decisions must also be taken regarding how to deal with incomplete answers. Making a home visit, writing to the respondent again, or telephoning, are all possibilities.

11.6.2.3 Clinical and laboratory examinations

If clinical and other examinations are to be undertaken, appropriate facilities should be arranged in advance. Such facilities can often be found in clinics, hospitals or schools. To encourage participation, the facilities should be located as close as possible to the participants' homes or places of work, or easily reached by public transport. Participants can be provided with bus tickets or reimbursed for their travel costs to and from the examination site. The facilities should be appropriate for people with special needs such as the disabled and the elderly.

11.6.2.4 Following study participants over time

Cohort studies often depend on regular contact with study participants over an extended period. Such studies are easier to undertake in communities where populations are relatively stable, or residents are legally required to register with the local authorities, or where a household registration system is in force. Most local authorities maintain records of the residents who live or lived in the area under their jurisdiction, including data on where residents came from and where they moved to. Conversely, communities with highly mobile populations, or without a household registration system, or in which registration with local authorities is not required, may be more challenging for a prospective cohort study. The duration of the proposed study and possible means of tracing participants if they move to another new area (such as names and addresses of next of kin or close friends) are also important considerations when deciding whether to undertake a cohort study in a particular community.

If follow-up relies on the extraction of information from vital statistics records, registries, hospital admission or discharge records, a check should be made to identify any changes that might occur during the follow-up period, and to determine whether these could influence the consistency of the data. For example, hospital admission policies could change over time, so that data based on these records would not be consistent. Consequently, investigators monitor whether these type of policies change during the follow-up period.

11.6.2.5 Reporting results to subjects

The extent to which study results are reported to individual participants will depend on what was agreed before the study was initiated and the nature of the findings. Informed consent is solicited before a study is started, so participants have the right to be informed of the study results.

If the number of participants is large and clinical or other examinations show that most of the findings are within normal clinical guidelines, it may not be necessary to report detailed results to each individual participant; however, the investigators still should inform individual participants that the findings are normal. In addition, the investigators should provide an assurance that clinically irregular findings will be reported to the individual, and/or their healthcare provider, as soon after detection as possible. The study team should stress from the beginning of the study that it cannot be held responsible for treatment of disorders detected during examinations.

Once the study has been completed and reviews carried out, the study team should report its findings to all relevant parties, including local authorities, institutions, and all participants. The study findings can be reported to the community residents at a meeting, presented in a summary report of the technical report using language and a writing style that is appropriate to the community, or disseminated through the mass media.

11.6.3 **Quality assurance**

Quality assurance is the process of ensuring the accuracy and precision of the study measurements by systematically following a number of procedures when designing the measurement instruments, preparing for data collection, applying the measurement instruments, and processing the resultant data. For an environmental epidemiological study, this means that all possible efforts have been made to reduce any potential errors or uncertainty in the findings. The basic elements of quality assurance planning include procedures for staff training, data collection, instrument calibration, instrument maintenance and inspection, laboratory practices, data management, and auditing of study activities. Strategies to assess and adjust for measurement error are discussed in Chapter 5. Armstrong *et al.* [4] compiled a list of strategies to enhance quality in measuring exposures, which is adapted as Table 11.5. The table makes clear that data collection consists of many steps and that error could be introduced at any of these.

Collaboration is recommended only with those laboratories that operate internal and external proficiency tests to demonstrate repeatability and reproducibility of performance. Such tests also enable comparison between laboratories so that systematic errors made by individual laboratories can be detected. A laboratory must adhere strictly to the quality assurance/quality control rules defined by recognized certifying agencies to obtain accreditation. Even if formal accreditation is not necessary for their activities, responsible laboratories use standard operating procedures that guarantee a high degree of quality control.

Table 11.5 Quality control procedures for data collection in epidemiological studies

---

Design of the instrument

Design of forms:

- Include all items needed to compute dose, timing of exposure, etc.
- Include adequate subject identifiers—at least an identification number and a check digit or alphabetic code on all forms.
- Make instructions clear and data collection items unambiguous.
- Use different typefaces for instructions, data collection items, and responses.
- Provide mutually exclusive and exhaustive response categories for closed-ended items.
- Make forms self-coding for simple items, e.g., data collector circles a number corresponding to the appropriate response category.
- Make response codes consistent within and across forms, e.g., 1 = no, 2 = yes.
- Provide for coding without loss of information, i.e., do not design forms so that continuous data are categorized at the coding stage.
- Do not require computation by data collectors.
- Design forms for direct entry of data into the computer.

Study procedures manual

- Always have a study procedures manual.
- Include at least the following in the study procedures manual:
  - description of the study in general terms
  - sample selection, recruitment and tracking procedures
  - informed consent and confidentiality procedures
  - data forms
  - general methods of data collection
  - item-by-item clarification of questions and responses, including special cases
  - editing procedures
  - coding instructions for items not self-coded on form
  - codebooks.
- Update manual and distribute updated pages whenever procedural changes are made.

Preparing for data collection

Pre-testing instruments:

- Have instruments reviewed by other researchers.
- Pre-test instruments on samples of convenience.
- Train data collectors and pre-test instruments on samples similar to study subjects.
- Identify problems through feedback from pilot-test subjects and data collectors and by monitoring data collection and make appropriate changes as early as possible.
- Review frequencies of responses to identify items with little variation in responses.

Training of data collectors:

- Discuss importance of complete and accurate data.

Table 11.5 (continued) Quality control procedures for data collection in epidemiological studies

- Review study manual.
- Practice data collection.
- Monitor initial data collection by each data collector.

Quality control during data collection

Supervision of data collectors:

- Assign cases and controls in a case-control study (or exposed and unexposed subjects, in a cohort study) in the same proportions to each data collector.
- Maintain ignorance of data collectors to status of subjects, as far as possible.
- Replicate some proportion of data collection (e.g., 10 percent of subjects) to identify fictitious data, items with poor reliability, data collectors with errors on certain items, etc.
- Compare the distribution of study variables among data collectors.
- Compare distributions of study variables over time.
- Address problems identified through monitoring immediately with the relevant data collector(s).
- Conduct staff meetings for retraining, discussion of problems, and motivation.

Editing and coding:

- Have data collectors edit data forms immediately to clarify responses and check for missing items.
- Have editor perform a second edit soon after data collection to check for missing items, inadmissible codes, inconsistencies among responses, illegible responses, etc.
- Have editor code open-ended questions and query those inadequately answered.
- Correct errors by call back to subjects (or check back to records).
- Have one staff member maintain an editor's log to ensure consistency of recording and coding of unanticipated responses, and to record comments and responses coded as 'other'.

Quality control during data processing

Key entry:

- Create a codebook with format and codes of 'raw' data items.
- Enter data contemporaneously with data collection.
- Double-enter (verify) all data.
- Edit data by computer by performance of range and logic checks contemporaneously with data entry.
- Correct errors and feed back findings of relevance to data collection.

Creation of new variables:

- Check and recheck the programming code used to create new variables.
- Check the correctness of new variables by manual computation from a sample of original records, whenever reasonably possible.
- Review distributions of original and created variables.
- Create a codebook with detailed descriptions of new variables created, including the original variables and programming code used to create them.

Adapted from Armstrong *et al.* [4].

A separate quality assurance procedure should be established for each set of data measurements that are to be collected. This should define:

+ **Calibration of study instruments**: this is performed in order to avoid systematic 'drift' in instrument readings and variability in measurement when more than one instrument is used. An external calibration device can be used for some instruments; e.g., a calibrating syringe can be used with spirometers when assessing lung function. If no external standard exists, a calibration curve has to be constructed on the basis of controlled conditions (e.g., using reference samples).

+ **Assessment of repeatability**: this refers to agreement between results of successive measurements carried out under the same conditions. Some procedures, such as pulmonary function tests, should be repeated 3–5 times, and the results of these must fall within a predefined range of variation if they are to be considered valid [see, for example, 5]. Environmental measurements can be validated by random collection and analysis of duplicate samples.

+ **Measurement reproducibility**: this refers to agreement between results of successive measurements taken under varying conditions (e.g., different operator, weather, place and time). If the measuring takes the form of an interview, reproducibility may depend on the thoroughness of interviewer training.

+ **Sensitivity, specificity and limits of detection:** this refers to measures of performance on the test relative to known true values. These measures are often determined by analyzing reference specimens with known values of the environmental or biological variable (e.g., serum specimens with known pesticide concentration).

Quality assurance procedures for dealing with these issues can be based to some extent on existing methodologies or guidelines. For example, if a collaborating analytical laboratory follows well recognized standard operation procedures, it may be possible to use the standard procedures in the study. Additionally, standard rules regarding the taking of measurements—for example methods for spirometry testing recommended by the American Thoracic Society [5]—can be included in the study protocol.

Besides instituting a quality assurance procedure for each measurement activity, a quality assessment of the entire study should be carried out on a regular basis throughout the study to detect any weak points. Follow-up action to remedy these weak points might include redirecting the study resources to where they are most needed (e.g., changing to a more expensive but more accurate measurement procedure), additional training, or modifying use made of equipment.

11.7 **Tools for data management and analysis**

Most of a study's activities involve defining the exposure and health outcome variables that are to be assessed and selecting the appropriate methods for measuring them. However, effort expended on these tasks may be wasted if the data collected are not correctly recorded and processed, or edited. Additionally, even after the data have been evaluated, and the results of the study presented, the data should not be discarded, since an opportunity for re-analysis may emerge after the investigation has been concluded. For example, a new hypothesis may be generated but must be tested by further analysis of the data. An attempt might also be made to expand the study by undertaking a follow-up investigation of the study group. Long-term secure storage, or archiving of the data, must therefore be assured.

Computing software

Most epidemiology studies involve a considerable amount of data collection and data processing and therefore use computers to store data. This text assumes that each team conducting an epidemiological study has access to a computer.

Recent advances in computer technology now make it possible to analyse almost any epidemiological study on a personal computer (PC). In addition, a wide variety of software is available for data entry, data analysis and graphical presentation of data on PCs. One useful package is EpiInfo, which is available from WHO and the US Centers for Disease Control and Prevention. This package is useful for data entry and editing, and can be used on portable computers in the field as well as on desktop computers. There are many other comparable packages but some of them are costly or less widely available. Statistical analysis programs include S+, R, WinBUGS, SAS, SPSS, and STATA.

When selecting software, the desired format of the final dataset must be considered. Most of the available statistical packages provide quite flexible data processing procedures and create data files suitable for easy input into their analysis programs. However, some analysis methods may not be available in the package used, or the intention may be to combine the dataset with other datasets, for processing elsewhere. In either case, it should be ensured that the data can be recorded in a format that is compatible with other software or hardware so that files can be exported if needed.

Linkage of data

In most environmental epidemiology studies, study subjects undergo several procedures, such as interviewing, medical examinations and laboratory tests. The data collected may be stored in different database files. All the information relating to each study subject must then be linked. Consistent use of each subject's identification number (ID) on all forms and questionnaires will facilitate this. If serial numbers are used, as in medical examinations or laboratory tests in clinics or hospitals, these should be recorded in a data entry book for cross reference with the subjects' ID numbers. Follow-up studies may require that the same subjects are re-examined one or more times. If so, each form used for a subject should be marked with that subject's ID number.

11.7.1 Data recording and storage

For the sake of simplicity, two principal methods of data entry can be distinguished: the information is collected by study participants or staff and recorded manually on prepared forms; or the information is directly recorded in a computer, as when computerized questionnaires or measuring devices equipped with an electronic digital recorder are used. In principle, the latter alternative involves fewer steps, which means that fewer opportunities for human error are created. It is also generally faster. However, it is not always practicable due to higher equipment costs. Nevertheless, whichever method is favored, the data processing software should be defined and selected at the study planning stage.

Effective data entry depends on well-designed study forms and questionnaires. In addition, the following steps should also be carried out using the data management:

1. **Data entry and formal checks.** These include verification of the type (text, logical, date or numerical), field length and range of values allowed for each variable. The software used for the data entry should detect inconsistencies and prompt the operator for correct data. Most databases or statistical packages can do these checks.

2. **Double data entry**. It is recommended that two operators enter the key data fields independently. Inconsistencies—detected due to misreading of unclear hard copy, for example—should be corrected to ensure that the computer record is compatible with the hard copy forms.

3. **Logic checks**. The logical links between the variables should be verified. For example, an error must have occurred if pregnancy complications have been entered on a record as the reason for the hospital admission of a male subject. If the error is not due to a typing mistake (which is the most common error), the data should be verified at the data source. For the above example this would mean consulting the hospital records. If data on one individual are collected on several occasions, the different data sets should be compared. However, changes in the values of the controlled variables do not necessarily indicate an error in recording or in data entry. They may be related to real changes in the studied parameters or to interview reporting errors. The latter are difficult to correct if the check is not conducted simultaneously with the interview. In extreme situations, the inconsistency of a record may indicate a mistake in the subject's identifier.

4. **Analysis of univariate distribution of each factor**. If the factors being investigated are continuous variables, outliers may be due to mistakes in data measurement or recording.

Only after the above checks have been completed and any errors have been corrected in the data file and on the forms (if the error occurred before data entry) can a data file be regarded as 'clean'. Running all the procedures again to verify that all corrections have been entered and were sufficient is often worthwhile. At each stage of data processing, backup copies of the data files should be made and stored independently of the working file.

11.7.2 **Data editing**

Often, the raw data collected at the beginning of a study must be transformed to create variables for additional analysis. Such transformations, or data editing, may consist of combining several variables to create a single, new, well-defined variable. The creation of a diagnostic category, 'chronic bronchitis', from a series of questions relating to the occurrence of cough and phlegm symptoms and their frequency and duration in recent years, would be an example. Other examples would be calculation of a 'body mass index' from data on body height and weight, or calculation of mean exposure values from a series of measurements performed over a period of time. For example, this could consist of calculation of the maximum daily 1-hour average concentration of an air pollutant such as ozone, based on measurements recorded by an automatic monitor every two minutes.

A general rule for data editing is that the original variables should be stored and remain accessible as the source of all newly created variables. If the definitions of transformed variables change, access to the original data may be crucial so that the revised transformed variable can be calculated. An example of inappropriate data reduction would be recording only the mean value of a series of measurements relating to air pollution; reconstructing the measurements' distribution or calculating the proportion of measurements that were higher than a certain level would not be possible.

11.7.3 Archiving and documentation

Several copies of the clean, edited data files should be stored. Currently, copying files from a hard disk to large capacity removal disks or a tape back-up drive is the most common means of storing data. Archived data should be documented so that even someone who did not work on the study can interpret the data correctly. This is crucial for the study review (audit) and for any re-analysis of the data. The study activities should also be thoroughly documented.

Some items relating to the data characteristics (e.g., definitions of code values) can be stored in the data analysis computer program file. However, a printed copy of the documentation should also be available. The documentation accumulated during the study should be prepared on the assumption that no decision is obvious.

In addition to a description of the basic methodology of the study, extensive documentation describing all of the study data management and analytical procedures and accounting for its results may also be required; for example, if various members of the study team conducted the data analysis, and the results were published in several different publications.

Confidentiality of information may be an issue if data on individuals is to be processed and stored. Identification of the subjects may be crucial for study purposes (e.g., to link exposure and health data, or to link health data derived from different sources), but open access to personal information may violate ethical rules of research. The identifiers used in a study should therefore be coded so that unauthorized identification of the study subjects is prevented. The simplest means of doing this is by separating personal information (names, exact address, date of birth, etc.) from the other information collected for the study, and storing it and the corresponding identifiers in a separate file to which access is restricted.

11.8 References

[1] Miettinen OS. *Theoretical epidemiology: principles of occurrence research in medicine.* New York: Wiley 1985.

[2] Ferris BG. Epidemiology Standardization Project (American Thoracic Society). *Am Rev Respir Dis.* 1978 **118**(6 Pt 2):1–120.

[3] Asher MI, Weiland SK. *The International Study of Asthma and Allergies in Childhood (ISAAC).* *Clin Exp Allergy.* 1998 **28**(Suppl 5):52–66; discussion 90–1.

[4] Armstrong BK, White E, Saracci R. *Principles of exposure measurement in epidemiology.* Oxford and New York: Oxford University Press 1992.

[5] American Thoracic Society. Standardization of spirometry, 1994 update. American Thoracic Society. *Am J Respir Crit Care Med.* 1995 **152**(3):1107–36.

Chapter 12

Stakeholder and participant involvement

Primitivo Rojas and Raymond Neutra

12.1 **Introduction**

Environmental epidemiology studies range from analyses of existing data, which involves no contact with study subjects, to sample surveys involving a few percent of a dispersed population where there is not a 'natural community' to involve, to disease registry or case control studies where an association of diseased persons may form a community, to particular geographical communities which experience unexplained disease clusters or unusual hazard exposures. For all of these studies there are potential policy implications of the results, and each type of study has different types of potential for stakeholder involvement.

When defined communities or affected stakeholders request that an epidemiological study be done to assess the effect of some suspicious environmental factor or are in search of the cause of a perceived disease cluster, the underlying reason for their request is not idle curiosity about epidemiological associations, but rather the hope that policy decisions will be taken and that they will benefit from the results of the epidemiological study. Even large-scale geographically dispersed surveys initiated for descriptive or analytical reasons have personal and societal policy implications in the minds of the persons being studied. Often, a community group or stakeholder wants to know if there is an association, not only so policy can be made, but to find a responsible party for a negative health outcome and to clean up the community. Alternatively, a community with members who perceive an unjust exposure or an excess risk of disease seeks to document its situation so that other communities could be spared a similar fate.

The question of whether stakeholders and lay people should be involved in the decision about whether an epidemiological study should be done is central to the public participation debate. Additionally, what questions should be asked in the research, how should the study be conducted, how should the analysis be done, and how the results will be used are often questions of importance to the communities in question. In environmental public health, history has shown that public participation is an important element of the decision-making process. Contributions made by the public participation process have helped lead public health institutions down the path of conducting better studies and ultimately have led to better public policy. The US National Institute of Environmental Health Science (NIEHS) has been supporting public participation in environmental health research since the 1990s. Much of the work they have supported has led to policy changes at the local, state, and federal levels.

Public participation is a necessary ingredient in political equality, legitimacy, accountability of government, and the social responsibility of citizens [1]. The International Association of Public Participation (IAPP) has developed a number of core values that anchor and guide the development and implementation of public participation efforts [2]. These efforts cover a wide spectrum of issues beyond environmental epidemiological studies. These core values can be modified and used by institutions that are willing to explicitly include public participation in the work that is being done, and were developed with broad international input to identify those aspects of public participation that cross national, cultural, and religious boundaries. The purpose of these core values is to help individuals and organizations make decisions that reflect the interests and concerns of potentially affected people and entities. These values are relevant both to scientific surveys and studies of specific concerned communities which would include biological monitoring and exposure assessment studies. The core values are:

1. The public should have a say in decisions about actions that affect their lives.
This public participation process:

2. Includes the promise that the public's contribution will influence the decision;

3. Communicates the interests and meets the process needs of all participants;

4. Seeks out and facilitates the involvement of those potentially affected;

5. Involves participants in defining how they participate;

6. Provides participants with the information they need to participate in a meaningful way; and

7. Communicates to participants how their input affected the decision.

12.2 Stakeholder involvement

Since a community is made up of many different publics, businesses, customers, management and labour, landlords, tenants, and various other constituents, the ethical frameworks and interests of a representative group of community stakeholders are diverse. In most instances, these stakeholders may not have thought through how the possible epidemiological study results might influence policy. An important first step is to identify the relevant stakeholders and involve them in a discussion concerning the policy decisions they would like to see carried out and the missing information that is keeping them from proceeding. One needs to consider what methods could lead to an effective outcome. Would one epidemiological study, combined with general knowledge, be likely to produce a degree of certainty that would be certified by the scientific community as 'establishing' a causal relationship? Would that degree of certainty be required by all stakeholders to adopt policy? Often times, these discussions lead to the realization that the results of an epidemiological study will not have the policy consequences the stakeholders had assumed, and that other courses of action would be more effective for pursuing their policy goals. In this instance, it is the ethical responsibility of researchers and public health agencies to provide recommendations for alternative activities, other than an epidemiological study, that could lead to an appropriate response to the problem. For example, when told that there would be no definitive proof of legal culpability from follow-up studies of 'multiple chemical sensitivity' after a train derailment and spill of toxic herbicides, residents of a rural community decided that further epidemiological study was not worth the effort or risk of further stigmatization of this resort community.

Requested environmental epidemiological studies are triggered by disease clusters, chemical or radiological accidents, or the discovery of unrecognized hazards such as hazardous waste sites or even naturally occurring hazards such as asbestos deposits. Often the community includes stakeholders whose business activities resulted in the exposure and who have a strong interest in not documenting any health effects. The business stakeholders may fear the consequences of being truly or falsely implicated. There is often a conservative, libertarian contingent in the community that is worried most about property values, publicity surrounding a study, and the risk of false incrimination. Another commonly identified group is the stakeholders who demand the study in the first place and are convinced that health has been damaged. They worry about falsely exonerating the exposure and are suspicious of the inherent conservatism of scientists, particularly government scientists.

There are a number of possible differences in approach and interpretation between epidemiologists and stakeholders. There may be disagreement about whether to conduct an epidemiological study in the first place or to continue it, or how to interpret initial results that differ from some group's expectations. There may be disagreements on how to format conclusions of the study with some stakeholders desiring a greater or lesser degree of certainty to warrant certifying a result as 'established'. There may be struggles over what to study and how to define the problem, as well as when to notify individuals of specific study results for which there may be no definitive interpretation. Requests for studies are thus characterized by mistrust among the stakeholders, and between stakeholders and environmental epidemiologists. Proceeding without an ethical and financial commitment to meaningful diverse stakeholder involvement in the decision-making process regarding a study can polarize and damage a community. Instead, information about the study and the potential results should be presented in a manner appropriate to the language and literacy level of the affected community. Additionally, the history and the cultural background of the community should be understood to determine how to best provide the information to the community.

In general, a stakeholder advisory committee is convened and meets intermittently with varying frequency over several years. The implications of various definitions of stakeholder are significant because they shape the attitude in which a convening organization perceives approaches and designs the process of participation. A more inclusive definition of stakeholders takes into account practical constraints and encourages a planning approach that facilitates the identification, prioritization, and involvement of direct and indirect stakeholders in the decision-making process.

There are a number of questions that typically arise in the process of choosing the stakeholders:

1. What is a fair composition of stakeholders? Is there a representative group of stakeholders that will assure the full range of results representing various interests, ethical rights, and duties, in order to best inform policy?

2. Given that 'experts' have values that influence their scientific judgments, what is the best composition of 'experts', so that the fairest characterization of the facts is presented to inform policy?

3. How should stakeholders and experts relate? Should there be one committee for both? Should there be two committees that interact?

12.3 Community-based participatory research in environmental health

There are number of different approaches to incorporating public participation in environmental health and public health in general. One approach, which is supported by many of the communities where studies have been conducted, is referred to as *Community-Based Participatory Research* (CBPR). The US NIEHS [3] defines CBPR as a methodology that promotes active community involvement in the processes that shape research and intervention strategies, as well as in the conduct of research studies. This approach to research upholds that public participation is a central and critical component to the research process. Foundations and government agencies have played leadership roles in promoting and funding CBPR. Nevertheless, reluctance still remains common, due to inherent difficulties in addressing the real concerns of community members (as opposed to a research agenda determined by individuals outside the community) and in laying the groundwork necessary for sustained community capacity building. Nina Wallerstein [4] provides a useful distinction in the two different historical traditions that inform CBPR. The northern tradition emphasizes participation for the purpose of the practical goal of improving a particular system. In contrast, the southern tradition is research with an openly emancipatory stance that challenges the idea that elite scientists have a monopoly for finding the truth and questions whether they should control the conduct of the study alone. The southern tradition is focused on activism toward more fundamental social change. Many CBPR scholars argue for more of a southern tradition. In a health study incorporating general public participation, the feedback and purpose of participation may be to inform the study design and focus. In contrast, a fuller expression of CBPR could possibly involve the community or interested stakeholders involved in the formation of the research question, the collection of data and the analysis and call to action from the findings.

Minkler *et al.* [5] recently discussed questions that can help determine if a project uses a community based participatory research approach. It may be helpful to think about these questions when planning and proposing your epidemiological research project. Some of those questions are:

1. Did the impetus for the research come from the community?

2. Is attention given to barriers to participation with consideration of those who have been underrepresented in the past?

3. Can the research facilitate collaboration between community participants and resources external to the community?

4. Do community participants benefit from the research outcomes?

5. Is there an explicit agreement between, or attention given to researchers and community participants, with respect to ownership and dissemination of the research findings?

6. Does the research project build on the strengths and resources within the community?

7. Does the research project facilitate collaborative, equitable involvement of all partners in all phases of the research?

The above questions are central to the concerns of advocates of *environmental justice.* The US Environmental Protection Agency (USEPA) provides the following short historical description of environmental justice:

> The environmental justice movement in the United States questions inequities in the permitting of waste incinerators and distribution of toxic waste sites. Activists maintain that these waste sites are disproportionately located in areas where low-income and people of color live. This growing issue deeply affects the people living in these communities who feel that they are faced daily with a diminishing 'quality of life,' as well as exposure to possibly significant health hazards [6].

Many US state agencies are creating policies and programs to address the issue of environmental justice including Tennessee, New York, Indiana, Minnesota, and California [7]. Many environmental justice advocates push for CBPR as the preferred approach to conducting research that involves the stakeholders in a meaningful way and that creates pressure to share more power in the research design and the ensuing action to resolve the problem at hand.

12.4 Planning and implementing public participation in studies

The process for deciding to conduct an epidemiological study involving public participation can vary from community to community. At any point in time there may be various epidemiological studies that are at different stages of development. Four of the possible stages are (1) proposed studies; (2) upcoming studies; (3) ongoing studies; and (4) completed studies. Ideally, the public participation process should start when the study is being proposed.

Planning an approach to a public participation effort will help increase the effectiveness of the effort. Thoughtful planning will help prioritize the opportunities that exist for public participation in the decision-making process to conduct the study, identify how the project will utilize a public participation approach in all the stages of the study, and allocate appropriate resources for public participation. The mechanism for applying public participation to a particular study needs to be compatible with the function of stakeholder input. IAPP has developed a tool called the Public Participation Spectrum. There are five goals that can help assess the level of participation that will be used and help determine the amount of planning and resources that need to be applied. These are:

1. **Inform:** to provide the public with balanced and objective information to assist them in understanding the problems, alternatives, and or/solutions.

2. **Consult**: to obtain public feedback on analysis, alternatives, and/or decisions.

3. **Involve**: to work directly with the public throughout the process to ensure that public issues and concerns are consistently understood and considered.

4. **Collaborate**: to partner with the public in each aspect of the decision including the development of alternatives and the identification of the preferred solution.

5. **Empower**: to place final decision-making in the hands of the public.

In order to meet these goals, investigators and stakeholders from the community can utilize the following steps:

1. Develop programmatic and process goals for the public participation process and define how success will be determined. Decide at what stage of the study the public participation process will begin.

2. Identify and address any constraints that may exist. Is there access to expertise in public participation? Is there institutional resistance to involving the public? How does one's institution define successful participation? What are the social, political, and cultural constraints that need to be taken into account? What are the language and literacy issues that need to be addressed?

3. Identify the relevant stakeholders. (For example, those worried about their health, those concerned with their individual rights and property, representatives of the responsible parties, local opinion leaders and politicians, and representatives of the general business community, etc.)

4. Identify stakeholders' attitudes to one another, their interests and needs, and their ethical frameworks; discuss what the research questions could be.

5. Discuss the possible outcomes of the study and the stakeholders' assumptions about what actions will be triggered by which actors. Develop a clear process in advance on how all information will be gathered and used to make decisions and who will make the decisions.

6. If a study is still desired, what hypotheses are to be tested? What methods will be accepted? What role will community members play? How can cooperation be assured? Is there money available for technical consultants to the community?

7. What are the possible results of the study? What kind of language will be used to express these possible results? What criteria will be used to interpret the patterns of evidence so that the community does not feel that the results have been presented in a way that advances one or the other possible agenda?

8. How does one assure that there is 'community informed consent' and that most stakeholders want the study to be performed and understand its potential consequences?

9. What format should be used to convey the final results to individual participants, the community itself, and the world beyond? Who will peer review the results? Can stakeholders select scientific or non-scientific members to the peer review committee? What mechanisms can be put in place to make sure that the study results will not be suppressed, delayed, or distorted?

10. What kind of participation is the epidemiologist willing to offer regarding any policy decisions that are made after the study has been completed? What effect can the stakeholders have on the outcome and direction of any policy decisions? How will the differences between the epidemiologists' focus to address a more defined research question be reconciled with the community's focus and desires to address concerns more broadly?

The answers to these questions are unique to each situation. Having as many stakeholders as possible in that discussion is recommended, to have early buy-in to the overall research process. Early on, there is often mistrust between community stakeholders and the investigator and among the stakeholders themselves. There may be intense negotiation around procedural matters to make sure the stakeholders' interests are protected and not co-opted. Trust and the ability to hear technical information usually take months to achieve and is earned by scrupulous fairness from all participants in the process. Participants must also be willing to spend many hours, days, and weeks investing in the process of listening to stakeholders' interests. Often, messages delivered early in the process can be truly 'heard' only much later in the process when trust has been established. This occurs after the group has weathered the successful negotiation of procedural issues early in the overall project. The public interest stakeholders often have fewer resources than the representatives of responsible parties or business groups. Ideally, there is a budget for travel, per diem, and salary replacement for time lost. Sometimes, one needs to budget for incorporating outside expert opinion trusted by the public interest stakeholders.

To have meaningful stakeholder involvement in a study, it is important to plan with one's budget. Some of the typical items to consider are shown in the blank Table 12.1. The costs of these items will vary according to project scope, geography, and other factors. It is important to plan for these items in your initial project budget. In a project such as the

Table 12.1 Items to be included in a budget for stakeholder involvement

PERSONNEL Position	Salary	Percentage FTE	Salary Cost	Fringe Cost	Total
Investigator					
Other personnel as needed (health educator, public participation specialist, etc.)					
SUBTOTAL					
NON-PERSONNEL					
Item			Item subtotal		
Travel (lodging, car rental, per diem, airfare, etc.)			_____		
Stakeholder meetings (meeting space, per diem, honorarium, health education materials, translations, etc.)			_____		
Other direct (facilities rent, office supplies, communications, printing and duplicating, training, consolidated data center, etc.)			_____		
SUBTOTAL					
TOTAL					

Dunsmuir case study which follows, dealing with a complex multi-year project, 20 percent of the budget can be spent on facilitating and supporting stakeholder participation and outreach.

Typically, epidemiologists do not have the skill set, background, or training for all the planning, relationship- and trust- building, education, and advocacy for institutional and community change that public participation sometimes involves. Individuals with a background in community development, health education, or social work are the most successful in this kind of work. The flow of this work fluctuates, with great intensity at the beginning and end of a study, and sometimes only intermittent input during the course of the studies.

If there is going to be appropriate public participation and appropriate responsiveness to the concerns of community members, there needs to be institutional, multidisciplinary commitment and support for public participation—it is the job of all the people working in public health (scientists, educators, and leadership) to further their understanding and expertise in developing effective public participation partnerships with communities and interested stakeholders. A case study is provided that elucidates some of the challenges and opportunities for conducting public participation.

12.5 **Dunsmuir case study**

12.5.1 Background of incident

On 14 July 1991, a large pesticide spill occurred when a train derailed in an area of Northern California near the town of Dunsmuir. Approximately 19 000 gallons of metam sodium (a herbicide) spilled into the Sacramento River. Most of the aquatic life was killed in a segment of the river that extended for about 45 miles downstream from the point of the spill. People near the river were exposed to the by-products of metam sodium, namely methylisothiocyanate (MITC) and hydrogen sulphide. Approximately 700 people sought medical services within a month after the train spill.

12.5.2 Concerns and divergent points of view of stakeholders

After the spill, a number of issues surfaced in Dunsmuir, a town of about 2100 people. The concerns included questions about short- and long-term health problems, transportation and regulation of hazardous chemicals, and the roles and responsibilities of different government agencies. Some residents were also concerned about obtaining proper medical treatment, and were receiving different opinions from their personal doctors and some of the lawyers and 'clinical ecologists' that were present. *Clinical ecologists* are physicians who believe in a physiological basis for 'multiple chemical sensitivity' (MCS) and use controversial laboratory tests to make the diagnosis. Representatives from 63 agencies at the local, state, and federal levels responded to this incident, which contributed to a sense of frustration, as residents were given mixed messages from different agencies. For example, residents were initially told they shouldn't worry about long-term health effects, yet a few weeks later, information became available that showed metam sodium may in fact cause birth defects.

After the spill, the town was socially transformed. As one local resident said, 'Everyone was mad. It's as if everyone took a dose of Dr. Jekyll's potion and drank it all at once.' The town became divided between those who believed the health concerns were legitimate and those who did not. This division carried over into other community issues, ultimately resulting in a recall campaign against the mayor and two city council members. From the economic perspective, the business leaders and other residents were concerned about the economic impact because the town relies heavily on tourism for hiking and fishing.

12.5.3 Stakeholder participation

The Environmental Health Investigations Branch (EHIB) of the California Department of Health Services was called in by the county health department to assist with the scientific assessment of the potential health effects from the spill and to facilitate community education. EHIB conducted two studies. One was a review of the medical records of some 700 people who consulted their doctors or emergency departments. Another was a door to door interview survey a year after the spill which compared the prevalence of allegedly new symptoms in community members who had been in town at the time of the spill to those who had not.

Before this second study was designed, health educators from EHIB conducted a community assessment to better understand the background, history, and composition of Dunsmuir and the surrounding community. Several meetings occurred at the beginning of the investigation to assess how EHIB could be responsive to the Dunsmuir community. EHIB met with the county health department, the chamber of commerce, representatives from the school district, local residents, environmental groups, and elected officials. One of the concerns voiced by one segment of the community was the potential for health problems and the belief that little effort was being done to characterize the extent of the impact on the health of the community. Other stakeholders were convinced that a health study would stigmatize this resort and provide credence to what they considered to be complaints by malingerers. An outcome of these initial meetings with the different stakeholders was the decision to conduct a door to door health survey in town to document the health effects reported within a month of the spill but under the guidance of a stakeholder advisory committee.

EHIB set informational and process goals for this first phase of involvement. The informational goals included educating the community about the chemicals and the health effects, and clarifying what the health department could and could not do so that there would be realistic expectations. The process goals involved creating positive relationships with community members and involving the community in the decision-making process. Different residents and groups were involved in the development and implementation of the survey. During this time a 'core' group of residents representing different points of view became the group EHIB continued to seek for advice. The lead epidemiologist and health educator spent much time attending community meetings to talk about the survey, hear concerns, and answer questions. They were present at meetings ranging from City Council meetings to a local club's Christmas potluck. Residents voiced their concerns about the impact of lawsuits, issues of confidentiality, who, how, and when the survey would be conducted, and potential impacts on the economy and its relationship to the spill. All these issues were discussed, and attempts to deal with all the problems early on and in a straightforward manner were made. This dialog with the different individuals provided an opportunity for EHIB to move forward with a process that incorporated the concerns of the community, but also allowed for the creation of a scientifically valid and sound survey. Overall, residents helped decide how the survey would be conducted, what types of questions would be included, and how to phrase the questions. By the time the survey was conducted everyone in town knew the interviewers were coming and 81 percent of the households participated.

Survey results were not available until a year later. During that year, the town continued to be divided. EHIB had hoped to form a formal community advisory group, but this was in part delayed by the conflicts in town, since residents did not want to serve on a committee with others whom they considered their enemies. The second phase of EHIB's involvement included releasing the survey results and determining whether to conduct follow-up studies. By that time in spring of 1993, EHIB formed a formal stakeholder advisory group. To accomplish this, the health educator polled a number of residents and asked who should be part of such a group to ensure that the health department had the opportunity to hear the different perspectives from the residents. After hearing these responses, the advisory group was formed and consisted of nine members who represented the city council, chamber of commerce (business leaders), local environmental groups, seniors, schools, people with health problems associated with the spill, and local medical care providers. An important task of this group was to consider how the results would be released and to review ahead of time the fact sheets, press releases and study summary to make sure that language was clear to lay people and was not constructed in such a way so as to be unduly alarmist or inappropriately reassuring. Release was given to representative stakeholders before a release was provided to the press.

12.5.4 Health impact of metam sodium

In a way, the survey results helped explain why some felt there had been no effects and some felt there had been. Eighty percent of residents present during the spill had experienced no ill effects at the time or one year later. However, the prevalence of people who had developed asthmatic symptoms and unpleasant symptoms triggered by perfumes, chemical odours, etc. after the spill was greater among those present at the time of the spill than among those who had been out of town. This difference was statistically significant. There was a doubling of the miscarriage rate, but there would have to have been a tenfold increase to reach statistical significance in this small population.

12.5.5 Additional research in Dunsmuir

After the survey was completed, one of the key questions before the advisory group was whether to conduct follow-up studies. From a scientific point of view, it would have been of interest to objectively assess all of the new asthma patients and to obtain a detailed description of those who claimed to have developed MCS. The stakeholder's advisory group members were concerned whether further study on the community would actually provide definitive proof that the new symptoms were due to the chemical spill. The answer was 'no'. They were also concerned about possible social and economic impacts that further study and media interest would create in their community. Some community members felt that the community was already moving toward being a healthier community, and that the effort to conduct more studies could stir up many difficult emotional issues that the community would now like to move past. It would also stigmatize the community and might interfere with the recovery of tourism. In the end, the advisory group recommended that no further studies be done in Dunsmuir but that EHIB convene a group of experts to advise on how to study MCS in other future chemical spills. They asked that EHIB certify the fish in the nearby river were safe to eat. This surprised some of the scientists on the project, but throughout the process the scientists had also been able to learn about the types of concerns the residents had regarding these studies. Once this recommendation was made, the advisory group was disbanded and EHIB's work in Dunsmuir was completed. After a review of chemical analyses of fish, the requested letter of reassurance was sent to the mayor, and EHIB obtained funds to convene an expert advisory committee to develop protocols for studying MCS after chemical spills.

12.5.6 Lessons learned

There are many elements that contributed to the overall success of this project. Through the community assessment, the discussion of expectations in the initial planning stage, the involvement of community members through informal (conversations, interviews) and formal (advisory group) mechanisms, the attention to group process and dynamics, and the shared decision-making all contributed to the satisfaction that both the community members and scientists felt about the project. EHIB also took an extra step to evaluate the participation process. The evaluation was conducted through informal discussion and a more formalized survey to find out what aspects of the process had been useful to stakeholders and had allowed them to participate in a fuller way. The results showed that the participants were generally satisfied with EHIB's work and their participation in the process. The results of the health survey had been descriptive and were not able to answer questions related to the specific cause of the health problems. However, residents had learned about the limitations of research studies, had a greater understanding about what research could and could not accomplish, and also believed that 'We all had tried our best.'

Lessons learned from this effort:

◆ **The importance of having a good understanding of the interests, history, and issues relevant to the community.** EHIB made sure that the composition of stakeholders represented a group of people that understood the issues that were relevant to the community overall. The stakeholders involved local officials, people who understood considerations about economic and tourism issues, providers from the medical community, those who had experience with the spill and members who could advocate for the needs and specific concerns of sensitive populations such as children and seniors.

- **The importance of involving the community in culturally appropriate ways and building credibility.** In order for the advisory group to feel comfortable talking to scientists, details such as the physical set up of meeting rooms, language used, how to refer to scientists and community members and how discussions are led, needed to be addressed.

- **The importance of providing the time and tools for the advisory group to develop a greater understanding of environmental health research methods and process.** In order to ensure stakeholder involvement, a health educator facilitated the advisory group and worked with the scientists to make the environmental health research more accessible to all stakeholders. Specific opportunities for input and decision-making were structured and coordinated into the participation process. This contributed to stakeholders feeling more ownership of the results and the process.

- **The importance of drawing on stakeholder expertise in framing study questions and questionnaires and reaching respondents.**

- **The importance of drawing on stakeholders in developing a strategy for releasing results and critiquing the intelligibility and any degree of bias of fact sheets and press releases.**

- **The importance of thinking through the implications of when community members decide for themselves whether research is or is not the most appropriate remedy.** The health educator on the project worked closely with the scientists to get institutional support for the advisory group to have more influence in the decision of whether or not research would be conducted. When the advisory group reached its decision, the researchers had to be ready and willing to give up control and move forward.

- **The importance for the researchers to be willing to be educated about the community perspective on the issue in question and to be in support of community decision-making.** Institutionally there was support for a strong decision-making role for the community. Part of the work that kept this support in place by all was the ability to 'keep the issue visible'. This was done by keeping in constant contact with community members and relaying questions and concerns to the scientists working on the project. This kept the scientists abreast of the level of interest and expectations from the community and helped the researchers better understand the negative effects of withdrawing their commitments to the community.

- **The importance of making the roles of the researchers and community members explicit and the nature of the collaboration clear.** In this case, EHIB used public participation methods by involving stakeholders in the development and implementation of the health assessment, and defined the composition and goals of the advisory group. In doing so, EHIB was able to define the process and ensure that the discussions fit within EHIB's scope of work.

- **The importance of how issues are defined and a shared responsibility for what is moved forward.** In this case, the community identified the problems and concerns about the overall effects of the spill. In turn, their concerns about exposures and the environment were turned into research questions that could be addressed by EHIB. EHIB defined the research project agenda, and the community members didn't advocate for other goals or challenge science or environmental policy-making, although these had been some of their earlier issues that some community members had wanted to address. It is unclear if the focus of education on the pros and cons of research and epidemiology served to neutralize their activism, although that was not the intent. Even within environmental health, other areas can be explored outside of the research agenda that help communities to tackle the issues at hand. Communities often benefit from understanding right-to-know principles, receiving information on environmental health toxicants, and understanding what options may exist for their community in light of an environmental health concern.

This case study illustrates the participation of stakeholders, their influence on the decisions about conducting epidemiological research and the importance of community participation in issues that affect the health and well-being of individuals and the communities in which they live. The public participation efforts helped researchers identify and respond to the concerns and values of the community. It also helped in the process of developing consensus and inclusion on the decision to not pursue further studies.

12.6 **References**

[1] Renn O, Webler T, Wiedemann PM. *Fairness and competence in citizen participation: evaluating models for environmental discourse.* Dordrecht and Boston, MA: Kluwer Academic 1995.

[2] International Association for Public Participation. IAP2 Core Values. 2006; available from http://www.iap2.org/displaycommon.cfm?an=4

[3] NIEHS. Environmental justice and community-based paricipatory research. Available from http://www.niehs.nih.gov/research/supported/programs/justice.

[4] Wallerstein N, Duran B. The conceptual, historical and practice roots of community based participatory research and related participatory traditions. In: Minkler M, Wallerstein N, eds. *Community based participatory research for health.* San Francisco, CA: Jossey-Bass 2003: 27–52.

[5] Minkler M, Blackwell AG, Thompson M, Tamir H. Community-based participatory research: implications for public health funding. *American Journal of Public Health.* 2003 **93**(8):1210–13.

[6] USEPA. *Environmental justice: region 5 history.* 2007; available from: http://www.epa.gov/envjustice/History.

[7] USEPA. *Environmental justice fact sheets.* 2006; available from: http://www.epa.gov/compliance/resources/publications/ej/ej_fact_sheets.html.

Chapter 13

Ethics and environmental epidemiology

Colin Soskolne

13.1 Introduction

Epidemiologists, as with other professionals, are paying increasing attention to the topic of ethics; that is, the norms of professional conduct. This is partly because publicly funded enterprises and agencies—many of which employ epidemiologists—need to be held accountable for the activities of their members. This said, it was only recently, in the mid-1980s, that epidemiologists introduced the discussion and consideration of ethics to their profession [1]. Environmental epidemiologists formally acknowledged this topic through the International Society for Environmental Epidemiology (ISEE), which stimulated discussion of ethical issues when it established its Standing Committee on Ethics and Philosophy in 1991.

Today, most professional groups and sub-specialty organizations have either a code of ethics, or a set of ethics guidelines, to which they and their membership are expected to adhere. These guidelines tend to be aspirational in nature (i.e., 'ought', as opposed to being prescriptive, i.e., 'should/must') and have often been developed by consensus through discussion among the leadership and members of the profession. On the other hand, the scientific ethic, being one that specifies what constitutes ethical conduct among scientists as a group, across all professions, is prescriptive. In this chapter, various aspects of both are explored to sensitize the reader to the branch of applied professional ethics.

For epidemiologists as a group, ethical concerns are broad; they range from the choice of research question through the conduct of studies, including the need to protect people who participate in epidemiological research. This concern exists regardless of whether the person participates directly in research through face-to-face interviews and examinations, or indirectly through the use of information about him or her, retrieved from medical, employee, or physician billing records. Ethical research with people requires of the researcher a duty (i.e., prescriptive) to inform people honestly of all possible risks and benefits that could arise as a result of their contribution of information about themselves to research. Ethical concerns and duties also extend through the design of studies to the communication and dissemination of the research findings.

This chapter focuses on ethical issues that are specific to environmental epidemiology. First, however, the reader must recognize that ethics stems from the discipline of moral philosophy (i.e., the study of human conduct and values), a branch of enquiry that, like other disciplines, has developed several theories to explain phenomena. One theory of applied ethics upon which environmental epidemiology depends is that of *utilitarianism*. According to this theory, actions are based on the principle of securing the greatest amount of good for the greatest number of people.

The development of ethics guidelines for epidemiologists has focused on the protection of the rights of the person being studied, and on the ethical conduct of the epidemiologist in relation to research funding and the reporting of findings. Equally important is the ethical responsibility of epidemiologists to carry out studies of potential health hazards as soon as they have been identified or suspected. A decision *not* to carry out a study may be unethical, particularly when the data needed for the study are readily available. For example, the data collected in medical surveillance programmes in industry could be used to establish new epidemiological knowledge about occupational health hazards, but few of these programs analyse the data in this manner. What then is the role of the environmental epidemiologist in such a situation? Ethics underlies the answer to this question.

13.2 **Ethical issues in public health**

13.2.1 **Applied considerations**

For environmental epidemiologists, ethical concerns are dominated by the overriding concern to ensure that the overall public good takes precedence over the special interests of any subgroup. This overriding concern is the foundation of the ethical theory of utilitarianism. It has particular import in epidemiology as a science that focuses on population health issues. This stands in contrast to clinical investigative work of relevance to any single patient for which other established ethics guidelines would apply.

There are two approaches to ethical analysis: one is based on *principalism* (i.e., principles); the other is based on *casuistry* (i.e., precedent established from prior case study analysis). A combination of the two can be helpful to the thoughtful epidemiologist for understanding the ethical components of any concern or tension that would normally arise in the everyday research and practice of environmental epidemiology.

Principalism derives from the Georgetown Paradigm, which recognizes four principles in ethics. They are:

1. Respect for *autonomy* (i.e., respect for persons to self-determination). This principle requires that individuals be honestly informed of the risks and benefits to be derived through their participation in a research study so that they are in a position to make as fully informed a decision as possible about their willingness, or not, to participate in the research;

2. *Beneficence* (i.e., the need to do good). This principle requires that the underlying intent behind any research in the environmental health area should be the attainment of public benefit;

3. *Non-maleficence* (i.e., the need to do no harm). This principle requires that no harm be intended through anyone's participation in epidemiological research; and

4. *Distributive justice* (i.e., the need for fairness, or equity). This principle requires that the distribution of any harms and benefits that could derive from an environmental epidemiological study should be equally shared, not only by those capable of implementing the findings from any study into policy, but also by those who have participated in the research (i.e., by those who will have taken whatever risks may have been associated with the research investigation itself).

Because principles often can be in conflict or in tension with one another, agreement from within the profession can be sought in resolving tensions among the four principles.

Several additional principles can be invoked in evaluating the ethical propriety of any particular action. In particular, principles from the sustainability literature (including the 'Polluter Pays' principle and the 'Precautionary Principle'), together with human rights articles have been combined to argue for the need to protect indoor air. More recently, four principles were brought together to assist the thoughtful researcher and policy-maker in justifying a public health intervention. These are the 'Harm Principle'; the 'Least Restrictive or Coercive Means Principle'; the 'Reciprocity Principle'; and the 'Transparency Principle' [2].

Casuistry, as an adjunct to principalism, provides the opportunity, through invoking in a thoughtful way the solution from an analogous ethical tension (i.e., the analysis of a case study), to assemble and prioritize those issues and principles that seem relevant to a current set of circumstances. It is based on the precedent of how a past ethical tension had been resolved. The real-world application of this approach can convey more understanding of the ethical deliberations to the practitioner. Hence, a combination of the two approaches of principalism and casuistry to ethical analysis can be quite revealing.

In summary, ethical concerns pervade each and every level of any environmental epidemiology study, from its design through its conduct, and then to the dissemination of its results. In addition, all aspects of environmental epidemiological practice have ethical dimensions. The need thus exists for professional accountability through behaviors that are honest in intent, that demonstrate integrity in the pursuit of science, and are rooted in humanitarian principles. It behooves environmental epidemiologists to be familiar with these arguments.

13.2.2 **Theoretical considerations**

Scientists and public health practitioners are expected to subscribe to the values of science that, in essence, include the pursuit of truth. This is most assured when scientists are impartial (i.e., objective) in their research and practice. The scientific ethic is one that specifies the duties of scientists, including their obligations to the participants of research, to society at large, to colleagues, and to the sponsors of their research. These duty-based ethics fall under the class of theories in ethics called deontology (i.e., duty-based ethics).

Professionals employed in the public health sector (i.e., practitioners and applied sciences researchers as opposed to basic sciences researchers) have the community's health interests to protect and uphold. They usually (normatively) invoke the utilitarian theory over any other theory of ethics. This theory requires that the greatest good be done for the greatest number of people, akin to the principle of beneficence (requiring that more good than harm be accomplished through public health action): it does not preclude the inclusion in the ethical discussion of public health ethics of other principles such as respect for autonomy, non-maleficence and equity. These other principles will manifest as contextual pillars, precipitated by the means employed for attaining the desired end of maximizing benefits from public health action. The utilitarian approach in public health sciences is consistent with those standards that derive from the values to which public health professionals have subscribed over many years. Hence, this approach is said to be normative.

Complimentary to the utilitarian theory of ethics is the *egalitarian* theory, which values all community members equally, with special concern for the most vulnerable members of society (e.g., children, the elderly, and traditionally marginalized communities). It upholds the principle of solidarity and measures the well-being of the group by that of the least well-off in the group. Its success is determined on the basis of equity in the distribution of harms and benefits associated with public health actions.

In contrast with both of these theories, the *libertarian* ethic has less utility within public health because it holds the individual more important than the community, thus making less attainable the greatest good for the greatest number of people. Consequently, public health practice draws for its actions primarily on the utilitarian theory of ethics (in contrast with the libertarian theory of ethics).

Under libertarianism, the just society protects the rights of property and liberty, allowing persons to improve their circumstances on their own initiative. Social intervention in the market—according to the libertarian theory—undermines justice by placing unwarranted constraints on individual liberty. Hence, libertarians hold the view that taxation for the redistribution of wealth is coercive and, therefore, inappropriate. Consequently, healthcare is not a right under this conception, and privatization in the healthcare system is a protected value.

The founders of, for example, confederation in the US, shared those human values allied more with libertarianism than with egalitarianism. This stands in stark contrast with the shared Canadian values that have favored egalitarianism in the founding days of the Canadian federation. Regardless of the country in which one is practising public health, an understanding of the collective value system and social context within which public health policy currently is practised will be relevant to any understanding or interpretation of both the public health-related policies and/or actions promoted by respective governments.

In addition to the ethics theories of deontology, utilitarianism, egalitarianism and libertarianism, relational ethics provides an approach that reminds us to consider the social context of all the players and stakeholders in any situation that precipitates an ethical enquiry. It addresses the relationships among the players in a situation. For instance, how community health officers relate to a community in posting an environmental health advisory can best be understood from the relational ethics perspective [3].

Laws govern public health whose tradition has been relatively faultless in protecting public health. Whether the laws relate to infectious diseases or to chronic diseases, public health professionals have an excellent track record of balancing the personal needs of individuals against the need to protect the common good. Personal needs include the right to personal privacy: public health professionals often have to make decisions in the face of tensions between the individual's right to privacy and the public's right to know of any potential health threat that the individual poses to a community.

Context in ethical analysis is critical. Regarding communicable diseases, because each pathogen has unique characteristics for transmission, the ethical public health professional will consider these characteristics. For example, host–parasite relations must be considered in recommending public health action, and these include: portals of entry and of exit, reservoirs in which the pathogen normally reproduces and multiplies, and its mode of transmission; and, for diagnostic testing, each of the determinants including the sensitivity, specificity, and predictive value of the test.

Because the public health enterprise constitutes a significant portion of any country's gross national product, it is subject to pressure from many vested interests. More specifically, because public health interventions can impact the financial interests of a variety of stakeholders, the public health professional has to remain vigilant of the pressures that could arise from recommendations in support of health policy. Because the tradition of public health professionals is to serve the public health interest, public health professionals can be held accountable for their actions in service of the public health interest. For this reason, above all others, ethics guidelines can be helpful as the basis for ethical decision-making in public health. They are designed to keep both researchers and practitioners faithful to the public health interest above any other interest.

13.3 Ethical and legal guidelines for research

Many academic and research institutions and government agencies use independent bodies to review the ethical aspects of research proposals that require the participation of human subjects (as voluntary participants). In a number of countries, the law protects the rights of individuals to privacy and requires that research participants provide 'informed consent'. Elsewhere, requirements are less strict or nonexistent.

Whatever the circumstances, environmental epidemiologists should adhere to the ethical codes for scientific research developed internationally such as those of the Council for International Organizations of Medical Sciences (CIOMS), or they should adapt them to local circumstances, whenever they carry out research involving people [4, 5]. Ethics guidelines or codes of professional conduct embrace concern not only for individual research participants and public welfare, but also for interpersonal conduct among professionals. For example, the *Ethical Guidelines for Epidemiologists* [6] of the Industrial Epidemiology Forum, and since then, those of the ISEE [7, 8] cover:

◆ obligations to research subjects/participants;

◆ obligations to society;

- obligations to funding agencies and to employers; and
- obligations to colleagues.

A statement known as the Toronto Resolution has attempted to identify those elements that each profession's ethics guidelines should include. The intention is to ensure that professions are cognizant of the broader social implications of their activities and that they should oppose:

- prejudice;
- activities that cause adverse environmental impacts;
- actions that threaten individual human rights; and
- actions that serve militarism.

The Toronto Resolution also stresses that professional guidelines should:

- explain clearly the principles underlying any specific guidelines;
- refer to measures to ensure the compliance of members;
- establish mechanisms for reporting violations of guidelines for protecting whoever reports a violation;
- anticipate consequences to participants and society from the profession's perspective;
- cover both applied and basic professional activities;
- specify procedures for peer review;
- urge that all basic research results be made universally available; and
- urge the dissemination of professional standards in order to encourage the 'socialization' of students of the discipline.

Summers *et al.* [9] have demonstrated that very few ethics guidelines, in fact, address these dimensions. Thus, they encourage professions to consider integrating these concerns into their respective specialized sub-specialty guidelines when next revising them.

13.3.1 Social responsibility to protect, inform and provide benefits

Environmental epidemiologists have a social responsibility to ensure that the work they undertake is beneficial to the communities and public they serve, and that the benefits of this work far outweigh any risks that may be involved.

Risk–benefit assessments of a proposed study should therefore take socio-cultural factors, such as cultural traditions and norms, as well as considerations of the relevance and importance of the research, into account. If a population does take some risk by participating in a study, any benefits that accrue following completion of the research should be available to that population and be affordable.

Each participant should be informed in detail of the study results that relate to him or her, and of the interpretation of these results. These results must be held strictly in confidence and should not be released, even to the family physician, unless prior written authorization has been obtained from the participant. The participant should have the right to be informed of any adverse medical conditions concerning him or her that were discovered during the study. An individual may benefit directly from participating in a study if, for example, a previously undiagnosed disease or susceptibility is detected. Alternatively, if no abnormality is found, the person may be reassured.

Conversely, informing participants that they have contracted a disease that cannot be treated effectively may be counterproductive. Likewise, if no abnormality has been found, the transient and limited value of a negative examination enhances the possible need for repeat examinations, and may not be appreciated. (These factors have been assessed in the area of screening.) Furthermore, job or insurance opportunities may be denied to people (i.e., research subjects) in whom abnormalities have been detected and reported. Issues relating to providing informed consent are elaborated on below.

13.3.2 Intergenerational equity, precaution, and sustainable development

Intergenerational equity is new to Western thinking, but old in First Nation's thinking. Some aboriginal communities in Canada uphold the Seventh Generation Principle, which concerns the consequences of present day decisions on the well-being of seven generations hence. Thus, any environmental decision today is evaluated on its impact for air, water, and soil quality, as well as food security dimensions, well into the future.

The notion of precaution is not new to epidemiologists yet it is vexing to industrial interests and, in turn, to politicians. Precaution simply requires that we inform policy so that harms should be minimized and ideally be prevented. The Precautionary Principle thus emerges. It places the burden of proof on those commercial interests claiming product safety by requiring evidence of safety in advance of allowing the product into the marketplace. Otherwise, the community has to take risks by virtue of access to new products that have not been fully tested in the marketplace. Of course, the analogous arguments are extended to broader policy interventions concerning massive projects, the benign nature of whose environmental consequences can never be assured.

These two concerns are being more recognized in the context of the sustainability debate. How certain can we be that development—as in economic growth—will not have calamitous consequences for the health and well-being of populations in the future? Uncontrolled growth is seen as having severe consequences for population health. One example of this is that of global warming through fossil fuel burning, resulting in climate change.

13.4 Scientific integrity, whistleblowers, and victimized colleagues

Epidemiologists are required to conduct unbiased research. They are meant to exercise objectivity in the interpretation of their findings. Epidemiologists employed in the different economic sectors (e.g., academia, government, unions, non-governmental organizations [NGOs], private consultants, and industry), and those who receive payment, through contracts and grants, to conduct their research, are all subject to conscious or unconscious pressures. The pressure that exists arises because science is not value neutral. Thus, biases creep in at every step in the process of scientific enquiry depending on one's implicitly or explicitly held values.

Some scientists hold the public interest dear, and they also will have the perception and insight to recognize when ill is being served. Perhaps they have a higher level of social conscience than most. When such people bring attention to such ills, they are seen as having blown the whistle, and usually on their employing agency, potentially resulting in their loss of employment. In recent years, public pressure has resulted in legislation that serves to protect whistleblowers from retribution levied by their employers.

The ISEE, in 1999, introduced a procedure to provide moral support to individuals who might perceive themselves as being unduly victimized for their work in the public health interest. The procedure serves to bring moral suasion to the perpetrators of such pressures. The procedure appears on the ISEE website (http://www.iseepi.org).

13.5 Advocacy and hired guns

Depending on the nature of the employing agency, groups with particular positions to uphold will employ the services of epidemiologists (often as consultants) to make a case that supports a particular position. Because epidemiological research is relatively 'soft', it is thus open to criticism. The maxim 'he who pays the piper calls the tune' relates strongly to consultants, whose advice can be biased to please the sponsor. People who engage in such work will rationalize their position as one of defending the fact that all science is refutable and that, by their critiques, science-based knowledge will advance.

Each of us, however, in claiming to be an epidemiologist, ought to be accountable to the ethics guidelines that require the public health interest to take precedence over any other interest. Yet guidelines are not enforceable in voluntary professional associations. Thus, moral suasion is all that can be extended to try to better protect the public interest.

To help epidemiologists recognize the biases introduced through various pressures, definitions have been drafted to help us understand the concepts of research suppression (or, oppression) bias, research repression bias, and funding bias. These are provided on the ISEE website (http://www.iseepi.org).

13.6 Confidentiality and privacy

In epidemiological research, confidentiality refers to safeguarding and protecting the privacy of research participants, and assuring that nominal medical information will not be disclosed to any third party. Without medical information, major epidemiological research could not be conducted, so access to medical information on individuals is essential. With this need for medical information, epidemiologists have self-interest in preserving confidence in their ability to indeed maintain people's privacy. If not, the public would not be as forthcoming with making personal information available for research purposes.

Furthermore, because people have the human right to privacy, researchers have an obligation in encouraging people to participate to respect and uphold this right. Thus, ethics guidelines require not only that health researchers ensure the privacy of all information gleaned for research, but also that health researchers obtain the information they need in an ethical manner through a truly informed process that includes assurances about the way in which personal privacy will be protected.

In many clinical investigations, a request for permission to disclose personal information can be made directly to the patient. The situation in other types of investigations may differ. Some epidemiological studies require that only existing or historical medical records of large groups of individuals be examined; no direct contact with individuals is needed for the purposes of the study. In this case, a request for permission to use personal information may be very difficult. Indeed, if individuals have relocated or perhaps died, it may be difficult, or impossible, to contact them to seek access to their medical records; attempting to do so could increase the cost and complexity of the study considerably, making the study less affordable. Moreover, if many individuals cannot be contacted, the participation rate may be much lower than for investigations that, from the outset, are based on contact with individual patients or cases. Such non-participation bias can greatly undermine the validity of a study, rendering it of questionable value.

Problems about confidentiality can be difficult to resolve. This is because the needs of a society as a whole may be unlike those of its individual members. An important example is in the use of existing medical records to conduct epidemiological investigations. In such instances, the benefits to society from the study's findings must be balanced against the potential loss of patient privacy. Even if the type of information that is to be obtained from the patient's medical record is relatively non-controversial (e.g., blood pressure), those handling the data might become privy to more sensitive information (e.g., psychiatric history, tests for venereal diseases, and genetic markers). If reasonable safeguards to protect personal privacy can be assured, the agreement of the appropriate hospital staff regarding access to medical records may be sufficient. To help ensure that the confidentiality of the medical records is not violated, those responsible for extracting the data can be required to take an oath to the effect that they will not disclose any information to a third party.

Confidentiality of information also relates to groups of people or specific populations. For example, it is sometimes necessary to avoid the precise identification of small groups of individuals, such as those who live in a defined area, or who constitute a specific minority. It may also be necessary to protect groups or doctors who are involved in the care of patients, and sometimes even medical institutions or the region served by them.

General concern about confidentiality can mean that access to medical information relating to individual patients is denied. This may occur even if the identities of patients and doctors have been removed—for example, if the information was originally collected for a different purpose and explicit consent for the currently proposed study was thus never obtained. However, if a physician and an Ethics Review Committee (or IRB) are convinced that obtaining access to medical records is justifiable, this problem may be resolved. Reasonable safeguards to protect the confidentiality of individual medical records can be provided and adequate assurance given that the information will only be used for aggregate statistical reporting purposes to serve the common good. In these instances, personal identifiers are often discarded after exposure and outcome data have been linked for analysis purposes.

Until relatively recently, society was safeguarded not only by the reluctance of many physicians to divulge personal information, but also by the fact that the means of accessing, transferring and linking information was not very sophisticated. Developments in computer technology have changed this picture dramatically, and the confidentiality of medical information stored on computerized information systems is giving rise to even more perplexing ethical questions. There is the legal question as to who 'owns' the medical records: the physician, the patient, or the health authority? Does ownership apply to the paper on which the record is written, or to the information itself? Further difficult questions relate to the legal right of access and the legal right to deny access to this information.

With litigation so strong in the US, the right of access to data collected by one team of researchers for use (i.e., re-analysis and reinterpretation) by another team has recently been addressed [10]. The question of safeguarding the privacy of the individual records takes on special concern in such circumstances.

13.6.1 Data accessionists and data protectionists

There are interest groups whose position is that no individually identifiable information should be made available to anyone, or to any entity. Even the periodic government census is deemed unacceptable by such groups. In contrast, there are groups, in particular researchers, that can demonstrate the great public good that comes from research that exploits individual records for research purposes.

It therefore behooves researchers to meet with these groups of data protectionists to acknowledge their concerns for the harms that can arise through disclosure of individual personal information. Also, most importantly, they must provide these people with the assurances they need that research data are treated with the utmost confidence, and that great social good derives from personal information used in medical and health research.

13.7 Policy of openness and stakeholder engagement

The leader of a study team has the duty, and indeed the responsibility, for making results (with their interpretation) available to the study participants, the public, policy- and decision-makers, and the scientific community. If the study had known design imperfections, all results would be prone to misinterpretation, and the epidemiologist must clearly indicate the unsatisfactory aspects of the study so that the public and decision-makers are not misled. Both the strengths and limitations of the work must be objectively presented in all forums. It follows that, as far as possible, all interested parties should be encouraged to contribute to debate concerning the interpretation of study findings.

Once a conclusion has been issued about the relation of a measurement of biological effect to a quantum of exposure, a broader dialogue can proceed. The epidemiologist should play the role of expositor in this dialogue, but should recognize that evidence that is being presented represents only one factor. When discussion extends beyond the realm of variables included in the epidemiological study to include, say, religious factors, the epidemiologist can speak only as an ordinary citizen unless confining attention to the variables studied.

Unfortunately, non-scientific factors can lead to a blurring of scientific evidence, and unnecessary concern may result. Examples would be when a study's sponsor attempts to influence the dissemination of results, or when an investigator incompletely discloses findings in the belief that the stakeholder or the potentially affected community may be upset about the findings. It would appear that the only way of systematically and correctly avoiding this situation is by a declared policy of openness on the part of the scientific team, and by as much exchange of scientific information as possible with a broad base of stakeholders. It is a duty that those responsible for measurements, assessments, and interpretations are committed to maintaining integrity in the pursuit of scientific information.

13.8 Communication with the public

A report of the results of a study must be prepared in precise, accurate, and objective scientific language. A simplified report for presentation to policy-makers, the public and in some cases, the mass media, is also often required. However, since the latter type of report will, by necessity, omit technical details, the risk of misinterpretation may be high. Scientists and epidemiologists who were involved in the original study should therefore review and approve any such material objectively. The presentation may need to make explicit delimitations of the epidemiological approach, and the need for support from additional studies before drawing firm conclusions.

An epidemiological investigation may produce a result based on descriptive or cross-sectional data analysis, but require the corroboration of a follow-up study, say, a case-control study. In the absence of the latter studies, the researchers would be faced with the dilemma of whether or not to publish the results of the initial analysis. The public could be alarmed by the initial finding, and so much so that repercussions ensue. For instance, property values may decline in an area in which a particular environmental contaminant has been detected, or people may move away from such an area. On the other hand, with-holding the information may be inappropriate. In most societies, it should be possible to explain the strengths and limitations of an initial finding so that any concern is placed in context, pending the outcome of a more definitive study.

13.9 Ethics review and informed consent

Commonly, an application for epidemiological research must be accompanied by proof that approval of the proposed study has been received from an appropriately constituted ethics review committee (see Chapter 11). Indeed, committees and boards such as ethics review committees and institutional review boards (IRBs), human subjects committees, research ethics boards, or ethics review committees are established in most North American medical institutions and public health agencies. Their job is to ensure that the public interest, and that of the eligible research participants in particular, is protected whenever any medical or health investigation is proposed. These committees generally comprise a layperson, and members from a variety of disciplines, such as medicine, science, law, theology and philosophy.

13.10 **ISEE ethics guidelines**

The International Society for Environmental Epidemiology (ISEE) was among the first in epidemiology to adopt ethics guidelines. These guidelines emerged from a multidisciplinary workshop in 1994, the proceedings of which were published in 1996 and subsequently were adopted in 2000. They can be found on the web page: http://www.iseepi.org/about/ ethics.html. This document has profound application importance and thus should be considered core reading for any trainee in environmental epidemiology; it lays out the normative behaviors that socialize students to assume the ranks of the profession.

13.11 **References**

[1] Soskolne CL. Epidemiology: questions of science, ethics, morality, and law. *American Journal of Epidemiology*. 1989 **129**(1):1–18.

[2] Upshur RE. Principles for the justification of public health intervention. *Can J Public Health*. 2002 **93**(2):101–3.

[3] Lambert TW, Soskolne CL, Bergum V, Howell J, Dossetor JB. Ethical perspectives for public and environmental health: fostering autonomy and the right to know. *Environmental Health Perspectives*. 2003 **111**(2):133–7.

[4] **CIOMS**. *International guidelines for ethical review of epidemiological studies*. Geneva: Council for International Organizations of Medical Sciences 1991.

[5] **CIOMS**. *International ethical guidelines for biomedical research involving human subjects*. Geneva: Council for International Organizations of Medical Sciences, World Health Organization 1993.

[6] Fayerweather W, Higginson J, Beauchamp T, eds. Industrial Epidemiology Forum's Conference on Ethics in Epidemiology. J Clin Epidemiol. 1991 44(Suppl I).

[7] Soskolne C, Light A. Towards ethics guidelines for environmental epidemiologists. *The Science of the Total Environment*. 1996 **184**(1,2):137–47.

[8] ISEE. *Ethics and philosophy*. Available from: http://www.iseepi.org/about/ethics.html].

[9] Summers C, Soskolne CL, Gotlieb C, Fawcett E, McClusky P. Do scientific and scholarly codes of ethics take social issues into account? *Account Res*. 1995 **4**(1):57–68.

[10] Neutra RR, Cohen A, Fletcher T, Michaels D, Richter ED, Soskolne CL. Toward guidelines for the ethical reanalysis and reinterpretation of another's research. *Epidemiology*. 2006 **17**(3):335–8.

Chapter 14

Health risk assessment

Nino Künzli and Laura Perez

14.1 From environmental epidemiology to public health risk assessment

Epidemiological studies usually result in estimates of the quantitative associations between environmental factors and health in humans. These risk functions—the odds ratio (OR), relative risk (RR), or a regression coefficient—are not of direct public health relevance. Such measures of risk do not take into account the absolute level of risk, the range or distribution of an environmental exposure, the health state of a population, or the distribution of susceptibility factors. Risk assessors need to translate this information into quantities relevant to policy makers and the public. As will be shown, environmental epidemiology can make important contributions to environmental health risk assessment procedures.

The term 'risk assessment' has various meanings and scientists from different disciplines may have partly different concepts in mind when using it; the meaning of the term may further be complicated in its translation into different languages. A simple definition states that *risk assessment* is the qualitative or quantitative estimation of the likelihood of adverse effects that may result from exposure to specified health hazards or from the absence of beneficial influences [1]. This definition does not distinguish risks of individuals from those in populations. Assessments of health risks of individuals are often called 'health risk appraisals' (HRA) or health hazard appraisals (HHA) and describe an individual's chance of becoming ill from selected causes. This chapter focuses on the assessment of environmental health risks in populations.

The *environmental health cycle* demonstrates the link between environmental epidemiology and public health risk assessment (Figure 14.1).

The environmental health cycle connects four main topics (or boxes). The first step consists of the identification of an environmental exposure (or a hazard) (box A). The central domain of environmental epidemiology and other environmental health sciences, e.g., toxicology, is to understand whether and how this exposure affects health (box B). Understanding these associations allows an assessment of the overall impact of the exposure on health in the population (box C). The procedures that combine and translate

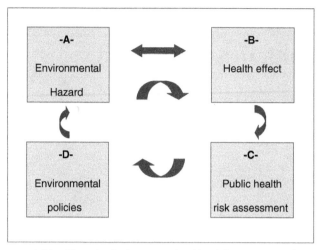

Fig. 14.1 Environmental health cycle. Environmental epidemiology assesses the association between A and B (arrow). Risk assessment combines this information to quantify risks on public health (C). Policies intend to improve the environment to protect health(D).

A and B into C are the subject of risk assessment. Ideally, this step may be used to shape science-based policies (box D) that eliminate or modify environmental exposures in a way that will be beneficial for health (box B). This step—namely risk management—is intended to reduce the public health burden attributable to the adverse exposure (box C). The concept of the environmental health cycle is also reflected in the specific definition of the classical risk assessment framework.

14.2 **Classical risk assessment framework**

Risk assessment is one component of a larger paradigm called risk analysis, which includes risk assessment, risk management, and risk communication. Risk analysis emerged only in the past 25 years when regulations on health and environmental risks started to be developed. The value of risk analysis is that it integrates social, cultural, economic, and political considerations to manage and communicate risk in policy decisions and implementation.

In the context of public health, *risk assessment* is the process of quantifying the probability of a harmful effect to individuals or populations from certain human activities. In most countries, the use of certain chemicals or the operations of certain facilities (e.g., power plants, manufacturing plants) are not allowed unless it can be shown that they do not increase the risk of death or illness above a certain threshold. For example, the US Food and Drug Administration (FDA) required in 1973 that cancer-causing compounds must not be present in meat at concentrations that would cause a cancer risk greater than one in a million lifetimes, meaning that the maximum number of new cases of cancer projected to occur in a population of one million people due to exposure to meat over a 70-year lifetime should not be more than one.

Risk assessment can be defined as a formalized basis for the objective evaluation of risk in a manner in which assumptions and uncertainties are clearly considered and presented. Risk assessment commonly involves multidisciplinary efforts among physical scientists, toxicologists, epidemiologists, biologists, mathematical modelers, and information specialists. Major categories of risk assessment include chemical, cancer, microbial, complex engineered systems, natural phenomena (seismic, flood), radiation (nuclear power), ecological, occupational, and economic. In environmental health, risk assessment is commonly used in occupational exposures, hazardous waste, air and drinking water contaminants, consumer products, and effluent discharges. In recent years, risk assessment has been used more broadly to study public health risk.

The risk assessment framework that is practiced most frequently today follows the 'Red Book' paradigm, which was promulgated by the US National Research Council in 1983 [2]. Risk assessment flows include the following steps:

1. hazard identification,
2. dose–response relationships,
3. exposure assessment, and
4. risk characterization.

Risk characterization is the culmination of the other steps (Figure 14.2).

Hazard and dose are considered in juxtaposition with exposure to determine risk or to determine what additional data are needed to calculate risk or to refine risk estimates. As shown in several examples, epidemiology may be a very relevant source of information in some or all steps.

14.2.1 **Hazard identification**

Hazard identification is the act of determining what the hazard is and its ability to cause harm. Thus it is the process of determining whether exposure to a chemical agent can cause an increase in the incidence of a particular adverse health effect (e.g., cancer, birth defects) and whether the adverse health effect is likely to occur in humans. For example, the elements involved in carrying out a hazard identification of a given chemical include the physical and

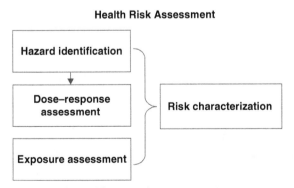

Fig. 14.2 The risk assessment classical framework.

chemical properties of the agent, the routes of exposure, the metabolic properties, the toxicological effects (animal and *in vitro* studies), the environmental fate, and the human toxicity and epidemiology data. An important step in hazard identification is the selection of key research studies that can provide accurate, timely information on the hazards posed to humans by a particular chemical or environmental exposure. Hazard identification does not provide information on the magnitude of the potential harm caused by it.

14.2.2 Exposure–response relationships

The exposure–response relationship is the quantitative relationship between the total amount of an agent absorbed by a group of organisms (or the study population) and the changes in the group in reaction to that agent. This information usually results from toxicological or epidemiological studies. In epidemiological studies, the 'dose' of an environmental factor may not be known. Thus, 'exposure' may be characterized more simply by using 'ambient concentrations' or other markers of the unknown exposure. Thus, risk assessments may be based on dose–response, exposure–response, or concentration–response relationships. The 'best' exposure–response relationships can be derived from single studies, or be a pooled estimate from several sources. Exposure–response functions derived for one situation (with e.g., specific pollutant mixtures) may not always be applicable in another situation or population. There is, for example, substantial heterogeneity in the size of the association between ambient air pollution and daily mortality all across the world. Derivation of exposure–response relationships for low levels of environmental exposures is particularly challenging. In many modern societies, however, low doses of agents tend to be the most prevalent.

Results of epidemiological studies are often expressed as a relative risk (RR) that compares the risk of developing diseases for exposed persons with the risk for less or unexposed persons. This value reflects the fact that many harmful agents are thought to increase the risk of disease in multiplying a background risk by a certain amount per unit of exposure, rather than in adding a fixed excess risk per unit of exposure.

In animal studies, the estimation of risk involves development of suitable dose–response data and extrapolation from the observed relationship to the expected response occurring at exposure levels relevant to humans. These extrapolations involve numerous assumptions and uncertainties which in most cases are predetermined by policy makers. As a rule, humans are considered more susceptible than animals. Typically, for studies of exposure to a chemical in animals, a dose–response analysis is developed and extrapolated to humans. If the effect studied is cancer, the result provided by the dose–response relationship is the probability of its occurrence.

14.2.3 Exposure assessment

Exposure assessment is the determination or estimation of the route, amount, frequency, and duration of exposure. In environmental epidemiology, the exposure assessment procedures are done for specific study populations. The target of exposure assessment in risk analysis is instead the total population, which in most cases may not be the population used in the epidemiological study. However, the exposure information provided by epidemiological studies is sometimes the 'best available' source of information for the risk assessment as well. Depending on the purpose of the project, exposed populations need to be characterized by age, sex and other parameters related to exposure (i.e., water or food intake). A commonly used measure of exposure in toxicological studies is the intake dose. This represents the amount of a given chemical at the exchange boundary and is expressed in mg/kg body weight/day. In epidemiological studies, environmental concentrations or some markers are often used as proxy measures of 'dose'. To translate these results into risk assessments it is important to derive the population distribution of the same type of 'exposure'.

14.2.4 Risk characterization

This is the final step in the evaluation. It is the description of the nature and probability or magnitude of the risk. Combining the results of the exposure assessment and the exposure–response assessment gives an estimate of the increased risk of disease for a specific exposure. It is thus a process in which hazard, exposure, and exposure–response information are evaluated. These evaluations determine the overall risk or whether an exposed population is at greater than expected risk of disease or injury. In risk characterization, the magnitude and nature of the increased risk for a given population is explored using either qualitative or quantitative approaches. Qualitative studies are generally descriptive and indicate that disease or injury is likely or unlikely under specified conditions of exposure. On the other hand, quantitative analysis provides a numerical estimation of risk based on mathematical modeling. For example, under given specific exposure conditions, it may be expected that one person per 1000 would develop a disease or injury.

14.3 Types of risk assessments

Depending on the context and questions to be answered, a range of terms is in use for the assessment of the public health risk of environmental factors, changes, or policies. An overview is given of the most commonly used terms and their typical context. It emphasizes that the use of these terms is not necessarily consistent across the literature. Terms are not distinctly defined and choices may reflect the goal, the context, or the main emphasis of a project (e.g., health, the environment, positive or negative effects, costs). However, data needs, methods, and challenges are common to the whole family of risk assessments.

14.3.1 Environmental impact assessment

Environmental impact assessments (EIAs) are often legally required to assess the impact of projects or policies on the environment. For example, the planning of a parking structure, a power plant, a dump site, or an airport expansion may come with the legal requirement to report the direct and indirect effects of the project on the quality of ecosystems (e.g., air, soil, water, noise). Some authorities require environmental impact reports (EIRs) to include an assessment of the effects on public health. Thus, EIRs may often include 'health risk (or impact) assessments' (see below).

14.3.2 Health impact assessment

While a health impact assessment may be part of the above mentioned EIA or EIR, the term health impact assessment (HIA) or 'public health impact assessment' has more recently been promoted by policy makers and legislators to put public health more broadly and explicitly at the center of risk analyses. At the European level, for example, Article 152 of the Amsterdam Treaty calls for the European Union to examine the possible impact of major policies on health. The term HIA has been tailored towards 'the estimation of the effects of a specified action on the health of a defined population' [3]. It is a combination of procedures, methods and tools by which a policy, program or project may be judged as to its potential effects on the health of a population, and the distribution of those effects within the population [4].

Thus, the assessment relates to a real or hypothetical future action (e.g., a policy, a project, a program), which may or may not be environmental in nature. For example, a UK city council aimed at reducing car use among staff [5], and the committed HIA had to assess potential health effects of related policies. Both classical environmental factors such as pollution and noise, as well as other pathways (accidents, physical activity, community severance), were taken into account in both qualitative and quantitative approaches. Recommendations regarding promotion of alternative modes of transport and the minimization of inequalities of the policy were stated. Another illustrative example is presented in Section 14.6.2.

14.3.3 Environmental risk assessment

An environmental risk assessment (ERA), also referred to as risk assessment or health risk assessment, is a process of identifying and quantifying the current or future adverse effects on human health and the environment caused by one or several chemical substances. ERAs are used to inform regulatory and program decisions to protect human health and the environment from risks of contamination and chemical accidents. For example, ERAs can be used to investigate whether measures (i.e., clean-up) are needed to limit the potential consequences on human health of chemical releases at waste sites. ERA, based on the risk assessment methodology, includes a comprehensive analysis of the dispersion of hazardous substances into the environment, the potential for human exposure, and a quantitative assessment of both individual and population-wide health risks associated with those levels of exposure. An illustrative example of a human health risk assessment of PCBs in sediments is presented in Section 14.6.3.

14.3.4 Public health burden assessment

A related type of risk assessment is based on the quantification of the expected health burden due to an environmental exposure (e.g., air pollution) in a specific population. These studies are sometimes referred to as health burden assessment, health impact assessment or health risk assessment. While the HIA mentioned previously may relate to either positive or negative impacts of an environmental factor, a health burden assessment may imply negative consequences of environmental (or other factors) on health. A prominent example is the WHO Global Burden of Disease [6, 7]. This study provides a comparative evaluation of the burden of disease attributable to a range of risk factors, both environmental and non-environmental. In contrast to a typical EIA or HIA, it is an assessment of the status quo rather than a specific policy or action. However, it comes with the inherent assumption that public health policies targeting any of the risk factors could lead to a partial or total reduction of the assessed burden. Several illustrative examples of public health risk assessments relating to the burden of disease due to air pollution, arsenic in groundwater and smoke exposure are presented later.

14.3.5 **Accountability studies—monitoring the effect of policies**

Accountability studies may not necessarily be considered risk assessments but are certainly worth mentioning at the interface of environmental epidemiology, public health risk assessment, and policy making. The term was first introduced by the Health Effects Institute (http://www.healtheffects.org) as a specific approach for assessing the health consequences of policies or actions that affect air quality. Similar to intervention studies, accountability studies attempt to directly evaluate the health changes that can be accounted for as a consequence of a change in environmental exposures. Thus, while risk assessments may primarily quantify the (hypothetical) health burden of some future action or policy, accountability studies intend to provide the quantitative evidence of a policy related change. Accountability studies may primarily use epidemiological approaches, thus all strengths and limitations as well as potential biases discussed in this book also apply to accountability studies. Accordingly, the results of an accountability study are not necessarily closer to the (immeasurable) truth than a classical risk assessment that uses existing information from various sources to quantify public health risk. Moreover, these studies are not yet very common. Studies that would evaluate the health benefits of a policy using controlled methods as in intervention studies are impossible to conduct in the environmental policy field; thus, accountability studies are in general evaluations of 'natural experiments' that happen due to a policy.

The coal ban implemented in Dublin in 1990 is an example of an environmental policy implemented to protect public health. The immediate and sustained positive effects on air quality were paralleled by a decline in mortality [8]. Thus, the accountability study was able to confirm the health benefit of the ban. The improved air quality observed as a consequence of the ban led to immediate reductions in death rates that were close to those expected from epidemiological investigations of the association between ambient air pollution and mortality [9].

While the Dublin example relates to one single policy, others have looked into the health benefits related to improvements in air quality that resulted from a non-specified broad range of policies. For example, air quality improved considerably in some, but not all, areas of Switzerland between 1993 and 2001. Repeated cross-sectional investigations in children have shown that bronchitis episodes decreased the most in those communities with the largest improvements in air quality but remained more or less the same in areas with little or no change in air pollution levels [10]. Epidemiological investigations implemented during and after the re-unification of Germany also documented the dramatic decline in air pollution in some former East German communities which was paralleled by substantial improvements in respiratory health in children [11, 12].

14.3.6 Health–benefit assessment and cost–benefit analysis

These terms are usually in use in risk assessment projects where the health burden of a hypothetical or true change in policy or action is quantified in monetary units. Such 'benefits' on the health side may be compared to the 'costs' of some action or policy to inform legislators and other decision makers (cost–benefit analyses; cost–effectiveness analyses). Health cost estimations are usually the last step of the health risk, burden, or impact assessment rather than an independent procedure. The risk assessment procedures quantify health effects (e.g., number of cases) attributed to an environmental factor or policy while cost assessors would attach a monetary value to each case of morbidity or death. Economists use various methods to estimate the direct and indirect costs of a health burden.

14.4 Quantitative methods to derive public health risk

While risk assessments may be qualitative only, quantitative analyses are particularly useful. There are different ways to quantify the risk or impact of an environmental exposure on public health. Choices may depend on data availability or the objective(s) of the project. We describe primarily two categories, namely the quantification of a number of attributable cases using epidemiological or toxicological data and measures that quantify the amount of time lost due to environmental hazards. The last section briefly summarizes methods to quantify costs.

14.4.1 Attributable numbers

The proportion of cases attributable to an environmental exposure can be estimated if we know the distribution of the exposure in the population of interest and the exposure–response relationship, which is often expressed as a relative risk (RR). The basic formula to derive the attributable fraction (AF) among the total population is the following:

$$AF_{pop} = \frac{p_e \times (RR - 1)}{\left(p_e \times (RR - 1) + 1\right)} = \frac{I - I_0}{I}$$

Where p_e represents the fraction of the population exposed to the (environmental) factor under investigation, and RR the (adjusted or unadjusted) relative risk, i.e., the exposure–response function between exposed and unexposed. In risk assessments where the total population is exposed (i.e., air pollution), p_e equals 1 and the above formula can be simplified respectively. Note that the attributable fraction is nothing other than the difference between the incidence (or prevalence) among the total population (I) and the unexposed (I_0), which is also called the excess risk, expressed as a proportion of the incidence in the total population.

Depending on the objectives, the AF can be related to a subpopulation rather than the total population. Alternative denominators are the occurrence of disease among the exposed, the unexposed, the diseased, or the diseased with the exposure. Table 14.1 summarizes the different measures of attributable risk and the most commonly but inconsistently

Table 14.1 Measures of potential impact among exposed and total population

Standard nomenclature[1]			Impact numbers[2]		
Description		Formula	Description		Formula
Attributable risk or excess risk	AR_{exp}	$I_1 - I_0$	Exposure impact number	EIN	$\dfrac{1}{AR_{exp}}$
Population attributable risk	PAR	$I - I_0$ alternative formula $AR_{exp} \times p_e$	Population impact number	PIN	$\dfrac{1}{PAR}$
Attributable fraction (exposed) or attributable risk percent or etiologic fraction among the exposed or relative risk reduction	AF_{exp}	$\dfrac{I_1 - I_0}{I_1}$ alternative formula $\dfrac{(RR-1)}{RR}$	Exposed cases impact number	ECIN	$\dfrac{1}{AF_{exp}}$
Population attributable fraction or population attributable risk per cent	AF_{pop}	$\dfrac{I - I_0}{I}$ alternative formulas $\dfrac{p_e \times (RR-1)}{p_e \times (RR-1)+1}$ $p_c \times AF_{exp}$	Case impact number	CIN	$\dfrac{1}{AF_{pop}}$

1. Same nomenclature as in Steenland and Armstrong [14].
2. Impact Number from Heller *et al*. [13].

I_1, Incidence of outcome among the exposed.

I_0, Incidence of outcome among the unexposed.

I, Incidence of outcome in the total population (exposed and unexposed).

RR, Relative risk.

p_e, fraction population exposed.

p_c, fraction cases exposed.

used terminologies [13, 14]. Figure 14.3 illustrates these concepts for both the attributable and impact numbers that are further described below.

AF among the exposed is expressed with the following formula:

$$AF_{exp} = \frac{(RR-1)}{RR} = \frac{I_1 - I_0}{I_1}$$

If the frequency of the health outcome is known in the target population (e.g., the incidence or prevalence of a disease), the risk may be expressed in terms of the number of attributable cases rather than fractions by multiplying the number of current cases among the respective population by the AF.

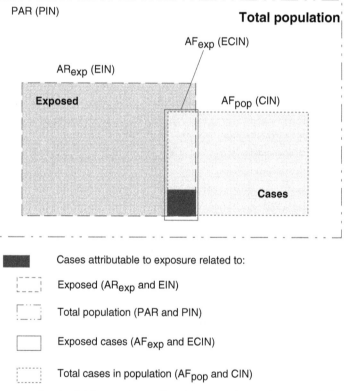

Fig. 14.3 Measures of potential impact for attributable cases. Square boxes mark the population to which the measure applies. PAR, population attributable risk; PIN, Population impact number; AR_{exp}, Attributable risk among exposed; EIN, Exposure impact number; AF_{pop}, Population attributable fraction; CIN, Case impact number; AF_{exp}, Attributable fraction among exposed; ECIN, Exposed cases impact number. Adapted from Heller *et al.* [13]. Reproduced with permission from Heller RF, Dobson AJ, Attia J, Page J. Impact numbers: measures of risk factor impact on the whole population from case-control and cohort studies. *J Epidemiol Community Health*. 2002 56(8):606–10.

Exposures to environmental hazards are often characterized on a continuous scale (e.g., in $\mu g/m^3$ or ppb for some air pollutants or water) where the simple distinction of 'exposed' versus 'non-exposed' may not be appropriate. In such cases, exposure distributions may be derived for several levels of exposure (or concentrations) and the above formula can be generalized for the AF_{pop} as follows:

$$AF_{pop} = \frac{\sum p_{ei}(RR_i - 1)}{\left[\sum p_{ei}(RR_i - 1) + 1\right]}$$

In this case p_{ei} is the proportion of persons exposed to level i of exposure and RR_i is the relative risk for each level of exposure against no exposure.

The above formulae make implicit assumptions about the level of 'no exposure' (or the reference exposure) which determines the size of the RR in the case of a dichotomous exposure or the number of exposure categories in the case of ordinal groups of exposure. These assumptions ultimately affect the quantified burden. Assessors have to define a reference exposure. 'Zero exposure' may be the obvious choice in some cases, such as environmental tobacco smoke. However, risk assessments for ubiquitous environmental hazards for which zero exposure may be impossible to achieve, may quantify the attributable burden above some non-zero reference level only. The often arbitrary choice of the reference level strongly influences the final result [15]. This must be taken into account in the evaluation and communication of results, and in comparison across studies. Examples to study this issue can be found in air pollution risk assessments where some projects may quantify the attributable risk of ambient air pollution concentrations above some 'natural background' [16] whereas others take into account only the burden due to concentrations above various air quality standards or policy scenarios [17].

Also, as seen in the formula, the proportion of people exposed to (some level of) exposure affects the total burden. Accordingly, in the case of environmental hazards with no thresholds of effect, the largest public health burden originates from improvements among those with low to moderate levels of exposure rather than among the (usually small) proportion in the upper tail of the exposure distribution. This apparent paradox needs to be carefully communicated to the public. An example from the air pollution policy domain is shown in Table 14.2 [17].

Ignorance of this paradigm may lead to the promotion of misleading and inefficient policies. For example, smog episodes, i.e., short periods with very high levels of ambient air pollution, regularly lead to the call for emergency policies to be employed during such days. However, the public health burden of such episodes is far smaller than the burden attributable to the many days outside of these periods where levels of ambient air pollution are much lower. Thus, air quality regulation should be focused on sustained reductions of pollution rather than expensive and inefficient emergency strategies. The latter are, however, more attractive for media and politicians alike, and as such come up in the discussion as a pattern as regular as the occurrence of summer and winter smog episodes.

Table 14.2 Estimated number of attributable deaths associated with a 5 µg/m³ decrease in ambient fine particulate matter (PM$_{2.5}$) concentrations in 26 European cities with >40 million inhabitants. Due to the tailed distribution of PM$_{2.5}$ across these cities, a reduction of PM$_{2.5}$ from 15 to 10 µg/m³ would have a 3-time larger benefit than a decrement from 25 to 20 µg/m³ in the annual mean.

	Decrease in ambient PM$_{2.5}$ concentrations (annual mean) from:		
	25 to 20 µg/m³	20 to 15 µg/m³	15 to 10 µg/m³
Potential reduction in death:			
Death per 100 000/year	11	23	35
in % of death	0.8%	1.7%	2.5%

Based on [17].

14.4.1.1 Impact numbers

Other measures that reflect the impact of a risk factor on the population have been proposed more recently [13]. These impact numbers are based entirely on attributable risks. They may be particularly appealing to communicate risks to policy makers, health-care providers, and consumers. Impact numbers are the reciprocal of the various types of attributable numbers (see Table 14.1). *Attributable numbers* simply communicate the number of cases attributed to a factor. *Impact numbers* provide instead the number of people with the disease for whom one case will be attributable to the exposure or risk factor. As shown in Table 14.1 and Figure 14.3, both quantities may relate to the total population or subgroups defined by exposure and disease. For example, if a risk assessment concluded that 38 percent of asthma exacerbations were attributable to ambient air pollution (attributable number), one may prefer to communicate that 'one out of 2.6 exacerbations' was caused by a preventable environmental factor (impact number).

14.4.1.2 Chronic and acute effects of environmental exposures in risk assessment

Some environmental hazards are typically seen as causes of chronic diseases (e.g., carcinogens in water, soil, or the air leading to cancer). Other agents are typically seen as triggers of acute or subacute health complaints, for example, death triggered by heat waves or the unloading of soy beans in the port of Barcelona that caused outbreaks of asthma attacks as allergens were spread all over the city during the process of unloading [18]. (Note that this famous example of an epidemiological investigation was followed by rigorous risk assessment and risk management processes. Since then, unloading has been carried out in closed systems to prevent related asthma attacks [19]). Risk assessments for either chronic or acute effects are generally derived using the above discussed methods. However, some environmental hazards may both contribute to the underlying pathologies that lead to chronic diseases and act as triggers of acute effects. In such cases, the above models need to be expanded to appropriately assess the overall public health risks of the combined acute and chronic effects.

Air pollution and asthma in children may be used as an example to demonstrate such a combined risk model. Ambient pollution is a known cause of acute exacerbations of asthma attacks [20]. While not yet conclusive, several studies suggest that air pollution, in particular emissions from traffic, may lead to the onset of asthma in children. In particular, children living in very close proximity to busy roads appear to have higher rates of asthma. Under such a combined causal model, air pollution may (1) increase the number of children with asthma, i.e., the pool susceptible to asthma attacks, and (2) cause exacerbations among the total pool of asthmatic children. The total burden of air pollution related asthma exacerbation (Tot PAR_{acute}) would thus be the total of three attributable proportions:

1. air pollution related exacerbations among those asthmatics that developed asthma due to air pollution (PAR1);

2. air pollution related exacerbations among asthmatics that developed asthma due to other causes (PAR2);

3. all exacerbations unrelated to air pollution among those who developed asthma due to exposure to air pollution (PAR3).

The equation for this model is the following:

$$\text{Tot } PAR_{acute} = PAR1 + PAR2 + PAR3$$

with the following components:

$$PAR1 = PAR_{chron} \times P_{acute} \times AF_{acute}$$

$$PAR2 = (Pop_{tot} \times P_{chron} - PAR_{chron}) \times P_{acute} \times AF_{acute}$$

$$PAR3 = PAR_{chron} \times P_{acute} \times (1 - AF_{acute})$$

where PAR_{chron} reflects the air pollution attributable number of prevalent asthma cases, P_{acute} the prevalence of the acute exacerbations among asthmatics, AF_{acute} the air pollution attributable fraction of exacerbations (derived with the standard formulas), Pop_{tot} the total population of children, P_{chron} the prevalence of the chronic disease and P_{acute} the prevalence of the acute condition among the population with the chronic condition (Pop_{chron}). The total of the three components is summarized in the following equation:

$$\text{Tot } PAR_{acute} = Pop_{tot} \times P_{chron} \left[AF_{chron} \times P_{acute} \times AF_{acute} \left(AF_{acute}^{-1} + AF_{chron}^{-1} - 1 \right) \right]$$

Although this model comes with a range of assumptions about the biology of chronic disease and its exacerbations that need careful evaluation, it probably better reflects the risk attribution of environmental hazards that contribute to both the underlying chronic disease processes and the triggering of acute exacerbations. Several chronic conditions such as asthma, chronic obstructive pulmonary disease, or atherosclerosis may fit into this model.

14.4.1.3 Carcinogenic risk

Cancer risk from environmental exposure is of particular concern for health and environmental authorities and thus is subject to many risk assessments. Any chemical for which there is sufficient evidence that exposure may result in continuing uncontrolled cell division (i.e., cancer) in humans or animals is considered a carcinogen. The number of cases attributable to such carcinogenic exposure is usually derived for specific populations. Due to the dominant role of toxicological studies in the assessment of carcinogenicity, cancer risk assessments are most often (but not necessarily) based on experimentally determined dose–response relationships [21]. The assumptions behind dose–response measures for carcinogenic compounds are that the exposure is equivalent to a whole lifetime (70 years), that there is no threshold, and that there is a linear relationship even at very low doses. Mainly three interrelated presentations of risks are encountered using toxicological information to assess risks:

1. The **unit risk**. This is the measure used for evaluating risks from chemicals in air or water. It represents the risk on a per unit concentration of chemical substance where human contact occurs, that is the quantitative estimate in terms of either risk per µg/L drinking water or risk per µg/m^3 air breathed. The cancer risk is derived by multiplying the unit risk by the continuous lifetime exposure concentrations in µg/m^3 in air and µg/L in water.

   The population cancer burden (N) for a specific population across all carcinogenic pollutants i in media j is calculated with the following formula:

   $$N = P \sum_i \sum_j UR_{i,j} \times C_{i,j}$$

   Where P is the population size, UR_i is the unit risk factor for pollutant i, and $C_{i,j}$ is the mean average concentration for pollutant i in media j. This represents the estimate of the lifetime mean exposure. Exposures of limited duration would be associated with a proportional reduction in cancer risk. The result of this calculation is an estimate of the number of cases expected from a 70-year exposure due to current levels. The expected annual number of cases attributable to the carcinogen would, thus, be N/70.

2. The **slope factor** (or cancer potency factor). This represents the increase in an individual's risk of developing cancer over a 70-year lifetime per unit of exposure where the unit of exposure is expressed as a dose in mg/kg/day. For example to estimate risks from exposure in food, one multiplies the slope factor (mg/kg/day), the concentration of the chemical in the food (ppm) and the daily intake (in mg) of that food. The total dietary risk is found by summing across all foods.

3. Risk can also be expressed as the concentration of drinking water or air concentration corresponding to a specific cancer risks (i.e., 1 in 10 000, 1 in 100 000 or 1 in 1 000 000). For example, the water concentration corresponding to a risk of 1 in 100 000 (E-5) given a water risk of 4.0E-5 µg/L is 2.5E-1 µg/L.

In contrast to the attributable risks, the carcinogenic risk approach explicitly integrates duration of exposure, namely a 'lifetime' (or 70 years). For other environmental diseases, the role of duration of exposure may not be clear or not be specified in the studies providing the risk functions.

14.4.2 Quantifying time: health-adjusted life year approaches

The impacts of environmental exposures on health described above are based on proba-bilistic risk measures and do not take into account the nature and the extent of environ-mental health effects. The impact of hazardous environmental exposures on human health involves premature mortality and morbidity but also adverse effects on the general quality of life. The development of Health-Adjusted Life Years (HALYs) originated from the desire to express the whole range of the health impact in a single integrated measure of risk [22]. Examples in the family of HALYs that combine diverging health effects in a single measure are Disability-Adjusted Life Years (DALYs), with Years of Life Lost (YLLs) and Years of Life Lost due to Disability (YLDs) as its components, and Quality-Adjusted Life Years (QALYs), which we describe below. More detailed resources are available on the WHO home page (http://www.who.int). Monetary estimates of risk also accomplish this goal (see below).

14.4.2.1 Years of life lost and years lost due to disability

The years of life lost (YLL) correspond to the number of deaths multiplied by the stan-dard life expectancy at the age at which death occurs. The formula for YLL is the follow-ing for a given cause, age and sex:

$$YLL = N \times L$$

where N is the number of deaths and L the standard life expectancy at age of death, expressed in years. The number of deaths due to an environmental risk factor corre-sponds to the 'attributable number of deaths' as derived in the previous sections; thus, YLL and related measures have similar data requirements with environmental epidemi-ology providing important information. The derivation of L, i.e., life expectancy, is straightforward from life tables.

As in the case of YLL, an incidence perspective is taken also for the calculation of years lost due to disability (YLD). To estimate YLD for a particular cause in a particular time period, the number of incident cases in that period is multiplied by the average duration of the disease and a weight factor that reflects the severity of the disease on a scale from 0 (perfect health) to 1 (dead). The basic formula for YLD is the following.

$$YLD = I \times DW \times L$$

where I is the number of incident cases, DW the disability weight, and L the average duration of the case until remission or death (years). The disability weights (DWs) seek to weight the disability of living with different diseases with the maximum possible weight being one. For example a late-stage cancer weights 0.81 but early stage bladder cancer weights 0.09. Weights are based on subjective judgments and reflect societal pref-erences of health states.

In its Global Burden of Disease evaluation, the WHO introduces an annual discount rate (r) of 3 percent in the YLD and YLL to down-weight the impact of death or disability at older ages. This is based on the theory that more distant years are less valuable.

For example, with this discount rate, a year of healthy life gained in 10 years' time is worth 24 percent less than one gained now. A number of people have argued that discounting should not be applied to future health gains or losses; discounting is rarely used by epidemiologists and demographers for summary health measures. The method to calculate YLD and YLL including the discount rate (r) is as follows.

$$YLD = \frac{I \times DW \times (1 - e^{-rL})}{r}$$

$$YLL = \frac{N}{r}(1 - e^{-rL})$$

14.4.2.2 Disability-adjusted life years

The disability-adjusted life year, or DALY, is a measure of the health burden that combines the concept of potential years of life lost due to premature death (YLL) with the inclusion of years of 'healthy' life lost due to poor health or disability. The DALY combines the time already lived with disability and the time lost due to premature mortality in one single measure (Figure 14.4) [22].

One DALY can be thought of as one lost year of healthy life and the burden of disease as a measurement of the gap between current health status and an ideal situation where everyone lives into old age free of disease and disability.

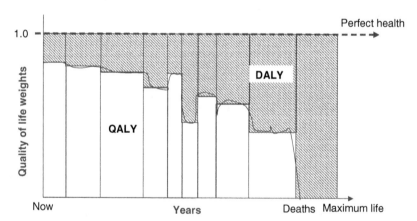

Fig. 14.4 Hypothetical life-path of health quality of life for an individual from now to death. The area under the curve (approximated by summing rectangles) is the QALYs accumulated by the person over this portion of their lifetime. The DALYs, the area lost from the ideal lifetime of living to the maximum life expectancy in full health, is the area above the life-path curve. Adapted from Gold et al. [22]. Reproduced with permission from Gold MR, Muennig P. Measure-dependent variation in burden of disease estimates: implications for policy. *Med Care.* 2002 40(3):260–6.

DALYs for a disease or health condition are calculated as the sum of the years of life lost due to premature mortality (YLL) in the population and the years lost due to disability (YLD) for incident cases of the health condition:

$$DALY = YLL + YLD$$

The derivation of DALYs relies on the abovementioned concept of *disability weights*. This was one of the major limitations and was subject to debates in its early use. The WHO Global Burden of Disease project is based on the use of DALYs, and efforts are being undertaken to harmonize the concepts and the calculations of DALYs. Compared to attributable cases, DALYs are a more integrated measure of risk burden. Table 14.3 presents the calculated world attributable mortality and DALYs obtained by the WHO Global Burden of Disease project and shows that the burden of some risk factors (i.e., environmental risk) differs when considering DALYs instead of mortality. Nevertheless, DALYs come with the disadvantages of additional data needs and further sources of uncertainties.

14.4.2.3 Quality-adjusted life years

Quality-adjusted life years, or QALYs, are often used as a measure of the benefit of an intervention. It is based on the number of years of life that would be added by the intervention. Each year of perfect health is assigned the value of 1.0 down to a value of 0 for death. If the extra years are not lived in full health, for example if the patient is confined to a wheelchair, then the extra life-years are given a value between 0 and 1 to account for this. For example, intervention A generates four extra years in health state valued at 0.75 (3 QALYs), and intervention B generates four extra years in health state valued at 0.5 (2 QALYS). Thus, intervention A generates one more QALY than intervention B. The weight assigned to a particular condition can vary greatly, depending on the population being surveyed. Those who do not suffer from the affliction in question will, on average, overestimate the detrimental effect on quality of life, while those who are afflicted have come to live with their condition [24]. Figure 14.4 visualizes the close relationship between DALY and QALY. While QALYs quantify the area under the curve of the quality of life value, DALYs count its complement, namely the degree of disability integrated over time.

Both QALYs and DALYs are designed to support resource allocation and to maximize the effectiveness of expenditures for health care or prevention. While the information can be useful to policy makers, one has to be aware of its limitations. For example, the use of QALYs in resource allocation decisions does mean that choices between patient groups competing for medical care are made explicit. Also, QALYs have been criticized because there is an implication that some patients will have reduced or no access to treatment for the sake of other patients. Gold *et al.* [22] describe in addition three main ethical limitations to these measures, which we summarize below. First, QALYs and DALYs fail to give priority to those who are the worst off. Distribution effects of resource allocation based solely on these measures will imply that those in most need because of their bad health or socially disadvantaged status will remain most in need. Secondly, these measures discriminate against people with limited treatment potential. For example, older persons and people with extensive disabling conditions with no treatment are considered 'bad investments' under this paradigm. This is because older people have a

Table 14.3 World attributable mortality and DALYs by risk factors as calculated in the World Health Organization Global Burden of Disease

Risk factor	Attributable numbers		% from total	
	Mortality (× 1000)	DALY (× 1000)	Mortality (n = 40 719 000)	DALY (n = 800 965 000)
Childhood and maternal undernutrition				
Underweight	3748	137801	9.20	17.20
Iron deficiency	841	35057	2.07	4.38
Vitamin A deficiency	778	26638	1.91	3.33
Zinc deficiency	789	28034	1.94	3.50
Other diet-related risks and physical inactivity				
Blood pressure	7141	64270	17.54	8.02
Cholesterol	4415	40437	10.84	5.05
Overweight	2591	33415	6.36	4.17
Low fruit and vegetable intake	2726	26662	6.70	3.33
Physical inactivity	1922	19092	4.72	2.38
Sexual and reproductive health risks				
Unsafe sex	2886	91869	7.09	11.47
Lack of contraception	149	8814	0.37	1.10
Addictive substances				
Tobacco	4907	59081	12.05	7.38
Alcohol	1804	58323	4.43	7.28
Illicit drugs	204	11218	0.50	1.40
Environmental risks				
Unsafe water, sanitation and hygiene	1730	54158	4.25	6.76
Urban air pollution	799	7865	1.96	0.98
Indoor smoke from solid fuels	1619	38539	3.98	4.81
Lead exposure	234	12926	0.57	1.61
Climate change	154	5517	0.38	0.69
Occupational risks				
Risk factors for injury	310	13125	0.76	1.64
Carcinogens	146	1421	0.36	0.18
Airborne particulates	243	3038	0.60	0.38
Ergonomic stressors	0	818	0.00	0.10
Noise	0	4151	0.00	0.52
Other selected risks to health				
Unsafe health care injections	501	10461	1.23	1.31
Childhood sexual abuse	79	8235	0.19	1.03

Source [23]. Reproduced with permission from the World Health Organization. *World Health Report 2002*. Annex Tables 11 and 12. Available at http://www.who.int/whr/2002/en/whr02_en.pdf.

limited number of years to gain, and because some illnesses may only improve to a limited degree. Third, these measures fail to account for qualitative differences in outcomes because of the way in which morbidity and mortality are aggregated.

While it is appealing to derive a single measure of burden, an inherent disadvantage is the 'black box' nature of these measures. Data inputs and the types of health outcomes included in the summary measures remain hidden. Environmental stressors may often affect a range of morbidities, and DALYs or related summary measures of risk depend on the number of outcomes considered in the risk assessment. This needs to be taken into account in the comparison of summary measures made across environmental factors or risk assessment studies.

14.4.3 Quantifying cost: benefits and effectiveness of environmental health policies

Monetary benefits of an intervention can be quantified by developing cost–benefit analysis or cost-effectiveness analysis. Cost–benefit analysis intends to translate all relevant considerations into monetary terms by giving money to both the costs of regulation (i.e., clean-up of contaminated soil) and the benefits of regulation, such as preventing diseases or saving a life. This part of the analysis can be very problematic because there are no natural prices for a healthy environment and economists have to derive these costs. The methods used consist of studying what people would be willing to pay for improving their security or reducing an environmental impact. The method called 'contingent valuation' is essentially a form of opinion poll where researchers ask a cross-section of the affected population how much they would be willing to pay to preserve or protect something that cannot be bought in a store [25]. An alternative method is based on what people are willing to pay from observation of their behavior in other markets [25]. For example, to assign a dollar value to risks to human life, economists usually calculate the extra wage—or 'wage premium'—that is paid to some workers who accept more risky jobs. If workers understand the risk and voluntarily accept a more dangerous job, then they are implicitly setting a price on risk by accepting the increased risk of death in exchange for increased wages [25]. Large discrepancies are found across cost–benefit assessments even between those conducted by the same authorities or agencies, e.g., within the US Environmental Protection Agency [26]. This must be critically evaluated and taken into account in the comparison of risk assessments which translate the health impact into monetary values.

Cost-effectiveness analysis is a method that helps select the best possible strategy or technique when resources are limited. Strategies can be compared by developing a cost-effectiveness ratio. It represents the price of the additional outcome purchased by changing from a current strategy or situation to a new one. If this price is below the wanted level the new strategy is considered cost effective. QALYs can also be used to assess the effectiveness of interventions. In this case the cost-effectiveness ratio will be the difference between the costs of two interventions divided by the difference in the QALYs they produce:

$$Cost-effectiveness\ ratio = \frac{cost_{Intervention} - cost_{current\ situation}}{effect_{Intervention} - effect_{current\ situation}}$$

14.5 **Uncertainties and limitations of risk assessment**

Environmental health risk assessment contributes increasingly to policy development, public health decision-making, the establishment of environmental regulations and research planning. Environmental health risk assessment also often plays an important role in cost-benefit analysis, cost-effectiveness analysis and risk communication. Epidemiology, toxicology, clinical medicine, and environmental exposure assessment all contribute information to the quantification of risk but are at the same time the source of a range of uncertainties that also affect the risk analyses.

An important uncertainty in quantitative risk assessment comes from the unit risk (i.e., dose–response) or exposure–response function to be used. Because, unlike laboratory experiments, epidemiology provides evidence based on studies of human populations under real-world conditions, epidemiology may be considered an optimal resource. Epidemiological studies avoid extrapolations across species and levels of exposures that are usually required for the use of animal data. However, epidemiological studies that report associations between measures of population health and the presence of hazardous factors in the environment require careful evaluation of the inherent limitations related to statistical power, bias, confounding, or uncontrolled effect modification. The selection of the appropriate risk function requires an evaluation of all available epidemiological literature [27].

Data from toxicological, clinical, and other areas of research often play a central role in the characterization of health hazards, the estimation of risks, and the understanding of causality. For many environmental factors, suitable epidemiological data may be lacking and thus risk analyses may rely solely on experimental knowledge. The time domain of the risk assessment and the relevant health outcomes also determine the level of uncertainty. Risk evaluations for environmental changes reaching far into the future may become inherently speculative. The public health risk for chronic outcomes with long latencies and pre-clinical phases is also more difficult to assess than consequences of exposures with immediate or subacute effects.

14.5.1 **Quantifying uncertainties**

As discussed above, risk assessments combine a range of quantitative and qualitative information from various sources which all have inherent uncertainties. In most cases, it is inevitable to generalize data and information derived from one source or population to the target population of the risk assessment. It is impossible to formally quantify all uncertainties in an integrated manner. Risk assessors have to communicate the key uncertainties and to discuss its potential implications on the final results. There are various options to provide a range of uncertainty around the 'best estimate'. The simplest method uses only the statistical uncertainty in the exposure–response function to provide an upper and lower bound of the burden associated with some exposure or policy. Typically, one may use the 95 percent confidence intervals of the risk function but other similarly arbitrary choices such as +/– one standard error of the estimate may be used.

Alternatively, in case of estimating attributable numbers, formulae are available to derive the confidence intervals of the attributable fractions directly. However, this approach integrates again only the uncertainty in the risk estimates (such as the RR or OR).

More sophisticated approaches may quantitatively propagate uncertainties across the various input data used in the derivation of the public health risk. This may include uncertainties in causality, the disease frequency, the population exposure distribution, the shape and slope of the exposure–response functions or the distribution of susceptibility factors.

14.5.2 Sensitivity analyses

The availability of simple and sophisticated approaches to quantify uncertainties should not cloud the fact that the nature of risk assessment is inherently imprecise, with many uncertainties not being quantifiable. This can be illustrated at the simple step of selecting the exposure–response or unit–risk function. While one may argue that the best estimate would be one derived in the target population, a meta-analytic estimate across all published response functions may be considered a more valid approach. However, meta-analyses imply that the environmental risk factors and the population characteristics assembled in all available studies are well representative for the target population. There are no 'final answers' to such unquantifiable questions of uncertainty. Sensitivity analyses are, thus, a useful element to address uncertainty. In the event of limited data it may even be the only option to give a quantitative or semi-quantitative estimate of the sensitivity of results to various assumptions made in the model. One may develop different scenarios where assumptions may be varied (e.g., as a function of different environmental policies or success rates of policies).

14.5.3 Comparability of risk analyses

One consequence of the various sources of uncertainties is the need to make many assumptions along the process of risk analyses. Different projects are likely to make different assumptions. If methods or assumptions differ between projects over time, across environmental hazards, or for different health outcomes, results may not be comparable across assessments. This can be a serious problem for policy makers as risk assessments may be used to set priorities in policy making.

The WHO Global Burden of Disease (GBD) project has undertaken important efforts toward standardization of methods [7]. However, there is still a long way to go, and comparability may even be limited across the 20 risk factors included in the GBD. The GBD applies common methods to derive the DALY but more proximal steps are more heterogeneous across the risk factors. The very different nature of these risks, ranging from ambient pollution to HIV standardizations, is inherently difficult.

14.5.4 Attributable risks versus preventable risks

While attributable risks and related measures are widely used in epidemiology and public health, one should not ignore their limitations. It is usually not possible to attribute 100 percent of cases to a set of known risk factors. Moreover, cases attributable to different exposures may add up to explain more than 100 percent of all cases. This is due to risk factors not being independent. The often made assumption that attributable cases reflect preventable cases is not necessarily correct. Risk factors compete with each other and the removal of one risk factor may lead to an advantage for another—thus, not all attributable cases will be preventable cases—or may at the same time reduce the susceptibility to another risk factor—thus, the preventable fraction may be larger than suggested by the attributable cases. The difficulty can be demonstrated with chronic diseases as the underlying cause for presenting acute episodes of morbidity such as asthma, chronic obstructive lung diseases, and others. For example, if ambient air pollution triggers myocardial infarction among those with pre-existing atherosclerosis [28], any preventive strategy that reduces the number of people with atherosclerosis would reduce the burden of air pollution related infarction, even if air quality remained the same. On the other side, if air pollution was an underlying chronic cause of the development of atherosclerosis, air quality regulation could prevent not only myocardial infarctions triggered by pollution but also a fraction of events triggered by any other cause as the pool of susceptibles—i.e., those with atherosclerosis—would become smaller.

The concept of attributable or preventable cases may be particularly difficult to communicate in case of mortality as death is ultimately not preventable. Risk reductions may postpone rather than prevent death. This is one reason why time-based estimates of risk may be the preferred choice (e.g., years of life lost) [29]. One should not neglect that they are based on the same data and assumptions, namely that the environmental exposure affects mortality rates. It is the increased mortality rates (or number of attributable deaths) that result in shortening of life expectancy. Risk assessments for single compounds—often based on toxicology—usually ignore synergetic or antagonistic effects of environmental exposures that most often consist in complex mixtures. It is in most cases impossible to reproduce real-life mixtures of exposures in experimental settings. Accordingly, risk assessments based on single pollutants may potentially underestimate the impact. This has, for example, been discussed in risk assessments of diesel particulate pollution where the sum of the risk related to the individual carcinogens identified in diesel particles may result in a smaller burden than an assessment based on integrated markers of diesel pollution, such as the ambient concentrations of black smoke (or 'soot') using epidemiological data [21]. As mentioned earlier, risk assessors often attach monetary values to the attributable burden derived in the assessment. This last step remains inherently incomparable, not only across regions or countries but even in risk assessments conducted within the same agencies where assumptions about the value of life may greatly differ [30].

14.5.5 **Risk assessment beyond science**

While the input data used in the risk or public health burden assessment originates from various sciences, the decisions evolving from risk assessments go far beyond science. Environmental epidemiologists involved in fields related to risk assessment must be aware of the boundaries between science and policy to be good advocates of current knowledge while acknowledging uncertainties. Table 14.4 is a non-exhaustive list of factors that may play a role in the decision-making process [15].

A minor albeit important part may be based on environmental epidemiology and toxicology. Risk perception or opinions about what represents an acceptable risk may play a major role. In the interest of public health, the risks versus benefits of the possible alternatives must be carefully considered. For example, it might well be that the emissions from hospital incinerators result in a certain number of deaths per year. However, this risk must be balanced against the available alternatives of no incineration (with the potential risk for spread of infectious diseases) or even no hospitals. Unless or until creativity and technological development offer superior methods for hospital waste disposal, the choice, based on risk assessment, must be that of the lesser evil. The result of a quantitative risk analysis is *per se* not sufficient to make an informed decision.

14.5.6 Precautionary principle

In the event of uncertainties and limited scientific evidence, the precautionary principle may play an important complementary role beyond quantitative risk assessment.

Table 14.4 Major criteria in judging the public health relevance of environmental exposure

Domain of judgment	Criterion
Exposure	Probability of exposure
	Intensity of exposure
	Frequency of exposure
	Duration of exposure
	Life period of exposure
	Number of people exposed
	Degree of choice (voluntary exposure?)
	Benefit of source that causes the exposure
Health effects	Type of health effects
	Degree and intensity of effect
	Size of effect (e.g., relative risk)
	Specificity of effect (other causes?)
	Acute versus chronic effect
	Frequency of health outcome among unexposed
	Reversibility of effect
	Acceptance of effect
	Cost of effects
Abatement/prevention	Number of susceptible among exposed
	Feasibility of abatement strategies
	Cost of abatement strategy
	Benefits of abatement strategy
	Specificity of the abatement strategy
	Reversibility of health problems
	Time of benefit of abatement
	Acceptance of abatement strategy
	Level of abatement (e.g., individual behavior versus structural)

Adapted from Künzli et al. [15].

The principle engenders the idea that if the consequences of an action are potentially severe or irreversible, the absence of full scientific certainty should not be used to prevent action. In practice the principle is most often applied in the context of the impact of human civilization or new technology on the ecosystem, as the environment is a complex system where the consequences of some kinds of actions are often unpredictable. The concept includes risk prevention, cost-effectiveness, ethical responsibilities towards maintaining the integrity of natural systems, and the fallibility of human understanding. It can also be interpreted as the transfer of more generally applied precaution in daily life (e.g., buying insurance, using seat belts or consulting experts before decisions) to larger political arenas.

14.5.7 Monitoring health and the environment to quantify risks

As shown in this chapter, public health risk assessment is based on the integrated use of population-based data about health and environmental factors. The availability and quality of such data ultimately determine the feasibility and validity of the risk assessment. Unfortunately this may often not be the case, thus regular monitoring of health and environmental risk factors must be promoted to accomplish the best possible science-based risk assessment. The use of standardized monitoring protocols and equipment is crucial to conduct risk assessments that are comparable across populations, regions, and over time. Long-term monitoring of environmental quality and population health may also set the grounds to evaluate the effects of policies that lead to changes in the environment and, thus, health (see Section 14.3.5 on accountability studies). Data from environmental monitoring networks may also be crucial for research in environmental epidemiology. Efforts to implement environmental health monitoring are therefore much welcomed. Information on major morbidities is largely lacking both in children and adults. Thus, while adverse effects of environmental factors might be well known, it may be very difficult to quantify the population risk as data on the distribution of the health conditions and/or the exposures may be lacking. For example, a major difficulty to quantify the GBD due to ambient air pollution was the complete absence of any air quality information in large areas of the world [31].

14.6 Illustrative risk assessment examples

This section provides five examples of various types of risk assessments conducted in the context of environmental health questions.

14.6.1 Public health risk assessments of ambient air pollution

The enormous increase in our understanding of the acute and long-term effect of ambient air pollution that emerged since the late 1980s triggered health impact questions from policy makers all around the world. The prevalent risk assessment methods rely on epidemiological information and the derivation of attributable cases [32]. However, some risk assessments for specific pollutants such as diesel particles employ the toxicology-based unit risk concept, combining the risk of the main carcinogenic substances contained in diesel exhaust [33].

The basic methods to translate epidemiological findings into attributable risks have been described in a World Bank report [32]. The emergence of new studies, in particular on long-term effects of air pollution, have led to expansions and updates of the methods [16, 21, 34]. While expert committees emphasized the need of further refinement of methods, and communications of uncertainties, the general concepts for the epidemiology-based risk assessment have been approved by US National Academy of Science (NAS) and the WHO and are widely applied for various purposes [4, 35].

14.6.1.1 The tri-national study

In light of Swiss research findings, the Swiss government was one of the first to call for a national health impact assessment of air pollution to estimate the healthcare costs of traffic-related air pollution. Policy makers decided to integrate external costs in the fees charged to heavy duty vehicles that pass through the Alps for international transit. The internalization of external costs became of interest for other European countries, and, as a consequence, the Ministries of Health and Environment of France, Austria, and Switzerland called for a tri-national health impact assessment. The assessment was based on epidemiological studies available as of 1996, including long-term effects of air pollution on mortality and various acute effects (cardio-respiratory hospital admissions, asthma attacks, bronchitis, restricted activity days). Ambient particulate matter (PM_{10}) were chosen as the marker of air pollution, and effects occurring below 7.5 $\mu g/m^3$ were ignored (reference level). Various pollution models suggested that more than 50 percent of air pollution was due to traffic. The study attributed some 6 percent of death to ambient PM_{10} and more than 3 percent to traffic related air pollution [16]. The economic evaluation of these risks estimated a burden of some 600–800 Euro per capita and year, driven to a large extent (75 percent) by costs assigned to the 40 000 attributable deaths [36].

14.6.1.2 California and US agencies

The USEPA and the California EPA regularly conduct health impact assessments and cost–benefit analyses employing the same or similar methods as mentioned above. The state of California conducted an extensive health impact assessment to evaluate the benefit of a more stringent $PM_{2.5}$ air quality standard [37]. Reductions of $PM_{2.5}$ were estimated to lead to substantial benefits in morbidity and mortality. As a consequence, an annual mean value of 12 $\mu g/m^3$ was adopted as the Californian air quality standard. This is one of the most stringent policies in the world and close to the guideline value of 10 $\mu g/m^3$ proposed by the WHO a few years later [38]. The USEPA uses the same risk assessment methods to assess the benefits of discussed or implemented new policies, e.g., the more stringent regulation of diesel technologies.

As scientific evidence increases, the health outcomes considered in the agencies' assessments increase and now include, for example, the effects of air pollution on infant mortality.

14.6.1.3 The APHEIS network

This cross-European risk assessment collaboration grew out of APHEA—Air Pollution and Health, a European Approach. APHEA was the first large-scale multi-city epidemiological investigation of the association between daily levels of ambient air pollution and daily mortality rates [9]. APHEA promoted the standardization of data collection and analysis procedures, and became a model for other large-scale multi-city studies. APHEIS was implemented to develop and distribute standard risk assessment approaches and tools to quantify the consequences of air pollution all across European cities to inform policy makers about these effects and the potential benefits of improved air quality.

14.6.1.4 Outdoor air pollution in the WHO Global Burden of Disease initiative

Ambient air pollution is one of the 20 risk factors considered in the GBD [6]. While the same methods were adopted as in other studies, the researchers were challenged by new uncertainties due to the limited availability of data in large parts of the world. Ambient air pollution was rarely monitored in Africa and parts of Asia, thus PM_{10} had to be estimated using information from mostly Western countries and proxies of pollution such as population density, industrialization, and other factors. Moreover, air pollution epidemiology was largely absent for most developing countries. Generalizability of response-functions from available US or European studies to Africa or megacities in Asia is somewhat speculative, and uncertainties are certainly larger in the GBD than in more local or regional air pollution risk assessment studies. This is described in Chapter 17 of the GBD and in a short article [31].

14.6.2 Health impact assessment and transportation policies

The relevance of health impact assessment in public policies is exemplified in a study by the WHO of transport land-use policies in Delhi, India [39]. This study showed that current transportation policies in mega-cities worldwide lead to major threats to health through traffic injuries, air pollution, noise, reduction in physical activities, and adverse impact on urban quality of life, but fail to take account of their impacts on poverty and social exclusion. In addition, these policies often neglect the access and transportation demands of the more economically disadvantaged groups of society, who rely mostly on public transportation, walking, and cycling. In this study, Delhi, the capital city of India, provided an example where the prior development of a health impact assessment could have been beneficial for the health of its inhabitants because current transport policies in Delhi are penalizing the least affluent groups of the population and making it more difficult for them to get to jobs, education, healthcare, amenities, and services [39].

14.6.3 Environmental risk assessment: risk of contaminated sediments for health

The USEPA is a leader in the development and use of environmental risk assessment as a tool to evaluate the likelihood and degree of chemical exposure and the possible adverse health effects associated with exposure to chemicals in soil, sediment, groundwater and air. An example of risk assessment that uses USEPA policy and guidance is the Human Health Risk Assessment for the Mid-Hudson River (Mid-Hudson HHRA). The HHRA quantitatively evaluated both cancer risks and non-cancer health hazards from exposure to polychlorinated biphenyls (PCBs) in the Hudson River, New York, USA, detected in fish, sediments, and river water in different phases of data collection and analysis. The contamination detected resulted from the discharge from approximately 1947–1977 of as much as 1.3 million pounds of polychlorinated biphenyls (PCBs) from different industrial manufacturing plants of the General Electric Company (GE) into the river. The final report on the risk assessments and other information related to the project can be found on USEPA's website (http://www.epa.gov/ hudson).

In this HHRA, as part of the exposure assessment, adults, adolescents, and children were identified as populations possibly exposed to PCBs in the mid-Hudson River due to fishing and recreational activities (e.g., swimming, wading), as well as from residential ingestion of river water. The exposure pathways identified in the Mid-Hudson HHRA were ingestion of fish, incidental ingestion of sediments, dermal contact with sediments and river water, and residential ingestion of river water. Different sources of data were combined to determine the ingestion rate, fishing and swimming frequency and other parameters required for the evaluation of exposure.

PCBs are a group of synthetic organic chemicals comprising 209 individual chlorinated biphenyls called congeners. Some PCB congeners are considered to be structurally similar to dioxin and are called dioxin-like PCBs. USEPA has classified PCBs as probable human carcinogens, based on a number of studies in laboratory animals showing liver tumors. Human carcinogenicity data for PCB mixtures are limited but suggestive. Based on this hazard identification, risks for cancer and non-cancer effects were evaluated for exposure to PCBs using dose–response functions derived from toxicological studies.

Results of the HHRA showed that under the reasonable maximum estimate (RME) scenario for eating fish, the calculated risk was approximately four additional cases of cancer for every 10 000 people exposed. This excess cancer risk was more than 100 times higher than USEPA's goal of protection of human health. For non-cancer health effects, the RME scenario for eating fish from the Mid-Hudson results in a level of exposure to PCBs that was 30 times higher than USEPA's reference level (Hazard Index) of one. Risks from being exposed to PCBs in the Mid-Hudson River through skin contact with contaminated sediments and river water, residential ingestion of river water for drinking water, incidental ingestion of sediments, and inhalation of PCBs in air were significantly below USEPA's levels of concern for cancer and non-cancer health effects.

The results of this risk assessment were the basis for decision-makers to request further development of clean-up strategies for the river from the polluter. Currently, a remediation plan consisting of removal of contaminated sediments from the river is being reviewed by USEPA, and dredging is expected to begin in 2007.

14.6.4 Burden of disease: groundwater arsenic in Bangladesh

Groundwater contamination caused by inorganic arsenic is a massive public health concern in Bangladesh. Since 1970, millions of hand-pumped tube wells have been installed with the initial intention to protect the population against the use of surface water contaminated with pathogens. This has led, however, to 95 percent of the country's

130 million residents becoming dependent on arsenic-impacted underground water. It is estimated that 25–57 million people in Bangladesh have suffered chronic exposure to arsenic, and because decades of exposure have already occurred, the exposed population is at an elevated risk of arsenic-induced health problems [40].

The degree and extent of risk mitigations is in part related to the burden of disease that can be expected from the exposure to arsenic and has been evaluated by quantitative risk assessment techniques by calculating the excess lifetime mortality rates for cancer [40]. In this risk assessment, measures of distribution of exposure, 'background' lifetime risks, and dose-specific relative risk estimates were combined. Arsenic exposure was ascertained through surveys and collection of groundwater samples from a subset of the population of Bangladesh. 'Background' mortality risks among the population were derived via life table methods using established mortality rates, and relative risks were used from studies conducted in Taiwan. The results indicated at least a doubling of lifetime mortality risk from liver, bladder, and lung cancers in Bangladesh owing to arsenic in drinking water. The results show that local and international governments should prioritize funding for reduction in arsenic exposure and develop a surveillance system for early diagnosis and treatment of arsenic-induced cancers in Bangladesh.

14.6.5 Environmental tobacco smoke exposure and legislation

Since the 1980s, there has been a growing body of epidemiological evidence linking environmental tobacco smoke (ETS) exposure to adverse health effects. Health impact assessments have been used by policy and public health regulators to develop legislation that prevents adverse health effects from ETS exposure. For example, a recent study estimated the health impact of workplace ETS in Europe [41]. ETS exposure in the workplace is a considerable concern for adult populations because of the time spent at the workplace each day. This study combined information on workplace ETS exposure for several countries in Europe and epidemiological studies on the effects of ETS exposure on respiratory and cardiovascular diseases in adults to derive population attributable fractions (i.e., the proportion of cases that would not be observed if exposure was absent) for each country. The results of the study suggested that the public health impact of ETS exposure at the workplace was substantial. For example, the proportion of lung cancer cases attributable to workplace ETS exposure in Spain, where no smoke-free workplace legislation was in place at the time of the study, was about 8 percent compared to 1 percent in Finland, which has had smoke-free workplace legislation since 1995 and for which current levels of ETS exposure are reduced. Many countries included in this study (i.e., Spain, France, Italy) have since passed smoke-free workplace legislation to reduce passive smoking in adult populations.

14.7 References

[1] Last J. *A dictionary of epidemiology*. Oxford and New York: Oxford University Press 1995.

[2] **National Research Council**. *Risk assessment in the federal government: managing the process*. Washington, DC: National Academies Press 1983.

[3] Scott-Samuel A. Health impact assessment – theory into practice. *J Epidemiol Community Health*. 1998 52(11):704–5.

[4] **World Health Organization**. *Health impact assessment: main concepts and suggested approach: a Gothenburg consensus paper, December 1999.* Copenhagen: WHO Regional Office for Europe 1999.

[5] Scanlon TJ, Lawrence L, Blair-Stevens T, Nichols S. A programme for Health Impact Assessment in Brighton and Hove. *Soz Praventivmed*. 2006 51(3):145–50.

[6] Ezzati M, Lopez AD, Rodgers A, Vander Hoorn S, Murray CJ. Selected major risk factors and global and regional burden of disease. *Lancet*. 2002 360(9343):1347–60.

[7] Murray C. *The global burden of disease* (Published on behalf of the World Health Organization and the World Bank). Cambridge, MA: Harvard School of Public Health 1996.

[8] Clancy L, Goodman P, Sinclair H, Dockery DW. Effect of air-pollution control on death rates in Dublin, Ireland: an intervention study. *Lancet*. 2002 360(9341):1210–14.

[9] Katsouyanni K, Zmirou D, Spix C, Sunyer J, Schouten J, Pönkä A, *et al*. Short-term effects of air pollution on health: a European approach using epidemiological time-series data. The APHEA project: background, objectives, design. *Eur Respir J*. 1995 8:1030–38.

[10] Bayer-Oglesby LG, Gassner M, Takken-Sahli K, Sennhauser FH, Neu U, Schindler C, Braun-Fahrländer C. Decline of ambient air pollution levels and improved respiratory health in Swiss children. *Env Health Perspect*. 2005 113(11):1632–7.

[11] Heinrich J, Hoelscher B, Frye C, Meyer I, Pitz M, Cyrys J, *et al*. Improved air quality in reunified Germany and decreases in respiratory symptoms. *Epidemiology*. 2002 13(4): 394–401.

[12] Heinrich J, Hoelscher B, Wichmann HE. Decline of ambient air pollution and respiratory symptoms in children. *Am J Respir Crit Care Med*. 2000 161(6):1930–6.

[13] Heller RF, Dobson AJ, Attia J, Page J. Impact numbers: measures of risk factor impact on the whole population from case-control and cohort studies. *J Epidemiol Community Health*. 2002 56(8):606–10.

[14] Steenland K, Armstrong B. An overview of methods for calculating the burden of disease due to specific risk factors. *Epidemiology*. 2006 17(5):512–9.

[15] Künzli N. The public health relevance of air pollution abatement. *Eur Respir J*.2002 20(1):198–209.

[16] Künzli N, Kaiser R, Medina S, Studnicka M, Chanel O, Filliger P, *et al*. Public-health impact of outdoor and traffic-related air pollution: a European assessment. *Lancet*. 2000 356(9232): 795–801.

[17] Boldo E, Medina S, LeTertre A, Hurley F, Mucke HG, Ballester F, *et al*. Apheis: health impact assessment of long-term exposure to PM(2.5) in 23 European cities. *Eur J Epidemiol*. 2006 21(6):449–58.

[18] Antó J, Sunyer J, Reed C, Sabria J, Martinez F, Morell F, *et al*. Preventing asthma epidemics due to soybeans by dust-control measures. *New England Journal of Medicine*. 1993 329:1760–3.

[19] Antó JM, Sunyer J. Epidemiologic studies of asthma epidemics in Barcelona. *Chest*. 1990 98 (5 Suppl):185S–90S.

[20] Pope CA, 3rd, Dockery DW. Health effects of fine particulate air pollution: lines that connect. *J Air Waste Manag Assoc*. 2006 56(6):709–42.

[21] Roosli M, Kunzli N, Schindler C, Theis G, Oglesby L, Mathys P, *et al*. Single pollutant versus surrogate measure approaches: do single pollutant risk assessments underestimate the impact of air pollution on lung cancer risk? *J Occup Environ Med*. 2003 45(7):715–23.

[22] Gold MR, Stevenson D, Fryback DG. HALYS and QALYS and DALYS, Oh my: similarities and differences in summary measures of population health. *Annu Rev Public Health*. 2002 23: 115–34.

[23] **World Health Organization**. *World health report 2002*. Annex Tables 11 and 12. Available at http://www/who.int/whr/2002/en/whr02_en.pdf.

[24] Philips C, Thompson G. What is QALY? Hayward Medical Communications, available at http://www.evidence-based-medicine.co.uk.2003.

[25] Ackerman F, Heinzerling L. Pricing the priceless: cost-benefit analysis of environmental protection. Georgetown Environmental Law & Policy Institute, available at http://www.law.georgetown.edu.2002.

[26] Kaiser J. Economics: how much are human lives and health worth? *Science.* 2003 299(5614):1836–7.

[27] Neutra RR, Trichopoulos D. The place of epidemiology in environmental decisions: needed support for the development of risk assessment policy. *Environ Health Perspect.* 1993 101 (Suppl 4):67–9.

[28] Peters A, Dockery DW, Muller JE, Mittleman MA. Increased particulate air pollution and the triggering of myocardial infarction. *Circulation.* 2001 103(23):2810–15.

[29] Miller BG, Hurley JF. Life table methods for quantitative impact assessments in chronic mortality. *J Epidemiol Community Health.* 2003 57(3):200–6.

[30] Kaiser J. Economics. How much are human lives and health worth? *Science.* 2003 299(5614):1836–7.

[31] Cohen J, Anderson R, Ostro B. Comparative quantification of health risks: outdoor air pollution. In: Ezzati M, Lopez A, Rodgers A, Murray C, eds. *Comparative quantification of health risks: global and regional burden of disease attributable to selected major risk factors.* Geneva: World Health Organization; 2003.

[32] Ostro B. *Estimating the health effects of air pollutants.* Policy Research Working Paper. Washington DC: The World Bank Policy Department Public Economics Division 1994.

[33] California Air Resources Board. *Public hearing to consider amendments to the ambient air quality standards for particulate matter and sulfates.* Sacramento, CA: Air Resources Board, California Environmental Protection Agency 2002.

[34] Künzli N, Medina S, Kaiser R, Quenel P, Horak FJ, Studnicka M. Assessment of deaths attributable to air pollution: should we use risk estimates based on time series or on cohort studies? *Am J Epidemiol.* 2001 153(11):1050–5.

[35] US National Research Council. Committee on Estimating the Health-Risk-Reduction Benefits of Proposed Air Pollution Regulations. *Estimating the public health benefits of proposed air pollution regulations.* Washington, DC: The National Academies Press 2002.

[36] Sommer H, Künzli N, Seethaler R, Chanel O, Herry M, Vergnaud J-C, *et al. An impact assessment project of Austria, France and Switzerland. Ancillary benefits and costs of greenhouse gas mitigation: Proceedings from an Expert Workshop.* New York: OECD 2000: 451–79.

[37] California Air Resources Board and the Office of Environmental Health Hazard Assessment. *Staff Report: Public Hearing to Consider Amendments to the Ambient Air Quality Standards for Particulate Matter and Sulfates.* Sacramento, CA: California Environmental Protection Agency 2002.

[38] World Health Organization. *Air quality guidelines for particulate matter, ozone, nitrogen dioxide and sulfur dioxide. global update 2005.*

[39] Tiwari G. Transport and land-use policies in Delhi. *Bull World Health Organ.* 2003 81(6):444–50.

[40] Chen Y, Ahsan H. Cancer burden from arsenic in drinking water in Bangladesh. *Am J Public Health.* 2004 94(5):741–4.

[41] Jaakkola MS, Jaakkola JJ. Impact of smoke-free workplace legislation on exposures and health: possibilities for prevention. *Eur Respir J.* 2006 28(2):397–408.

Chapter 15

Using integrated assessment to analyze and forecast the future effects of global environmental change

Pim Martens and Maud Huynen

15.1 Introduction

Global environmental changes are a manifestation of a larger pattern of change in the scale and intensity of human affairs. Global climate change is one of the most widely discussed of these global environmental changes. In 1996, the UN Intergovernmental Panel on Climate Change (IPCC) concluded that human-made changes in the global atmosphere were probably already beginning to change world climate [1]. During 1997 and 1998, global temperatures reached their highest levels since record keeping began in the mid-nineteenth century. Overall, ten of the twelve hottest years of the twentieth century occurred after 1988. During the late 1990s and turn of the century, it seemed that world weather patterns were becoming more unstable, more variable. In 2001, the IPCC firmed up its conclusion that human-induced climate change was already occurring and raised its estimation of the likely range (1.4–5.8°C) of temperature increase during the twenty-first century [2].

The impact of climate change and other environmental changes on population health poses significant challenges to scientists. The exploration of these systems-based risks to human health seems far removed from the methods usually discussed in textbooks of epidemiology and public health research. Only a few textbooks consider the more system-based health risks of environmental changes, such as those by Aron and Patz [3], Martens and McMichael [4] and Lindgren *et al.* [5]. Yet the wider public and policy decision-makers are seeking from scientists useful estimates of the likely population health consequences of these great and unfamiliar changes in the world.

Clearly, there is a major task for health scientists in this area. This chapter seeks to identify the nature and scope of the problem, and to explore the conceptual and methodological approaches to studying these relationships, modeling their future realization, providing estimates of health impacts, and communicating the attendant uncertainties. It will focus on one of the key approaches to exploring the relationships between global environmental changes and human health: integrated assessment modeling.

15.2 **Global environmental changes and their potential health impacts**

The main global environmental changes, of a kind that were not on the agenda a quarter-century ago, are summarized below [adapted from 6].

Climate change

During the 1990s, the prospect of human-induced global climate change became a potent symbol of the unprecedented large-scale environmental changes. Since 1975 average world temperature increased by approximately 0.5°C, and climate scientists generally thought this was the beginning of the anticipated climate change due to human-induced greenhouse gas accumulation in the lower atmosphere [2]. Weather patterns in many regions displayed increasing instability, and this may be a foretaste of the increasing climatic variability that is foreseen by many climate change modelers. The direct health effects of climate change include temperature-related effects (e.g., heat stress) and the effects of extreme weather events like storms and floods. Indirect effects include vector-borne diseases (e.g., malaria, Lyme disease), water-borne diseases (e.g., cholera, exposure to blue algae), food-related diseases (e.g., food availability, Salmonella) and health effects related to changes in air quality (e.g., pollen-induced allergies, ground level ozone increases).

Stratospheric ozone depletion

Meanwhile, higher in the atmosphere, a separate problem exists. Depletion of stratospheric ozone by human-made industrial gases such as chlorofluorocarbons (CFCs) has been documented over several decades. The stratospheric ozone layer acts as a protective radiation shield that intercepts most of the harmful UV radiation in the UVB band. As a result, the declining levels of stratospheric ozone are believed to increase the ambient levels of damaging UVB radiation, resulting in a higher risk of cataracts, skin cancer and a weakened immune-system response. Terrestrial levels of ultraviolet (UV) radiation are estimated to have increased by around 5–10 percent at mid-to-high latitudes since 1980. This problem is now projected to peak around 2010–20. Simulation models estimate that European and North American populations will experience an approximate 10 percent excess incidence of skin cancer in mid-twenty-first century [7, 8].

Loss of biodiversity

The loss of biodiversity is another major global environmental change. Biodiversity refers to the variability of genes, species and ecosystems, and maintaining a certain level of biodiversity is necessary for healthy ecosystem functioning and the provisions of ecosystem goods and services to mankind. Compromising these functions could result in loss of genetic or medical resources, disruption of biological control of diseases and negative impacts on food and water supplies. However, the pressures on biodiversity (e.g., habitat loss, over-exploitation, pollution and biotic changes) are still rapidly increasing throughout the world. As the human demand for space, materials and food increases, so populations and species of plants and animals around the world are being extinguished at an accelerating rate—apparently much faster than the five great natural extinctions that have occurred in the past half-billion years since vertebrate life evolved. The problem is not simply the loss of valued items from nature's catalog. It is, more seriously, the destabilization and weakening of whole ecosystems and the consequent loss of their products and their recycling, cleansing and restorative services. Meanwhile, 'invasive' species are spreading into new non-natural environments via intensified human food production, commerce and mobility. One example: the spread of water hyacinth in eastern Africa's Lake Victoria, introduced from Brazil as a decorative plant, has provided a microenvironment for the proliferation of diarrheal disease, bacteria and water snails that transmit schistosomiasis [9].

Freshwater supplies

Scarce and unclean water supplies are critical public health problems in much of the world. Approximately 40 percent of the world's population, living in 80 countries, now faces some level of water shortage, and this percentage is only expected to increase as agricultural, industrial and municipal water demands often greatly exceed the rate of natural recharge. In all continents, freshwater aquifers are being depleted of their 'fossil water'. Health risks of diminished fresh water supplies include reduced availability of water for consumption, washing or sanitation, which is strongly related to many intestinal infectious diseases (e.g., cholera). Water scarcity is, of course, also linked to reduced food supplies. Additionally, water shortages are likely to cause tensions and conflict over coming decades [10]. For example, Ethiopia and the Sudan, upstream of Nile-dependent Egypt, increasingly need the Nile's water for their own crop irrigation. So, health effects could be the result of armed conflict as well as the deterioration of water quality and reduced food supply.

Persistent organic pollutants

Many long-lived and biologically active chemicals have become widely distributed across the globe. Lead and other heavy metals are present at increasing concentrations in remote environments. Some of the worst pollutants are synthetic chemicals, particularly the group known as persistent organic pollutants polychlorinated biphenyls (POPs). These include halogenated hydrocarbons, dioxins and organochlorines such as DDT and polychlorinated biphenyls (PCBs). They are highly toxic in the environment, do not break down easily under natural circumstances and tend to accumulate up the biological food chain until they pose risk for human health. For example, their concentrations are increasing in polar mammals and fish and in traditional human groups that eat them. Exposure to low concentrations derived from the environment and food chain can pose chronic health risks (e.g., cancer, endocrine disruption), but the long-term implications of low-level exposure are still not fully known.

15.3 **Challenges to population health research**

The great majority of researchers are *empiricists* by training and tradition, studying the past and the present via direct observation. By definition, empirical methods cannot be used to study the future. To the extent that the advent of global environmental changes obliges scientists to estimate future impacts, should current or foreseeable trends continue, then empiricism must be supplemented by predictive modeling. Epidemiologists, whose primary task is to identify risks to health from recent or current behaviors, exposures or other circumstances, are oriented to asking questions about health impacts several decades hence.

These contextual difficulties aside, population health scientists must find ways to estimate the potential health consequences of current social and environmental trajectories. Not only is this an interesting scientific task, but—crucially—it will assist society to seek a sustainable future. Clearly, elucidating these risks to population health from environmental changes such as long-term changes in global climatic patterns, depletion of stratospheric ozone and biodiversity loss poses a special research challenge. For a start, these environmental changes entail unusually large spatial scales. They also entail temporal scales that extend decades or further into the future. Some entail irreversible changes. While some direct impacts on health would result—such as the health consequences of increased floods and heatwaves due to global climate change, or increases in skin cancer due to ozone depletion—many of the impacts would result from the disruption of the ecological processes that are, for example, central to food-producing ecosystems or to the ecology of infectious-disease pathogens. That is, many of the causal relationships are neither simple nor immediate.

15.3.1 Concepts

A fundamental characteristic of this topic area is the pervasive combination of *complexity* and *uncertainty* that confronts scientists. Policy-makers, too, must therefore adjust to working with incomplete information and with making 'uncertainty-based' policy decisions. Several aspects of the complexity and uncertainty of this research domain are dealt with specifically in three of the subsequent sections. Those aspects are: (i) complexity and surprises, (ii) uncertainties, and (iii) determinants of population vulnerability, and adaptive capacity, to these environmental changes. Chapter 16 deals with scientific uncertainty in the policy making process in detail, and the reader is referred to that chapter for an in-depth discussion.

Complexity and surprises

Predicting the impact of a changing world on human health is a difficult task which requires an interdisciplinary approach drawn from the fields of evolution, biogeography, ecology, environmental science, epidemiology and social sciences, and relying on various methodologies such as integrated assessment modeling (see below) as well as historical analysis, among others. When even a simple change occurs in the physical environment, its effects percolate through a complex network of physical, biological and social interactions that feed backward and forward. Sometimes the immediate effect of a change is different from the long term effects, and sometimes the local changes may be different from the region-wide alterations. The same environmental change may have quite different effects in different places or times. Therefore the study of the consequences of environmental change is a study of the short- and long-term dynamics of complex systems.

In addition, there is increasing evidence that natural ecosystems are able to cope with a certain degree of disturbance without shifting into a different state. As a result of this ecosystem resilience, they rarely respond to gradual change in a gradual way, often resulting in 'ecological surprises'. It is, for example, believed that ecosystems have the capacity to deal with partial losses in their biodiversity without consequences for their functioning [11]. It is only when a threshold in the losses of biodiversity is reached that the provision of ecosystem goods and services suddenly decreases with often irreversible biological, social and economic consequences. Thus, it is still difficult to predict how much biodiversity or what key species need to be preserved in order to secure healthy ecosystem functioning, and it is, therefore, very challenging to anticipate such surprises.

Uncertainties

The prediction of environmental change and its health impacts encounters uncertainties at various levels. Some of the uncertainties are of a scientific kind, referring to deficient understanding of actual processes: for example, knowing whether or not increased cloud cover arising because of global warming would have a positive or a negative feedback effect. Some of the uncertainties refer to the conceptualization and construction of mathematical models where the specification of linked processes may be uncertain or where key parameter values are uncertain. Some uncertainties are essentially epistemological, referring to what we can and cannot reasonably foresee about the structure and behavior of future societies, including for example their future patterns of emissions of greenhouse gases. Finally, there is of course the familiar source of uncertainty that arises from sampling variation, which leads to the need for confidence intervals around point estimates.

Vulnerability and adaptation

Human populations vary in their vulnerability to health hazards like climate change. A population's vulnerability is a function of the degree of climate change, the extent to which a health outcome is sensitive to climate change and of the capacity of the population to adapt to new climate conditions. The vulnerability of a population depends on factors such as population density, level of economic development, food availability, local environmental conditions, pre-existing health status, and the quality and availability of public healthcare.

Adaptation refers to actions taken to lessen the impact of the (anticipated) climate change. There is a hierarchy of control strategies that can help to protect population health. These strategies are categorized as: (i) administrative or legislative; (ii) engineering, or (iii) personal (behavioral). Legislative or regulatory action can be taken by government, requiring compliance by all or by designated classes of persons. Alternatively, an adaptive action may be encouraged on a voluntary basis, via advocacy, education or economic incentives. The former type of action would normally be taken at a supranational, national or community level; the latter would range from supranational to individual levels. Adaptation strategies will be either reactive, in response to observed climate impacts, or anticipatory, in order to reduce vulnerability to such impacts.

15.3.2 Research methods

Next to the conceptual challenges we have to face, the assessment of the risks to population health from global environmental change requires several complementary research strategies. Research into the health impacts of these environmental changes can be conducted within three domains, and there are a variety of methods than can be used within each domain. The three categories of research are:

- The use of historical and other analog situations which, as (presumed) manifestations of existing natural environmental variability, are thought likely to foreshadow future aspects of environmental change. These empirical studies help to fill knowledge gaps and strengthen our capacity to forecast future health impacts in response to changing environmental–climatic circumstances.

- The seeking of early evidence of changes in health risk indicators or health status occurring in response to actual environmental change. Attention should be paid to sensitive, early-responding, systems and processes.

- By using existing empirical knowledge and theory to model future health outcomes in relation to prescribed scenarios of environmental change. This is referred to as integrated assessment.

Analog studies
Empirically-based knowledge about the relationship between climate and health outcomes is a prerequisite to any formal attempt to forecast how future climate change is likely to affect human health. In fact, we cannot know in advance the exact configurations of the future world. Indeed, we should assume that in some respects the future will be unlike the present, both in its overall format and in the component relationships between now-familiar variables which, in future, will occur at unfamiliar levels. Nevertheless, our best guide to foreseeing the future is to have studied and understood the past and present.

For example, one can identify the contemporary climate of geographically distinct locations (e.g., the Bordeaux region in France) that can be used as an analog for the future climate of the target location (e.g., south-west England). Such an approach is called a spatial analog and relies on the assumption that an observed relationship between health and climate in a certain geographical area can be applied to other geographical areas to represent the effect of climate change at some point in the future. Other types of analogs that can be identified are event analogs (e.g., El Niño and situation analogs [4]).

Empirical studies of early health effects
If recent global climate trends continue and it becomes more certain that this process is the beginning of anthropogenic climate change, then epidemiologists must seek early

evidence of impacts on health. Such things as patterns of heat-related deaths, the seasonality of allergic disorders, and the geographic range and seasonality of particularly climate-sensitive infectious diseases can be expected to begin to change.

There is good evidence of climate-related changes in the distribution and behavior of animal species both within Europe and elsewhere. For example, the northern limit of the distribution of important tick vectors has moved north in Sweden between 1980 and 1994. Further analysis shows that changes in the distribution and density of that tick species over time have been correlated with changes in seasonal daily minimum temperatures [5]. However, there is little evidence yet of changes in human population health that can be attributed to the observed recent changes in climate (principally the warming that has occurred over the last 20 years).

Geographical information systems and remote sensing

Remote sensed (RS) data from weather satellites can be used to monitor changes in temperature and precipitation in order to predict continental and global patterns of disease outbreaks. Higher resolution satellite data can be used in a landscape epidemiological approach to modeling patterns at local to regional scales. A comprehensive model of disease risk due to, for example, climate change should incorporate the temporal aspects of the climate models integrated with the spatial forecasting made possible by the use of geographic information systems (GIS) technologies and spatial analyses. RS and GIS technologies provide unprecedented amounts of data and data management capabilities.

Monitoring

A range of national, regional and international organizations routinely collect relevant data, most obviously those monitoring environmental conditions, and (usually separately) health status. While these systems constitute a potentially powerful resource, most were implemented for purposes other than studying environmental change effects on health. *Monitoring* is the continuous or repeated observation, measurement and evaluation of health and/or environmental data for defined purposes, according to prearranged schedules in space and time, using comparable methods for sensing and data collection. Environmental change and health monitoring should be directed towards the following aims:

1. early detection of the health impacts of global environmental change;
2. improved quantitative analysis of the relationships between environment and health;
3. improved analysis of vulnerability;
4. prediction of future health impacts of environmental change, and validation of predictions; and
5. assessment of effectiveness of adaptation strategies.

From the above, it becomes clear that monitoring will also be an important component in the other methods mentioned earlier.

15.4 **Integrated assessment of human health impacts**

15.4.1 **Integrated assessment modeling**

In modeling population dynamics, fertility modeling approaches are widely accepted but only recently have existing mathematical techniques been introduced in the broader health area [e.g., 12, 13]. Usually, regression techniques are used to explore the relations between broad health determinants, like literacy, income status, nutritional status, water supply and sanitation, education and medical services, and the health status measured in healthy or total life expectancy. However, these regression techniques can only give suggestive evidence on the causes of population and health changes. Statistical models to estimate future fertility and health levels are based on extrapolation of past and current data. They operate on a short time horizon and are static in terms of specifying the dynamics behind changing fertility and health patterns. Therefore, there is a need for integrated approaches that take into account the simultaneous occurrence of multiple risk factors and diseases, as well as cause–effect relationships. Such an integrated approach cannot be used in the clinical area on an individual basis but is appropriate at the population level.

Rotmans and de Vries [14] presented an integrated systems approach to population and health. A generic model was designed which simulates the driving forces (socio-economic and environmental factors), fertility behavior and disease-specific mortality, burden of disease and life expectancy as well as the size and structure of the population, and a number of fertility and health policies. The major objective of the population and health model is to simulate changes in morbidity and mortality levels under varying social, economic and environmental conditions. Hilderink [15] elaborated on this modeling framework and developed the PHOENIX model.

A second but related example is the MIASMA framework, which is designed to describe the major cause and effects relationships between atmospheric changes and human population health [16]. The model focuses on climate change (in terms of changes in temperature and precipitation) and ozone depletion (in terms of changes in UVB radiation). Under varying climate and ozone regimes, changes in the dynamics and distribution of vector-borne diseases are simulated (malaria, schistosomiasis and dengue), changing patterns of skin cancer incidences, and changing mortality levels as a result of thermal stress.

15.4.2 **Integrated scenario analysis**

Scenarios are descriptions of possible futures that reflect different perspectives on past, present and future developments with a view to anticipating the future [17]. Scenarios do not provide predictions of future outcomes; rather, they outline (quantitatively, qualitatively or both) various possible futures in order to provoke reflection and debate about events and circumstances that may need to be faced. Even contemplating different possible future outcomes may induce people to reconsider and modify their present activities in view of a different, preferred outcome. For scenarios to be credible, they should be transparent and internally consistent views of the world [17].

Scenario analysis has evolved significantly over the past decades. In their early days, scenarios were used primarily as planning and forecasting tools, displaying a rather mechanistic and deterministic worldview. Currently scenario analysis supports a more open form of exploration [18].

Scenarios as aids to decision-making can be useful tools to:

- articulate our key considerations and assumptions: scenarios can help to imagine a range of possible futures if we follow a key set of assumptions and considerations;
- blend quantitative and qualitative knowledge: scenarios are powerful frameworks for using both data- and model-produced output in combination with qualitative knowledge elements;
- identify constraints and dilemmas: exploring the future often yields indications for constraints in future developments and dilemmas for strategic choices to be made; and
- expand our thinking beyond the conventional paradigm: exploring future possibilities that go beyond our conventional thinking may result in surprising and innovative insights.

Depending on how scenarios are produced and developed, they can have several limitations:

- lack of diversity: scenarios are often developed from a narrow, disciplinary-based perspective, resulting in a limited set of standard economic, technological, and to a lesser extent, environmental assumptions;
- extrapolations of current trends: many scenarios do have a 'business-as-usual' character, assuming that current conditions will continue for decades, excluding surprises;
- inconsistent: sets of assumptions made for different sectors, regions, or issues, are often not made consistent with each other;
- not transparent: key assumptions and underlying implicit judgments and preferences are often not made explicit, nor are factors which are exogenous and which ones are endogenous, or to what extent societal processes are autonomous or influenced by concrete policies.

Nowadays, scenarios as powerful exploratory tools can be used to paint pictures of possible future outcomes based on changing assumptions. In a sense, they can be used to promote considerations on capacity building for adaptation and mitigation in the face of climate change, by broadening and deepening the mindset of stakeholders involved in a process of exploring possible futures. To the best of our knowledge, scenarios which relate human health to global and environmental changes are scarce. Some examples do exist, however, of national attempts at envisioning changes to the health system using scenario-based approaches [see 19]. And some global scenario studies exist that describe changes in human health in a globalizing world [20, 21].

15.5 Critical methodological issues in integrated assessment of human health

When dealing with complex, long-term issues surrounded with uncertainties, integrated assessment (IA) models and scenarios seem to be appropriate tools. Even a simplified but integrated model can provide a useful guide to complex issues and complement highly detailed models that cover only some parts of the complexity of disease epidemiology.

However, to improve the health risk assessment by means of integrated assessment, there are several key methodological issues that need our attention. First of all, there is a clear need to validate highly aggregated assessment models on a local or regional scale. The equations within a global model may well be inappropriate for particular local conditions. Second, the unavoidable uncertainties introduced within these models must be treated adequately. Third, quantitative and qualitative approaches need to be combined to obtain a better understanding of the complex human–environment interactions. Finally, although IA modeling deals with a variety of processes on different spatial and temporal scales, there is hardly any experience in linking different scale levels. In the sections below, the focus will be on these issues related to integrated assessment modeling.

15.5.1 Validation in the absence of good data

Validation is defined here as the procedure for testing the adequacy of a given (mathematical) model [22]. With respect to the validation of integrated models, however, there are two major problems. First, complete validation of simulation models is impossible, because the underlying systems are never closed, i.e., lacking essential components [23].

Second, validation is often not possible because the requisite data and scientific knowledge are not available. One of the problems often encountered in applying process-based models in less developed countries is that the models, often adequately validated in the data-rich developed world, are found to be ill suited or poorly calibrated for use in the less developed countries. A paucity of data for validation generally means that data-demanding models can often not be used in such circumstances, and reliance has to be placed on less data-demanding models [24]. Unavailability of data necessitates reliance on simplified assumptions to generate an initial framework for analysis; this framework can be used to focus interdisciplinary communication on assessing health risks and identify priorities for future research. Although the use of such assumptions and simplifications potentially decreases the quantitative accuracy of the assessment, it should still allow for adequate prioritization and estimation of relative risk [25].

Validation can be divided into different types [26, 27]. Data (or pragmatic) validation requires concordance of the model's projections with observational data sets; this concordance can often be assessed by 'testing' the model on historical data sets. However, as mentioned above, the relative inaccuracy and imprecision of ecological and epidemiological data places limits on the model's testability in this way. Conceptual validation requires that the hypotheses and the theoretical structures of the model reasonably describe the perceived real world. This implies that the model structure, relations, parameters and dynamic behavior reflect the prevailing theoretical insights and the key facts relating to that part of reality that the model is supposed to represent.

Although the underlying model relationships may reflect the prevailing theoretical insights well (e.g., the use of the basic reproduction rate or its derivatives to estimate malaria transmission dynamics), this does not necessarily mean that a conceptually valid model will make accurate projections. It remains difficult to validate the highly aggregated outcomes of the global models.

15.5.2 Cumulating uncertainties

Any exploration of future developments inevitably involves a considerable degree of uncertainty. Because of the cross-disciplinary character of IA, it includes many different types and sources of uncertainty. Because IA-models are end-to-end approaches, they also contain an accumulation of uncertainties. Uncertainties may arise from incomplete knowledge of key physiological, chemical and biological processes. Many uncertainties are of a socio-economic nature—related to people's behavior—and reflect inadequate knowledge with respect to the driving forces of human behavior.

Various attempts have been made to classify the different types and sources of uncertainty. Morgan and Henrion [28] distinguish uncertainty about empirical quantities and uncertainty about the functional form of models, which may have arisen from: subjective judgment; disagreement among experts; systematic errors; approximation; and inherent randomness. Funtowicz and Ravetz [29] classified uncertainties in three categories: (i) technical uncertainties (concerning observations versus measurements); (ii) methodological uncertainties (concerning the right choice of analytical tools); and (iii) epistemological uncertainties (concerning the conception of a phenomenon).

Here, the various types and sources of uncertainty are aggregated into two categories [22] (Figure 15.1).

1. Scientific uncertainties arise from the degree of unpredictability of global climate change processes and their impact upon human health, and may be narrowed as a result of further scientific research or more detailed or appropriate modeling. These uncertainties include, for example, incomplete knowledge about the relationships between precipitation patterns and mosquito abundance.

2. Social and economic uncertainties arise from the inherent unpredictability of future geopolitical, socioeconomic, demographic and technological evolution. An example of these future eventualities is trends in urbanization and levels of poverty, which affect the vulnerability and response of human populations to global changes.

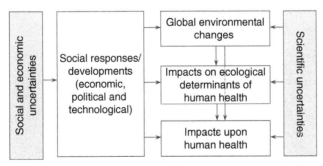

Fig. 15.1 Layers of uncertainty underlying the health impact assessment of global environmental change.

Whatever classification is chosen, the various types and sources of uncertainties in IA-models need to be addressed in an adequate manner. One way of presenting uncertainties is by specifying a set of future scenarios, where the scenarios selected are expected to span a range of plausible, representative futures. The Intergovernmental Panel on Climate Change (IPCC), for example, adopted this approach for its greenhouse gas emissions scenarios. The difficulty with this approach is that it doesn't give an indication of the cumulative uncertainty as well as the origin and meaning of the uncertainty range.

Another approach is the probabilistic method, using a (subjective) probability distribution for empirical quantities. In this method a large numbers of inputs are specified as probability distribution functions, and a number of repeated model runs are done to determine the uncertainties surrounding the output(s). The major difficulty with this method is that it requires specific knowledge about the nature of the distribution functions and the number of runs required. Furthermore, the usage of probability density functions is merely useful to address technical uncertainties. These techniques are not suitable for analyzing methodological and epistemological uncertainties, which primarily arise from subjective judgments and fundamental disagreement among experts. Another problem is that classical uncertainty analysis methods only address uncertainties in model inputs and neglect the interactions among multiple, simultaneous uncertainties which are crucial in IA. Therefore new methods are needed, for example methods in which not only parameters but also relationships within the model are varied (according to the bias and preference of a particular perspective) [30, 31].

15.5.3 Blending qualitative and quantitative knowledge

In most frameworks for IA—including those related to human health—quantitative and qualitative knowledge are considered and treated as mutually exclusive. For instance, usually those aspects of a problem or concern that are not well known, or about which there is only vague and qualitative knowledge, are left out in the modeling process. This means, however, that we miss crucial links in the causal chains that form archetypal patterns of human–environment interactions. Quantitative rigor therefore prevents IA from being comprehensive, in the sense of studying all relevant aspects of a complex problem. It is therefore illusory to think that the full complexity of human–environment interactions could be integrated into a formal, quantitative modeling framework. IA thus needs modeling frameworks that are combinations of quantitative and qualitative approaches, from the perspective that they complement each other.

15.5.4 A matter of scale

One of the most critical issues in IA modeling is that of aggregation versus disaggregation. The problem of modeling the impacts of global (environmental) change processes on human health is that it has to cope with a variety of processes that operate on different temporal and spatial levels and that differ in complexity.

First, IA modeling has to connect disciplinary processes that differ by nature: physical processes, monetary processes, social processes, and policy processes. Because of the multitude of disciplinary processes to be combined, a simple as possible representation of disciplinary knowledge is preferable. There is, however, no unifying theory on how to do this. In addition, the processes to be linked are usually studied in isolation from each other. This isolation is needed as part and parcel of the classic model of scientific progress and discovery. However, when the constraints of isolation are removed, there are a variety of ways in which to connect the reduced pieces of disciplinary knowledge. This manifold of possible integration routes, for which there is no unifying theory, is one of the reasons why quality control is so difficult to achieve in IA modeling. For instance, in order to link the reduced pieces of disciplinary knowledge in a systemic way, one can use elements from classical systems analysis, or the method of system dynamics, or a sequential input–output analysis, or a correlation-based approach, or a pressure-state-impact-response approach.

Second, IA modeling has to deal with different spatial scale levels. One of the ultimate challenges in IA modeling is to connect higher scale assessments with lower scale ones. So far, there has been hardly any experience with playing around with scale levels in IA modeling. Down-scaling or up-scaling the spatial level of a model has profound consequences. This is related to the question to what extent the processes considered are generic, or spatially bound in character. In other words: does a relationship at one scale hold at larger or lower scale levels?

Third, IA modeling is faced with a multitude of temporal scales. Short-term needs and interests of stakeholders have to be considered. However, biogeochemical processes usually operate on a long time scale, whereas economic processes operate on short to medium timescales. Another challenging aspect of IA modeling is to interconnect long-term targets as specified as a result of analyzing processes operating on longer term time scales, with short-term goals for concrete policy actions. Unfortunately, there is not yet a sound scientific method to achieve this, and thus far, only heuristic methods have been used.

The trend in current (IA) modeling is to move toward greater and greater disaggregation, assuming that this yields better models [32]. In general, it is difficult to know when to stop building more detail into an IA model. Past decades of model building have shown that small and transparent models are often superior in that they provide similar results to large models faster and offer ease of use. In this respect, it is useful to distinguish between *complicated* and *complex* models. Complicated models are models that include a variety of processes, many of which may be interlinked. If incremental changes in these processes generally lead to incremental changes in model output, one can conclude that the dynamics of the model are almost linear and not complex at all. The more complicated the model, the higher the possibility of errors and bugs. It requires thorough testing to pick up most if not all errors and bugs, an activity, which is, unfortunately, heavily underrated. Complex models, however, contain relatively few processes, but incremental changes in these processes may result in considerable changes in the results of the overall model. This non-linear behavior, due to the inclusion of feedbacks, adaptation, self-learning, and chaotic behavior, is often unpredictable.

Practically speaking, this means that disaggregation of IA models has profound consequences for the dynamics of the model. Breaking down a global model into various regions requires that the regional dynamics be dealt with in an adequate manner. Current regional

IA models use grid cells or classes for representing geographical differences and heterogeneities in regional IA models. However, they do not capture the regional dynamics with regard to population growth and health, economic development, resource use or environmental degradation, let alone regional interactions through migration and trade.

15.6 The way ahead

The advent of global environmental change, with its complexities, uncertainties and substantial displacement into the future tense, brings new challenges and tasks for science, public and policy. The advent of this research task also poses a political and moral dilemma. Many serious and continuing local environmental health hazards are being faced. Poor populations around the world are exposed to unsafe drinking water, microbiologically contaminated or, in the case of Bangladesh, containing toxic levels of arsenic. Environmental lead has been widely dispersed in the modern world, via industry, traffic exhausts and old house-paints; it continues to blight intellectual development in children. Urban populations face continuing hazards from air pollution. Persistent organic pollutants being spread. All of these environmental health issues must continue to command our attention. Yet, now, we must also extend the agenda of research and policy advice to include the larger-framed environmental change issues as emerging hazards to the health of current and future populations.

We are entering a century in which science must increasingly engage in issues relating to the processes and consequences of changes to ecological systems, be they the systems of the natural biosphere, the biophysical systems of global climate, or the increasingly large and complex social systems in which we live out our lives. During the last decades, IA models have proven themselves as legitimate and powerful approaches to complex issues. Particularly in the climate change debate, IA models have contributed by exploring impacts of climate change and evaluating mitigation and abatement strategies. IA models have also provided useful information on balancing the carbon budget, the role of sulphate aerosols, and on various aspects of land use. Integrated assessment modeling of human health is one of the latest branches of the IA tree.

However, there is still a long way to go before IA models will be fully accepted by the scientific modeling community on the one hand, and by the decision-making community on the other. Therefore, an ultimate challenge for IA modeling is to build up scientific and political credibility. To improve both scientific and political credibility of IA models, IA scholars should enhance IA models, improve the communication with disciplinary scientific and policy-making communities, and enrich and augment communication techniques.

As the *full* complexity of the interactions between global developments and human health cannot be satisfactorily reduced to modeling, what is the role of such modeling? Despite the difficulties and limitations of the modeling process, models first of all draw attention to the potential health impact of these global changes. Second, they may indicate the relative importance of the factors that influence these outcomes. This enhances public discussion, education and policy-making. However, an even more important is the role (integrated) modeling plays in the systematic linkage of multiple cause and effect relationships based on available knowledge and reasoned guesses. This should increase our understanding of the health impacts of global changes and identify key gaps in data and knowledge needed to improve the analysis of these effects.

15.7 **References**

[1] **IPCC.** *Climate change 1995: impacts, adaptations and mitigation of climate change: scientific-technical analyses.* New York: Cambridge University Press 1996.

[2] **IPCC.** *Climate change 2001: the scientific basis.* Cambridge: Cambridge University Press 2001.

[3] **Aron JL, Patz JA, eds.** *Ecosystem change and public health.* Baltimore, MD: The Johns Hopkins University Press 2001.

[4] **Martens P, McMichael A, eds.** *Environmental change, climate and health: issues and research methods.* Cambridge, UK: Cambridge University Press 2002.

[5] **Lindgren E, Tälleklint L, Polfeld T.** Impact of climatic change on the northern latitude limit and population density of the disease-transmitting European tick *Ixodes Ricans. Environmental Health Perspectives.* 2000 **108**:119–23.

[6] **Martens P, McMichael AJ, Patz J.** Globalisation, environmental change and health. *Global Change and Human Health.* 2000 **1**(1):4–8.

[7] **Slaper H, Velders GJM, Daniel JS, de Gruijl FR, van der Leun JC.** Estimates of ozone depletion and skin cancer incidence to examine the Vienna Convention achievements. *Nature.* 1996 **384**:256–8.

[8] **Martens P, den Elzen MGJ, Slaper H, Koken PJM, Willems BAT.** The impact of ozone depletion on skin cancer incidence: an assessment of the Netherlands and Australia. *Environmental Modeling and Assessment.* 1996 1(4):229–40.

[9] **Epstein PR.** Climate and health. *Science.* 1999 **285**:347–8.

[10] **Gleick P.** *The world's water: the biennial report on freshwater resources 2000–2001.* Washington DC: Island Press 2000.

[11] **Schwartz MW, Brigham CA.** Linking biodiversity to ecosystem function: implications for conservation ecology. *Oecologica.* 2000 **122**:297–305.

[12] **Weinstein MC, Coxson PG, Williams LW, Pass TM, Stason WB, Goldman L.** Forecasting coronary heart disease incidence, mortality and cost: the coronary heart policy model. *American Journal of Public Health.* 1987 **77**:1417–26.

[13] **Martens P.** *Health and climate change: modeling the impacts of global warming and ozone depletion.* London: Earthscan Publications Ltd 1998.

[14] **Rotmans J, de Vries HJM, eds.** *Perspectives on global change: the TARGETS approach.* Cambridge: Cambridge University Press 1997.

[15] **Hilderink H.** *World population in transition: an integrated regional modeling framework.* Amsterdam: Thela Thesis 2000.

[16] **Martens P.** *MIASMA: Modeling framework for the health impact assessment of man-induced atmospheric changes – CD ROM. Electronic Series on Integrated Assessment Modeling (ESIAM), Vol 2.* Bussum, The Netherlands: Baltzer Scientific Publishers 1999.

[17] **Parry M, Carter T.** *Climate impact and adaptation assessment.* London: Earthscan Publications Ltd 1998.

[18] **Berkhout F, Hertin J, Jordan A.** Socio economic futures in climate change impact assessment: using scenarios as 'learning machines'. *Global Environmental Change.* 2002 **12**(2):83–95.

[19] **Murray G.** Alternative future paths for Ontario hospitals. In: Dopson S, Mark AL, eds. *Leading health care organizations.* London: Palgrave MacMillan 2003: 196–213.

[20] Martens P. Health transitions in a globalising world: towards more disease or sustained health? *Futures*. 2002 **37**(7):635–48.

[21] Martens P, Huynen MMTE. A future without health? The health dimension in global scenario studies. *Bulletin of the World Health Organization*. 2003 **81**(12):896–901.

[22] Rotmans J, Asselt MBAv, Bruin AJd, Elzen MGJd, Greef Jd, Hilderink H, *et al*. *Global change and sustainable development*. Globo Report Series No. 4. Bilthoven, The Netherlands: RIVM (National Institute of Public Health and the Environment); 1994. Report No. 461502004.

[23] Oreskes N, Shrader-Frechette K, Belitz K. Verification, validation, and confirmation of numerical models in the earth sciences. *Science*. 1994 **263**(February):641–6.

[24] Carter TR, Parry ML, Harasawa H, Nishioka S. *IPCC technical guidelines for assessing climate change impacts and adaptations*. London: University College London; 1994.

[25] Patz JA, Balbus JM. Methods for assessing public health vulnerability to global climate change. *Climate Research*. 1996 **6**:113–25.

[26] Rodin EY, ed. *Mathematical modeling: a tool for problem solving in engineering, physical, biological and social sciences*. Oxford: Pergamon Press 1990.

[27] Rykiel EJ. Testing ecological models: the meaning of validation. *Ecological Modeling*. 1996 **90**:229–44.

[28] Morgan GM, Henrion M. *Uncertainty – a guide to dealing with uncertainty in quantitative risk and policy analysis*. New York: Cambridge University Press 1990.

[29] Funtowicz SO, Ravetz JR. *Uncertainty and quality in science for policy*. Dordrecht, The Netherlands: Kluwer 1990.

[30] van Asselt MBA. *Perspectives on uncertainty and risk: the PRIMA approach to decision support*. Dordrecht, The Netherlands: Kluwer 2000.

[31] Janssen M. *Modeling global change: the art of integrated assessment modeling*. Cheltenham: Edward Elgar Publishing Limited 1998.

[32] Rotmans J, van Asselt MBA. Integrated assessment modeling. In: Martens P, Rotmans J, eds. *Climate change: an integrated perspective*. Dordrecht, the Netherlands: Kluwer Publishers 1999: 239–75.

Chapter 16

The role and limits of epidemiology in policy arguments

Raymond Neutra

16.1 Introduction

For the purposes of this chapter, 'environmental health policy arguments' is taken to refer to arguments related to decisions about ongoing practices with regard to the physical and chemical environment that are likely to affect rates of disability, disease and death in the human population. This chapter will focus on ways that etiological epidemiology enters into the policy process. The many ways that descriptive epidemiology can be used to inform policy will not be covered here, for it has been admirably discussed elsewhere [1].

Upstream decisions about such things as investment in rail versus freeways may not be primarily motivated by health concerns, yet they profoundly affect health and thus qualify as environmental health policy. Downstream decisions about such things as automobile emission standards are motivated by health concerns and clearly qualify. It will be argued that the positions on policy of those who have a stake in decisions (stakeholders) are influenced by: their particular interests (how each option affects *their* pocket book and *their* health), their concerns about the costs and benefits to society at large, and very importantly, the ethical frameworks (ideology) that they bring to bear on the policy question at hand. There is no technically correct way to resolve differences in interest or conflicts about ideology. In a democracy, these are resolved through some kind of political process, hopefully one with a level playing field. Interestingly, adherents to the different ethical frameworks described below have preferences, not only for certain types of environmental policy options but also for certain styles of arriving at decisions. Politicians tend to use health scientists as gatekeepers to the initiation of policy discussions (Is there a health problem here requiring a policy decision, yes or no? If you aren't virtually certain don't embroil me in a policy argument!). However, health facts are only part of the environmental health policy-forming process; costs, interests and ideologies are often more influential. Furthermore, most stakeholders use the 'precautionary principle' and do not require a proof of harm 'beyond a reasonable doubt' to decide if a potential health risk warrants a policy decision. So, the epidemiologist can profoundly affect whether stakeholders are properly informed as they engage in the political processes that will ultimately form policy by:

- the format that the epidemiologist uses to frame his or her degree of certainty of a hazard;

- the transparency of the argument he or she uses to explain what warranted that degree of certainty; as well as

- the display of facts about who is exposed and who is particularly sensitive to that exposure.

These matters are the topic of this chapter.

16.2 Upstream and downstream policies

If one follows the strands of the causal web backward from disturbed health through immediate environmental causes to antecedent conditions, one finds that upstream decisions about land use, economic organization, investment in energy, transportation and agricultural technologies and the like are the ultimate causes of the downstream environmental conditions that originally influenced the risk of ill-health. Epidemiologists typically study the consequences of these downstream effects on health, but increasingly in health impact assessment (see Chapter 14), environmental epidemiologists will be asked to review the literature of downstream epidemiology to list the possible effects of upstream policy decisions and to estimate their approximate magnitudes and impacts on different segments of the population so that the health consequences of these decisions can be considered along with other societal pros and cons. Examples of upstream decisions that can impact health might include whether or not to put in a new dam that could alter vector habitat, choosing to subsidize sprawl and the automobile rather than denser in-fill development, or locating chemical industry sites near residences.

16.3 Stakeholders' ethical frameworks drive informational needs and policy preferences

16.3.1 Ethical frameworks

Making policy in the face of uncertainty is characteristic of many public health issues. However, stakeholders often come to the table, at least for the purposes of the problem at hand, with different ethical frameworks (ideologies). They use these in approaching problems that involve both voluntary and involuntary exposures. Many arguments about policy choices are really arguments about ethical frameworks. Ethics is the domain of discussion of what is good and what is right. The classification of ethical frameworks used here is an adaptation of classifications used by others [2, 3].

Utilitarians

Economists, engineers, epidemiologists and regulatory agencies often use a predominantly results-oriented, *utilitarian* framework. Anyone using this framework considers his or her options for a number of criteria. The criteria focus on expected good and bad results that would flow from choosing each considered option. The utilitarian chooses the option that produces the best balance of 'goods'. In order to find the option with the best balance of goods, the utilitarian stakeholder may assign dollar values to tangible criteria, such as project costs, or even to esthetic consequences or quality-adjusted years of human lives saved. When stakeholders using this approach end up advocating different courses of action because they have different interests, the utilitarian resolves the conflict by choosing the solution that aims at producing the 'best possible results for the most individuals at the least cost'. Sometimes this ignores the interests of a substantial minority in society.

Duty ethicists

On many issues, members of the general public do not adhere to the utilitarian framework. Often they adhere either to a *duty ethics* framework that tries to fulfill positive duties to others or to protect rights. Politically, liberal stakeholders on the left tend to emphasize the duty of the state to protect and nurture the weak, vulnerable and disadvantaged. They advocate precautionary expenditures in the health, environment and education sectors [4]. Politically conservative stakeholders on the right tend to emphasize the duty of the state to protect one's community from hostile insiders or outsiders. They advocate precautionary expenditures with a low degree of certainty about threats in the criminal justice and military sectors to punish insiders and outsiders who offend. Duty ethics pays little if any attention to the cost of complying with duties. It has been said that one ought to honor one's mother and father even if it is not cost-effective to do so!

Libertarians

Another variant of duty ethics is espoused by stakeholders who adhere to a 'non-interference' (or *libertarian*) framework, which places emphasis on so-called negative rights—the rights of the individual and his property to be free from governmental interference. Conservative duty ethicists and libertarians tend to resist government expenditures on environmental programs on ideological grounds and sometimes adopt a 'virtual certainty required' scientific standard for taking any environmental health action. Adherents to utilitarianism, duty ethics and libertarianism are all focused on human individuals. From these frameworks, the physical environment derives its importance from its role in the welfare of a collection of individual human beings. Even the utilitarian who aims at the 'best possible result for the most individuals at the least cost' arrives at this determination by conceptually adding up the results of each individual in society. This focus on the individual arose in Europe during the Renaissance and the Enlightenment.

Communitarians

The *communitarian* frameworks provide a strong alternative to this individualistic approach. They are oriented toward creating a certain kind of community in which 'community' may include non-human species, or even an ecosystem. For some variants of the communitarian frameworks, the ecosystem has 'rights' that are independent of human rights. *Traditional communitarian* values are generally defined by a moral elite group of elders. For example, among the Old Order Amish, an orthodox Protestant group in America, elders decide for the community which technologies should be adopted as compatible with a sustainable Christ-like community atmosphere [5]. This is the decision framework that operates in much of the non-Western world and is followed by fundamentalist religious groups even in modern Western countries. The less traditional *relativist communitarians* believe that each community, through some political process, defines the principles of what is good for the community and which options to pursue (usually a qualitative ethical analysis).

Ethics of care

Recently, feminist thinkers have advanced an *ethics of care*, which might be said to ask the question, 'How would you want to treat everyone in society if you imagined yourself as everyone's mother?'[3, 6]. This approach would pay attention to the particularities of a situation; would not be as driven by rigid adherence to the abstract principles favored by men [7]; would not assume that everyone ought to be treated equally; and would focus on results but not with the cold impartiality of utilitarianism [8].

16.3.2 Frameworks and policy preference

Adherents to diverse frameworks might prefer different policy options. For example, suppose a municipality that owned its own electrical utility decided that it was probable that electric and magnetic fields (EMFs) from power lines and appliances were hazardous and wanted to do something about it. The utilitarians in town might recommend that the municipal utility pay for the most cost-effective measures to reduce exposure, even if the responsible source itself was not mitigated. For example, they might decide to buy up enough old, high-exposure electric blankets and replace them with no-exposure eider down quilts to prevent as much disease as the power grid would supposedly be causing.

The adherents to the duty ethics framework might point out that the minority of people living next to the power grid would still be at unequal risk. Some, but not all, of them might invoke a strong form of the Precautionary Principle—that expensive avoidance policies would be warranted on the basis of a few credible scientists suspecting a small risk that violates the safety of even a small group of people. They might say that following the precepts of environmental justice, there is a special duty to protect this group if it were particularly vulnerable to EMFs, had less access to medical care or had been unfairly singled out for EMF exposure on the basis of low-income levels, race or previous exposures to other hazards. From this perspective, environmental agents like EMFs should be treated as 'guilty until proven innocent'. They would question the underlying assumption which is frequently found in cost–benefit analysis: young, rich, healthy lives of this generation are worth more than elderly, poor disabled lives of future generations [9]. Therefore, those advocating this framework would propose that the people living near the power lines should be protected by modifying the lines to lower fields, even if it were more expensive than buying up old electric blankets. They might also invoke the duty of the utility to clean up its own mess at its own expense.

The libertarian adherents to 'non-interference' might oppose both of these options because they involve involuntarily taxing the many for the benefit of the few. Regardless of the degree of confidence in the existence of an EMF hazard, they might prefer a 'right to know' information program that would require the labeling of transmission towers, rental agreements and documents during home sales to allow the free market and voluntary actions of those who were concerned to solve the problem.

Adherents to a communitarian framework might focus on a solution that fit some set of duties and rights of the community as a whole. The elders of the traditional Old Order Amish decided that electricity and all the appliances that go with it and the dependence it brings on the surrounding godless society was something to be avoided, except in refrigerators in the cow barn [5].

16.3.3 Epidemiological facts required by different ideologies

Utilitarians, who are interested in the best results for the most people, tend to focus on the population burden of ill health (e.g., the population attributable risk) as a parameter of interest. If there is uncertainty about whether an epidemiological association is truly causal, the utilitarian is willing to weight the observed effect by one's degree of certainty that it is causal to get a kind of 'expected effect'.

Duty ethics adherents focus on the individual lifetime theoretical added risk of the most highly exposed (which is based on the epidemiologist's attributable risk among the exposed). This is because the duty ethics framework and the law tend to focus on protecting the individual from risks that are more than *de minimis* (one added case per million lives in some American regulations). The duty ethics policy framework adherents will be particularly interested to learn if an exposure is distributed unfairly in the population, or if disadvantaged groups are more vulnerable to an exposure. These epidemiological facts about who is exposed and who is particularly vulnerable are often ignored in the design or in the reporting of epidemiological studies. To be relevant to the societal formation of policy, these facts need to be documented. For example, as part of a power line policy analysis [10], a geographic information system (GIS) analysis was done to determine what proportion of transmission lines run through residential areas and if poor neighborhoods or neighborhoods of color were disproportionately impacted (they were not).

16.3.4 Frameworks and preferred process and analysis

The traditional communitarians (let the elites decide) and the libertarians (let each individual and the market decide) favor nonpolitical processes for making policy. The social justice ethicists, relativist communitarians, ethics of care adherents, and the utilitarians recognize that some political process will be necessary for making decisions but the political process can take many guises. It could range from direct democracy through referendums, the usual kind of representative democratic and administrative procedures, to some special democratic procedure that provides special resources to 'level the playing field' and assures that representatives of powerful *and* powerless stakeholders, properly informed, play equal roles in making a decision, or at least a policy recommendation through ad hoc juries, science courts or the like. Table 16.1 summarizes the ethical frameworks, their focus of attention, the type of policy analysis they favor and the forum they favor for making a decision.

16.3.5 **Interests influence the choice of framework**

Stakeholders often try to satisfy more than one ethical framework in choosing a course of action, either because a particular stakeholder sees the merit in several frameworks or because adherents to individual frameworks bargain with each other to find solutions that attend to more than one framework. It should be noted that in real life, a self-interest that overrides any ethical concern for the common good is often at work. Usually stakeholders motivated by selfish interests invoke arguments from one of the above frameworks that address the common good to advance their case. It should also be acknowledged that a given stakeholder, while tending to adhere to one or the other policy or ethical framework most of the time on the basis of philosophical sympathies, may shift frameworks from issue to issue or even on the same issue, depending on his or her interests and the ratio of opportunity and risk presented by the options being considered. Margolis [11] has argued that we have all developed shortcut paradigms to deal with different combinations of opportunity and risk. When faced with a potential risk that offers us no benefit or opportunity, we use the 'better safe than sorry' paradigm. This is true no matter how uncertain the hazard or how small the probability of its affecting us. Under this paradigm only two possibilities are salient—the unattractive risky option and 'anything but that' option. As soon as the risk is accompanied by opportunity, or its avoidance is accompanied by inconvenience or cost, we tend to flip to the 'Is this a good deal?' paradigm. This 'flipping' has something of the quality of the transition between two perceptions of the famous visual illusion drawing that can either be perceived as an old lady or a duck. Once flipped into the duck perception, it is hard to imagine how one could have seen an old lady. Margolis gives the example of the New York parents who were enraged that the school district had endangered their children by not removing asbestos cladding from pipes in their schools ('better safe than sorry'). When the school administrators announced that schools would be closed in the fall to remove the asbestos and reopened for compensatory months in the summer, the parents were outraged that they were being inconvenienced and required to find childcare in response to such a trivial risk ('Is this a good deal?'). Margolis believes that stakeholders derive their paradigms from their perceived narrow interests and that they advance arguments about moral duties, unfair exercise of power, untrustworthy behavior of government and their concerns about involuntary exposures to dreaded agents as an afterthought and justification. While policy makers must be alert for stakeholders who adjust their policy frameworks to conform to and justify their narrow parochial interests, it is clear that financial interests are only part of the story, and that the concept of ethical frameworks helps to

Table 16.1 Ethical frameworks and their characteristics

General Class	Framework	Main focus	Concerned with cost and efficiency?	Concerned with which subgroup is at risk?	Preferred style of analysis	Favored decision forum
Duty/Rights	Traditional communitarian	Preservation of community	No	Yes	Qualitative ethical	Ethical elite decides
	Relativist communitarian	Preservation of community	No	Yes	Qualitative ethical	Some 'level playing field' democratic process
	Social justice	Individual positive rights and duties	No	Yes, focuses on lifetime added risk	Qualitative ethical	Special 'level playing field' process
	Libertarian	Negative rights, autonomy, freedom from interference, 'right to know'	No	Only if HE is at risk	Left to each individual	'Right to know' lets each individual and the market solve the problem
Results	Utilitarian	Best results for the most individuals at the least cost	Yes, costs are important	No, focuses on population attrib. risk	Quantitative analysis of costs and benefits	Experts provide analysis options to political forum
	Ethic of care	Compassionate results	No	Yes	Flexible, qualitative ethical	Democratic process

explain many public policy conflicts. There is no technical solution for choosing between these ethical frameworks [12], or for choosing a course of action when there are winners and losers in all of the possible courses of action. A democracy handles differences in interests and differences in ethical frameworks through the political process. It can be helpful in those political discussions to recognize when differences in ethical frameworks are driving the discussion because sometimes policy adjustments can address those ethical concerns. Bernstein *et al.* [13] present some practical guidance to contending stakeholders who wish to reach an environmental health policy despite the fact that they have different interests, ethical frameworks and perceptions of the scientific facts. Special resources and plenty of time are needed if all stakeholders are to have access to the policy process.

On a sobering note for epidemiologists, Sabatier and Jenkins-Smith [14] believe that policies are formed when stakeholders and government officials who share similar duty ethics frameworks form alliances. They then use technical and utilitarian 'best results' arguments to justify their preferred course of action. These alliances may require political work for many years to achieve their desired policy goals. This suggests that research into facts, of which epidemiology is an example, is often only marginally influential and sometimes may only be used as window dressing late in the policy process.

16.4 **A basic policy question**

Many environmental health policy questions can be formulated in the following way:

> All other things being equal, how certain must we be of how much ill-health before we would opt for cheap or expensive protective alternatives?

As we have already pointed out, the adherents to different policy frameworks prefer to approach questions such as these in different ways, with or without formal quantitative analysis.

Since the utilitarians will do an elaborate quantitative analysis of the various options available for addressing the problem at hand, and it is in this style of analysis that epidemiological information plays the greatest role, I examine this role through the lens of that kind of analysis. In a later section we consider the role of the epidemiologist in the more qualitative styles of policy analysis. The utilitarians would tend to represent the problem as a decision tree with a decision node branching between inaction, cheap and expensive protective practices, and with probability nodes representing the degree of certainty about the health consequences of the several courses of action. Ashford [15] has suggested that the consequences should be considered separately from the viewpoint of each of the main stakeholders, while the classical utilitarian considers the problem as if society was either one hypothetical 'person' or one large happy family, averaging over the divergent interests of the 'family members' to achieve the best possible results for the majority of individuals at the least cost. Rawls [16] has said that the 'fault of the utilitarian doctrine is that it mistakes impersonality for impartiality', where impersonality is ignoring the separate interests of individuals and impartiality is recognizing them as

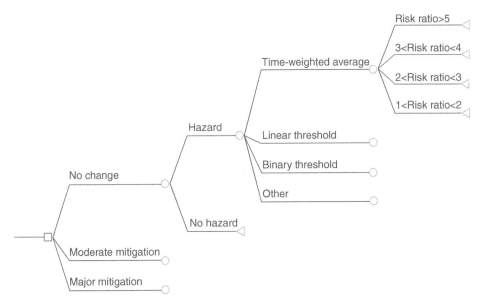

Fig. 16.1 Example of a utilitarian decision tree partially dependent on epidemiological information.

separate but deciding not to give particular weight to one's own interests in designated situations.

Figure 16.1 represents a schematic tree that requires the epidemiologist to specify the probability of a health hazard from magnetic fields from transmission lines that might result from the status quo, cheap, or expensive remedial actions. The epidemiologist must also specify the probability that varying exposure metrics are relevant and how probable are different types of dose–response curves. Each of the courses of action has costs and consequences including death, property value impacts, reliability of the power grid, etc. [17].

16.5 **What epidemiologists can and cannot bring to the decision tree**

The epidemiologist can bring some but not all of the ingredients needed for the contending stakeholders to work out an answer to the solution to a decision tree such as that in Figure 16.1. Listed below are the ingredients potentially brought by the epidemiologist. The items with an asterisk are ones of particular interest to adherents to the social justice duty ethics, communitarian and ethics-of-care frameworks:

- Based on the biological and epidemiological literature and community suspicions, which health conditions should be considered?
- What are the background-, age-, sex- and race-specific rates of these diseases?
- What is the probability that various exposure metrics are biologically relevant?

- What is the distribution of these exposure metrics in the population (including facts about unequal exposures to disadvantaged populations)?*

- How would inaction, or cheap or expensive remedial action shift the probability of exposure in the population (paying attention to facts about likely consequences to disadvantaged populations)?*

- What is the shape of the dose–response curve?

- What changes in added lifetime risk to highly exposed individuals from the several options are suggested by the epidemiological results?*

- What changes to the population burden of ill health from the several options are suggested by the epidemiological results (considering how the options influence the population exposure distribution)?

- Do the epidemiological results suggest a special vulnerability to exposure among disadvantaged populations?*

- What is the epidemiologist's degree of certainty that the epidemiological associations are largely causal in nature?

For most situations, the answers to many or all of these questions are quite uncertain. Even in the ideal situation, the epidemiologist only brings information about the probability nodes in the decision tree, but has no special expertise on the costs or the proper values to be assigned to the consequences that flow from pursuing the various options. Nor does the epidemiologist have any unique expertise in performing the kind of ethical analysis that would appeal to adherents of the duty ethics, communitarian, ethics of care or libertarian ethical frameworks. As an ordinary citizen of the society to which he or she belongs, the epidemiologist has the right and indeed duty to weigh in on these issues, but one should not assume that policy decisions hinge only on the probabilities about which the epidemiologist has expertise. Although there is controversy about whether an epidemiologist should be an advocate and always argue for the healthiest option [18, 19], everyone would agree that it is the epidemiologist's duty to provide the information needed by stakeholders formatted in a way that facilitates policy discussion.

16.6 **Alternative framings of the basic policy question**

Stirling and Gee [20] point out that researchers are often faced with situations in which they are hard-pressed to express their certainty about the hazardousness of an agent or the estimated rate of disease among those exposed to different levels of that hazard. This is particularly true of upstream decisions, or generic decisions about which procedures to follow with a class of new products. For example, when the US Federal Drug Administration decided that all drugs must pass efficacy and safety tests prior to going on the market and must be subject to post-market surveillance for unforeseen untoward side-effects, it would have been difficult to answer the question, 'How certain must we be of how much ill health before we opt for this full-blown system?' Stirling and Gee argue for generic precautionary strategies of flexibility, surveillance and intermittent re-evaluation in situations like this.

16.7 Formatting conclusions to accommodate different frameworks

Instead of saying, 'There is no conclusive evidence that *x* is safe or dangerous', a graduated format such as the one used in the California EMF risk evaluation [21] provides a

Table 16.2 Graduated Risk Format used in the California EMF Risk Evaluation.

Degree of certainty	
Is Agent X at the 95th percentile exposure home or at work safe, or does Agent X increase the risk of …….. to some degree?	*Degree of willingness to certify causality on a scale of 0 to 100*
Certify with virtual certainty that it increase the risk to some degree	>99.5
Strongly certify that it increases the risk to some degree	90 to 99.5
Prone to certify that it increases the risk to some degree	60 to 90
Close to the dividing line between certifying or not certifying that Agent x increases the risk to some degree	40 to 60
Prone to certify that it does not increase the risk to any degree	10 to 40
Strongly certify that it does not increase the risk to any degree	0.5 to 10
Certify with virtual certainty that it does not increase the risk to any degree	<0.5

From Neutra and Delpizzo [21].

more informative format. On a scale from 0 to 100 we demarcate 'willingness to certify causality-zones' such as 'prone to certify as hazardous' or 'certify with virtual certainty'. Using the term 'willingness to certify' makes clear the nature of the social transaction that is documented on this scale. It is not announcing a state of mind (belief) or measuring some Platonic quality of nature (probability); it is making a judgment according to an orderly procedure (certification).

The degree of certification in this table, that agent *x* increases the risk of disease *y* 'to some degree', is *not* the probability of getting the disease if one is highly exposed. Thus, one can be virtually certain (99 on a scale of 100) that asbestos adds to the baseline 1/100 000/year risk of mesothelioma without implying that 99 percent of those exposed to asbestos will develop mesothelioma. To minimize that misunderstanding, expressing the certainty as a percentage was avoided. A number within the degree of certainty zone in the table is also different from the number that the tort lawyer and workman's compensation board would like to have: 'How certain are you that this particular patient's disease was caused by the exposure to agent *x*?' One might be virtually certain (99 on a scale of 100) that agent *x*, at high exposures, increases risk of disease *y* by a factor of 1.2, but that doesn't mean that one is virtually certain that this exposed patient derived his disease from his exposure to agent x. Greenland [22] has written about what inferences can and cannot be drawn from epidemiological evidence to make claims about individual patients. To minimize confusion with that tort lawyer's certainty, the scale was not cut at 50 and terms such as 'more likely than not' or 'beyond a reasonable doubt', which are conventionally used to refer to a particular patient, were not used.

16.8 The structure of causal reasoning by epidemiologists

Two questions must be asked: 'How can one move from patterns of observed evidence to claiming a degree of 'willingness to certify causality?' and 'How can we display the evidence and our reasoning so that it is transparent and understandable to stakeholders who want to use and evaluate our judgments as part of the policy process?'

An epidemiological argument can be broken down into the same elements that Toulmin [23] has discerned in scientific, legal, management and aesthetic arguments. First, one has the 'grounds', the pattern of observed results from a series of 'evidentiary tests', along with how certain one was *a priori* that this factor was a credible component cause. One then has some inferential criteria that warrant upward or downward changes in one's degree of certainty on the basis of the results of the evidentiary tests. These inferential criteria (or warrants) in turn have some well-known factual *backing*. Finally, one has the acknowledgement of some caveats or *rebuttals* to the warrant. An argument making a claim about diagnostic certainty could be diagrammed, as in Figure 16.2 [21].

Now follows a discussion of some of the components of the argument as they apply to the epidemiologist, starting with some observations on the factual grounds.

16.8.1 The grounds

16.8.1.1 Fair and policy-neutral displays of evidence and description of evidentiary tests

An important element of the evidentiary grounds of an epidemiological argument is a transparent display of the body of evidence. For example, one might graphically display the relative risks observed in a series of studies along with their confidence intervals and the meta-analytic summary with its confidence limits. Another element of the grounds would be a series of interpretative evidentiary tests done on the study or studies being evaluated. Thus, one test might be, 'Is that meta-analytic rate ratio, indistinguishable from 1.00, is it moderate or is it well above the detection limit?' Suppose that the 'test result' was 'it is well above the detection limit'. When we get to the inferential warrant, we will have some guidance as to what one may infer from such a rate ratio.

One must be careful to describe the results of these evidentiary tests in policy-neutral language. The language that is often used to describe the pattern of evidence upon which we ground our reasoning carries hidden policy preconceptions:

'The meta-analytic association between the agent and the disease was *weak*' instead of, 'The meta-analytic association between the agent and disease was *just detectable given the size and quality of*

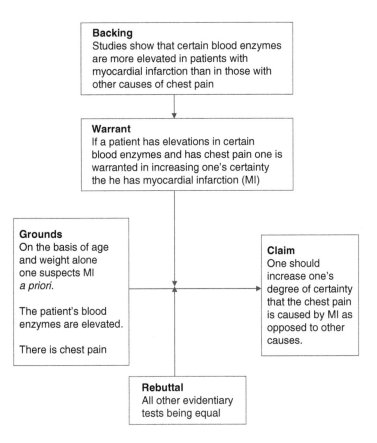

Fig. 16.2 The structure of an argument supporting a diagnostic claim.

the studies available.' The adjectives *weak* or *small* suggest the association, if real, would be unimportant, while in fact any association that 'even an epidemiologist can see' is likely to be of regulatory significance if it turns about to be causal in nature. The preferred wording anchors the size relative to methodological considerations.

Sometimes language is used to describe a body of evidence that could easily be misunderstood. For example, the phrase, 'There is *no evidence* that agent *x* causes disease *y*' does not reveal whether it means:

- 'No one has ever studied whether agent *x* causes disease *y*';
- 'Only literature of poor quality exist to date, and they do not suggest that agent *x* causes disease *y*';
- 'There is an abundant quantity of mechanistic, toxicological and epidemiological studies which meets and exceeds the usual standards of methodological quality, and all of the studies fail to demonstrate an association between agent *x* and disease *y*'.

When describing a body of evidence, we should be careful to characterize its volume, its quality, its consistency, and the size and direction of the observed effect relative to the power and quality of the studies to detect any effect.

16.8.1.2 Initial (*a priori*) credibility

The other component of the grounds is the initial or *a priori* credibility of the hypothesis that *x* could be a component cause of disease *y* on the basis of evidence available prior to knowing the results of this particular series of studies. In the diagrammed example, the doctor was influenced by *a priori* knowledge of the prevalence, in her area, of the various causes of acute chest pain and the age and weight of the patient prior to getting the results of the blood test.

Epidemiologists rarely make their *a priori* judgments explicit, yet disagreements about these judgments are at the root of many epidemiological controversies. For example, some physicists, on the basis of basic thermodynamic principles applied to simplified models of biological systems, are so convinced that the magnetic fields from power lines are incapable of producing physiological change that no amount of epidemiological evidence can outweigh their low *a priori* degree of certainty. Thomas Bayes, an eighteenth-century mathematician, recognized the importance of the *a priori* degree of certainty [24]. His insights suggest to start with some initial degree of certainty that an agent is capable of being harmful based on knowledge about agents in general. Evidence is then accumulated on this specific agent, and this may change the degree of suspicion or certainty.

16.8.2 The warrant

This brings us to the inferential criteria that one uses to evaluate the evidence and warrant any changes of certainty from one's initial (*a priori*) position. Many epidemiological arguments arise because the protagonists have not specified ahead of time what changes in their certainty they think the potential results of evidentiary tests warrant. Here, it will be argued that the hypothesis for which the observed pattern of evidence is most likely warrants the greatest increase of certainty from whatever its initial credibility was. This brings us to Bayes' theorem.

16.8.2.1 Bayes' theorem

As evidence builds, the degree of certainty of harm gets updated, but at any point in time that updated degree of certainty also depends on how suspicious we were initially. This idea is expressed mathematically by a simple version of Bayes' theorem [25]. (See Greenland [26] for a general discussion of Bayes' theorem and probability in epidemiology.)

$$\text{Prior Odds} * \text{Relative Likelihood of Evidence} = \text{Posterior Odds}$$

The first term of the Bayes' theorem is the prior odds, that is, the odds that a given hypothesis is thought to merit *a priori*, before examining the evidence. In this document it is called 'the prior' because it is based on evidence available prior to the current evaluation.

The second term, the 'relative likelihood,' is a multiplier, calculated (or qualitatively discussed) after scientific evidence has been collected and evaluated. The term relative likelihood is most properly restricted to the case where one compares the statistical likelihood of a result under one specific hypothesis relative to that under another hypothesis, usually the null hypothesis that x does not cause y. The term is used more broadly here. The relative likelihood expresses the likelihood of the observed pattern of evidence if the suspected agent did indeed cause disease, divided by the likelihood of that pattern if that agent did not cause disease.

The third term, the posterior odds, is the product of the first two and represents the odds of the risk being true after considering the prior evidence as well as our evaluation of the new evidence. Medical diagnosis is an example where the likelihood of evidence from medical history, physical examination and a series of laboratory test results taken in combination are evaluated for each of several possible diagnostic causes of the patient's problem. A degree of certainty is developed about the several possible causes of a patient's illness by considering both the relative likelihoods of the pattern of evidence and the prior odds of the diagnostic entity being present. While the idea of relative likelihood has increasingly entered into medical education [27], Musen *et al.* [28] point out that several approaches that have been taken to reduce this process to a computerized automatic procedure have not been successful. Similarly, epidemiological causal inference, which involves evaluating and weighting the results of evidentiary tests on epidemiological, toxicological, physiological and medical evidence, is still a matter of professional judgment.

16.8.2.2 Warrants, stated or unstated, have ethical content

Many controversies about what can be concluded from epidemiological evidence are really controversies about unstated warrants. For example, if there were some evidence that failed to provide toxicological experimental support to an hypothesis that a pollutant caused disease and yet there was a moderate epidemiological association to support it, people might opt for one of two warrants: (a) 'Moderate epidemiological associations unsupported by good toxicological experiment should not modify one's degree of certainty', or (b) 'Moderate epidemiological associations, even unsupported by good toxicological experimental evidence, ought to increase one's degree of certainty to some degree.' The choice between these two warrants should depend on a backing that is evidence based. In fact there are several examples of agents now known to cause disease in humans that for many years had no animal toxicological results to consider, and, indeed, some examples for which no good animal model for toxicology was ever found. Yet this moderately supportive pattern of epidemiological evidence is more characteristic of true hazards than of non-hazards. This backing evidence would support the warrant: 'Moderately supportive epidemiology, even in the absence of toxicological support, justifies an increased willingness to certify causality to some degree.'

Those whose certainty stays fixed until incriminating toxicological evidence arrives to support the epidemiology (warrant (a)) would point out that supportive epidemiological and toxicological evidence is highly unlikely among non-causal agents and that this pattern conveys a high *relative likelihood*, when present, which ought to boost confidence a great deal.

'That's fine' argue the advocates of warrant (b). 'But what if the toxicological evidence has not arrived? Your warrant is prone to falsely exonerate agents because you won't admit to the moderate relative likelihood conveyed by unsupported epidemiological evidence. Your warrant favors polluters while my warrant favors victims of pollution!'

'That's one way to put it,' retorts the enthusiast for toxicology, 'One could also say that your warrant favors intrusive bureaucrats and greedy tort lawyers!'

Scientists are trained to use strict warrants so as to avoid crying wolf. This practice minimizes wasting scarce scientific time on fruitless lines of investigation and protects scientific careers but may not always be appropriate when 'letting the wolf into the village' will jeopardize the public's health [29].

Scientific inferential warrants have ethical implications. They and their backing should be made explicit and the consequences of adopting them made clear.

16.9 **Conclusion**

If an environmental epidemiologist is interested in affecting environmental policy with etiological results, he or she should remember several things: Defects in the environment that impair health are usually due to large upstream non-health sector policy decisions related to land use, transportation, etc. As the environmental epidemiologist uncovers causal relations and thinks of remedies, he or she should look back to antecedent causes as well as proximate ones. Some but not all environmental health policy questions can be formulated in the following way: *How certain must we be of how much ill health before we would adopt cheap or expensive protective actions?* Stakeholders will answer this question on the basis of their interests and the ethical framework that they bring to bear on the problem at hand. While utilitarians favor quantitative cost-effectiveness or cost-benefit evaluations of the available courses of action using decision trees and expert consultants, and will favor cost-effective courses of action, duty ethicists, communitarians, and care-based ethicists prefer easily understood qualitative ethical analyses with substantial political participation by stakeholders. This latter group will favor solutions that meet ethical standards with less concern for cost. Libertarians mistrust government analyses and politically imposed solutions and favor voluntary market-based solutions. The choice of policy is largely driven by interests and ideology and only partly by the information about the probability of disease or death that the epidemiologist brings to the discussion. If the epidemiologist aspires to participate in the policy process, he would do well to understand the basics of utilitarian and ethical analyses as well as his own discipline. While the intellectual roots of nineteenth-century epidemiology are utilitarian in nature, the epidemiologist has the duty to provide information about the degree of certainty of hazard, extent of illness, and exposure in ways that accommodate the information needs of these different kinds of stakeholders. Displaying one's degree of certainty about hazardousness in a graduated fashion rather than as a dichotomy between 'virtually certain' and 'not virtually certain' accommodates a wider range of stakeholders. Revealing facts about who gets exposed and who is more sensitive to exposures is of interest to the duty ethicists in the policy argument. Clearly elucidating the factual grounds and the inferential assumptions that warrant a claimed degree of certainty about a hazard allow more stakeholders to understand what the epidemiologist has brought to the discussion. A Bayes-influenced style of epidemiological argument is one approach to this kind of transparency. Transparency helps stakeholders cope with dueling experts as they participate in a political process to make environmental health policy. The first Buddhist Japanese emperor, Shotoku Taishi, in 604 AD said, 'When big things are at stake, the danger of the error is great. Therefore, many should discuss and clarify the matter together so the correct way may be found' [30]. This advice is still well founded.

16.10 **References**

[1] Spasoff RA. *Epidemiologic methods for health policy*. New York: Oxford University Press 1999.

[2] Brown D. Ethics, science and environmental regulation. *Environ Ethics.* 1987 **9**:331–49.

[3] Roberts MJ, Reich MR. Ethical analysis in public health. *Lancet.* 2002 **359**(9311):1055–9.

[4] Lakoff G. *Moral politics: how liberals and conservatives think, 2nd edn.* Chicago, IL: University of Chicago Press 2002.

[5] Scott S, Pellman K. *Living without electricity*. Intercourse, PA: Good Books 1990.

[6] Baier A. *Moral prejudices: essays on ethics.* Cambridge, MA: Harvard University Press 1994.

[7] Gilligan C. *In a different voice: psychological theory and women's development.* Cambridge, MA: Harvard University Press 1982.

[8] Flanagan OJ. *Varieties of moral personality: ethics and psychological realism.* Cambridge, MA: Harvard University Press 1991.

[9] Ackerman F, Heinzerling L. *Priceless: on knowing the price of everything and the value of nothing.* New York: New Press 2004.

[10] von Winterfeldt D, Eppel T, Adams J, Neutra R, DelPizzo V. Managing potential health risks from electric powerlines: a decision analysis caught in controversy. *Risk Anal.* 2004 **24**(6):1487–502.

[11] Margolis H. *Dealing with risk: why the public and the experts disagree on environmental issues.* Chicago, IL: University of Chicago Press 1996.

[12] Lave L. Benefit-cost analysis: do the benefits exceed the cost in risks, costs and lives saved, getting better results from regulation. In: Hahn RW, ed. *Risks, costs, and lives saved: getting better results from regulation.* New York: Oxford University Press 1996: 104–22.

[13] Bernstein B, Florig H. *Managing magnetic fields in California public schools.* Oakland, CA: Public Healh Institute, 2001.

[14] Sabatier P, Jenkins Smith H. The advocacy coalition framework. In: Sabatier PA, ed. *Theories of policy process.* Boulder, CO: Westview Press 1999: vi.

[15] Ashford N. Implementing a precautionary approach in decisions affecting health, safety and the environment: risk technology alternatives and tradeoff analyses. In: Freytage E, Jakl T, Loibl G, Wittmann M, eds.*The role of precaution in chemicals policy.* Vienna: Diplomatic Academy 2002: 128–40.

[16] Rawls J. *A theory of justice, revised edn.* Cambridge, MA: Belknap Press of Harvard University Press 1999.

[17] von Winterfeldt D, Eppel T, Adams J, Eppel T, Nair I. *The powergrid and land use policy analysis. Final Draft.* Available at http://www.dhs.ca.gov/ehib/emf/pwrgrdfd.html.

[18] Rothman KJ, Poole C. Science and policy making. *American Journal of Public Health.* 1985 **75**(4):340–1.

[19] Weed DL, McKeown RE. Science and social responsibility in public health. *Environmental Health Perspectives.* 2003 **111**(14):1804–8.

[20] Stirling A, Gee D. Science, precaution, and practice. *Public Health Rep.* 2002 **117**(6):521–33.

[21] Neutra RR, Delpizzo V. Transparent democratic foresight strategies in the California EMF Program. *Public Health Rep.* 2002 **117**(6):553–63.

[22] Greenland S. Relation of probability of causation to relative risk and doubling dose: a methodologic error that has become a social problem. *American Journal of Public Health.* 1999 **89**(8):1166–9.

[23] Toulmin SE. *The uses of argument, updated edn.* Cambridge, UK and New York: Cambridge University Press 2003.

[24] Hacking I. *An introduction to probability and inductive logic.* London: Cambridge University Press. 2001.

[25] Weinstein MC, Fineberg HV. *Clinical decision analysis.* Philadelphia, PA: Saunders 1980.

[26] Greenland S. Probability logic and probabilistic induction. *Epidemiology.* 1998 **9**(3):322–32.

[27] Sackett DL, Sackett DL. *Clinical epidemiology: a basic science for clinical medicine, 2nd edn.* Philadelphia, PA: Lippincott Williams & Wilkins 1991.

[28] Musen M, Shahar Y, Shortliffe EH. Clinical decision support systems. In: Shortliffe EH, Perreault LE, eds. *Medical informatics: computer applications in health care and biomedicine, 2nd edn.* New York: Springer 2001: 573–83.

[29] Neutra R. Should one start or continue a line of research? Stakeholders' interests and ethical frameworks give different answers. *Annals, AAPSS.* 2002 **584**(1):125–34.

[30] Sansome G. *The First Japanese Constitution.* Tokyo: The Asiatic Society. 1938.

Further information

Organizations

International Society for Environmental Epidemiology

The International Society for Environmental Epidemiology (ISEE) (http://www.iseepi.org/) provides a forum for the discussion of problems unique to the study of health and the environment. With membership open to environmental epidemiologists and other scientists worldwide, ISEE provides a variety of forums for discussions, critical reviews, collaborations and education on issues of environmental exposures and their human health effects. These include annual meetings, newsletters, workshops and liaisons with academic, governmental, intergovernmental, nonprofit and business institutions.

International Society of Exposure Analysis

The International Society of Exposure Analysis (ISEA) (http://www.iseaweb.org/) was established in 1989 to foster and advance the science of exposure analysis related to environmental contaminants, both for human populations and ecosystems. The membership promotes communication among all disciplines involved in exposure analysis, recommends exposure analysis approaches to address substantive or methodological concerns, and works to strengthen the impact of exposure assessment on environmental policy.

World Health Organization

The World Health Organization (WHO) (http://www.who.int/) is the directing and coordinating authority for health within the United Nations system. It is responsible for providing leadership on global health matters, shaping the health research agenda, setting norms and standards, articulating evidence-based policy options, providing technical support to countries and monitoring and assessing health trends.

Main journals

Environmental Health Perspectives http://www.ehponline.org/
Epidemiology http://www.epidem.com/
Journal of Exposure Science and Environmental Epidemiology
http://www.nature.com/jes/index.html
Occupational and Environmental Medicine http://oem.bmj.com/

For searching scientific papers

Pubmed (Toxline and Medline) http://www.ncbi.nlm.nih.gov/entrez/query.fcgi

Books

Toxicology

JA Timbrell. *Principles of Biochemical Toxicology, 3rd edn.* London: Taylor & Francis, 2000. ISBN 0748407375. [new edition due in 2008]

CD Klaassen. *Casarett & Doull's Toxicology: The Basic Science of Poisons, 7th edn.* New York: McGraw-Hill, 2008. ISBN: 978-0-07-14751-3

Epidemiology

J Last. *A Dictionary of Epidemiology, 4th edn.* New York: Oxford University Press, 2001. ISBN 0195141687.

R Bonita, R Beaglehole, T Kjellström. *Basic Epidemiology, 2nd edn.* Geneva: World Health Organization, 2006. ISBN 9241547073.

K Rothman, S Greenland, T Lash. *Modern Epidemiology, 3rd edn.* Philadelphia: Lippincott Williams & Wilkins, 2008. ISBN 9780781755641.

H Checkoway, N Pearce, D Kriebel. *Research Methods in Occupational Epidemiology, 2nd edn.* New York: Oxford University Press, 2004. ISBN 019092422.

P Elliott. *Spatial Epidemiology: Methods and Applications.* Oxford and New York: Oxford University Press, 2000. ISBN 0192629417.

Disease

L Rosenstock, M Cullen, C Brodkin, Carrie Redlich. *Textbook of Clinical and Environmental Medicine, 2nd edn.* Philadelphia: Elsevier Saunders, 2005. ISBN 0721689744.

W Rom, S Markowitz. *Environmental and Occupational Medicine, 4th edn.* Philadelphia: Lippincott Williams & Wilkins, 2007. ISBN 0781762995.

J LaDou. *Current Occupational and Environmental Medicine, 4th edn.* New York: McGraw-Hill, 2007. ISBN 0071443134.

Exposure Assessment

MJ Nieuwenhuijsen (ed.). *Exposure Assessment in Occupational and Environmental Epidemiology.* Oxford: Oxford University Press, 2003. ISBN 0198528612.

E White, BK Armstrong, R Saracci. *Principles of Exposure Measurement in Epidemiology: Collecting, Evaluating, and Improving Measures of Disease Risk Factors, 2nd edn.* Oxford and New York: Oxford University Press, 2008. ISBN 9780198509851.

Risk Assessment

VT Covello, MW Merkhofer. *Risk Assessment Methods. Approaches for Assessing Health and Environmental Risks.* New York: Plenum Press, 1993. ISBN 0306443821.

WH Hallenbeck. *Quantitative Risk Assessment for Environmental and Occupational Health, 2nd edn.* Boca Raton, FL: Lewis Publishers, 1993. ISBN 0873718011.

M Robson, W Toscano. *Risk Assessment for Environmental Health.* San Francisco: Jossey-Bass, 2007. ISBN 9780787983192.

P Ricci. *Environmental and Health Risk Assessment and Management: Principles and Practices.* Dordrecht: Springer, 2006. ISBN 1402037759.

Statistics

M Bland. *An Introduction to Medical Statistics, 2nd edn.* New York: Oxford University Press, 2000. ISBN 0192632698.

B Rosner. *Fundamentals of Biostatistics, 6th edn.* Belmont, CA: Thomson-Brooks/Cole, 2006. ISBN 0534418201.

DA Savitz. *Interpreting Epidemiologic Evidence: Strategies for Study Design and Analysis.* New York: Oxford University Press, 2003. ISBN 01980195108408.

DG Kleinbaum, LL Kupper, A Nizam, KE Muller. *Applied Regression Analysis and Multivariable Methods, 4th edn.* Belmont, CA: Duxbury Press, 2007. ISBN 9780495384984.

General

ST Holgate, J Samet, HS Koren, R Maynard. *Air Pollution and Health.* London: Academic Press, 1999. ISBN 0-12-352335-4.

R Carson. *Silent Spring.* London: Penguin Books, 1962. ISBN 0-14-013891-9.

AJ McMichael. *Planetary Overload.* New York: Cambridge University Press, 1993. ISBN 0-521-55871-9.

T Colborn, D Dumanoski, J Peterson Myers. *Our Stolen Future.* London: Abacus, 1996. ISBN 0-349-10878-1.

J Thornton. *Pandora's Poison: Chlorine, Health and a New Environmental Strategy.* Cambridge, MA: MIT Press, 2000. ISBN 0-262-20124-0.

R Evans. *Gassed.* London: House of Status, 2000. ISBN 1-84232-071-8.

Index

Printed in the USA
CPSIA information can be obtained
at www.ICGtesting.com
CBHW071025310124
3873CB00010B/25